Newly Compiled
actical English-Chinese Library
Traditional Chinese Medicine
英汉对照）新编实用中医文库

neral Compiler-in-Chief Zuo Yanfu
主编 左言富
nslators-in-Chief
u Zhongbao Huang Yuezhong Tao Jinwen Li Zhaoguo
编译 朱忠宝 黄月中 陶锦文 李照国（执行）

Compiled by Nanjing University of Traditional Chinese Medicine
Translated by Shanghai University of Traditional Chinese Medicine
南京中医药大学 主编
上海中医药大学 主译

CHINESE ACUPUNCTURE AND MOXIBUSTION

中国针灸

Examiner-in-Chief	Yang Zhaomin
Compiler-in-Chief	Zhao Jingsheng
Vice-Compilers-in-Chief	Liu Yueguang
	Hu Kui
Translators-in-Chief	Li Zhaoguo
	Chen Renying
Vice-Translators-in-Chief	Xu Qilong
	Tian Kaiyu

主　审 杨兆民
主　编 赵京生
副主编 刘跃光
　　　 胡　葵
主　译 李照国
　　　 陈仁英
副主译 徐启龙
　　　 田开宇

BLISHING HOUSE OF SHANGHAI UNIVERSITY
TRADITIONAL CHINESE MEDICINE
海中医药大学出版社

Publishing House of Shanghai University of Traditional Chinese Medicine
530 Lingling Road, Shanghai, 200032, China

Chinese Acupuncture and Moxibustion
Compiler-in-Chief Zhao Jingsheng Translators-in-Chief Li Zhaoguo Chen Renying
(A Newly Compiled Practical English-Chinese Library of TCM General Compiler-in-Chief Zuo Yanfu)

ISBN 7-81010-667-8/R·633 paperback
ISBN 7-81010-682-1/R·647 hardback

Printed in Shanghai Xinhua Printing Works

图书在版编目(CIP)数据

中国针灸/赵京生主编;李照国,陈仁英主译.—上海:上海中医药大学出版社,2002
(英汉对照新编实用中医文库/左言富总主编)
ISBN 7-81010-667-8

Ⅰ.中… Ⅱ.①赵…②李…③陈… Ⅲ.针灸学-英、汉 Ⅳ.R245

中国版本图书馆CIP数据核字(2002)第039168号

中国针灸 主编 赵京生 主译 李照国 陈仁英

上海中医药大学出版社出版发行 (蔡伦路1200号 邮政编码201203)
新华书店上海发行所经销 上海新华印刷有限公司印刷
开本 787mm×1092mm 1/18 印张 22.666 字数 542千字 印数 6 601—8 700册
版次 2002年10月第1版 印次 2005年6月第3次印刷

ISBN 7-81010-667-8/R·633 定价 84.50元

Compilation Board of the Library

《(英汉对照)新编实用中医文库》编纂委员会

Translation Committee of the Library

Advisors Shao Xundao Ou Ming

Translators-in-Chief Zhu Zhongbao Huang Yuezhong Tao Jinwen

Executive Translator-in-Chief Li Zhaoguo

Vice-Translators-in-Chief (Listed in the order of the number of strokes in the Chinese names)

Xun Jianying Li Yong'an Zhang Qingrong Zhang Dengfeng Yang Hongying Huang Guoqi Xie Jinhua

Translators (Listed in the order of the number of strokes in the Chinese names)

Yu Xin	Wang Ruihui	Tian Kaiyu	Shen Guang
Lan Fengli	Cheng Peili	Zhu Wenxiao	Zhu Yuqin
Zhu Jinjiang	Zhu Guixiang	Le Yimin	Liu Shengpeng
Li Jingyun	Yang Ying	Yang Mingshan	He Yingchun
Zhang Jie	Zhang Haixia	Zhang Wei	Chen Renying
Zhou Yongming	Zhou Suzhen	Qu Yusheng	Zhao Junqing
Jing Zhen	Hu Kewu	Xu Qilong	Xu Yao
Guo Xiaomin	Huang Xixuan	Cao Lijuan	Kang Qin
Dong Jing	Qin Baichang	Zeng Haiping	Lou Jianhua
Lai Yuezhen	Bao Bai	Pei Huihua	Xue Junmei
Dai Wenjun	Wei Min		

Office of the Translation Committee

Director Yang Mingshan

Secretaries Xu Lindi Chen Li

《(英汉对照)新编实用中医文库》编译委员会

Approval Committee of the Library

《(英汉对照)新编实用中医文库》审定委员会

Foreword I

As we are walking into the 21st century, "health for all" is still an important task for the World Health Organization (WHO) to accomplish in the new century. The realization of "health for all" requires mutual cooperation and concerted efforts of various medical sciences, including traditional medicine. WHO has increasingly emphasized the development of traditional medicine and has made fruitful efforts to promote its development. Currently the spectrum of diseases is changing and an increasing number of diseases are difficult to cure. The side effects of chemical drugs have become more and more evident. Furthermore, both the governments and peoples in all countries are faced with the problem of high cost of medical treatment. Traditional Chinese medicine (TCM), the complete system of traditional medicine in the world with unique theory and excellent clinical curative effects, basically meets the need to solve such problems. Therefore, bringing TCM into full play in medical treatment and healthcare will certainly become one of the hot points in the world medical business in the 21st century.

Various aspects of work need to be done to promote the course of the internationalization of TCM, especially the compilation of works and textbooks suitable for international readers. The impending new century has witnessed the compilation of such a

序 一

人类即将迈入21世纪,"人人享有卫生保健"仍然是新世纪世界卫生工作面临的重要任务。实现"人人享有卫生保健"的宏伟目标,需要包括传统医药学在内的多种医学学科的相互协作与共同努力。世界卫生组织越来越重视传统医药学的发展,并为推动其发展做出了卓有成效的工作。目前,疾病谱正在发生变化,难治疾病不断增多,化学药品的毒副作用日益显现,日趋沉重的医疗费用困扰着各国政府和民众。中医药学是世界传统医学体系中最完整的传统医学,其独到的学科理论和突出的临床疗效,较符合当代社会和人们解决上述难题的需要。因此,科学有效地发挥中医药学的医疗保健作用,必将成为21世纪世界卫生工作的特点之一。

加快中医药走向世界的步伐,还有很多的工作要做,特别是适合国外读者学习的中医药著作、教材的编写是极其重要的方面。在新千年来临之际,由南京中医药大学

series of books known as *A Newly Compiled Practical English-Chinese Library of Traditional Chinese Medicine* published by the Publishing House of Shanghai University of TCM, compiled by Nanjing University of TCM and translated by Shanghai University of TCM. Professor Zuo Yanfu, the general compiler-in-chief of this Library, is a person who sets his mind on the international dissemination of TCM. He has compiled *General Survey on TCM Abroad*, a monograph on the development and state of TCM abroad. This Library is another important works written by the experts organized by him with the support of Nanjing University of TCM and Shanghai University of TCM. The compilation of this Library is done with consummate ingenuity and according to the development of TCM abroad. The compilers, based on the premise of preserving the genuineness and gist of TCM, have tried to make the contents concise, practical and easy to understand, making great efforts to introduce the abstruse ideas of TCM in a scientific and simple way as well as expounding the prevention and treatment of diseases which are commonly encountered abroad and can be effectively treated by TCM.

主编、上海中医药大学主译、上海中医药大学出版社出版的《(英汉对照)新编实用中医文库》的即将问世，正是新世纪中医药国际传播更快发展的预示。本套文库总主编左言富教授是中医药学国际传播事业的有心人，曾主编研究国外中医药发展状况的专著《国外中医药概览》。本套文库的编撰，是他在南京中医药大学和上海中医药大学支持下，组织许多著名专家共同完成的又一重要专著。本套文库的作者们深谙国外的中医药发展现状，编写颇具匠心，在注重真实，不失精华的前提下，突出内容的简明、实用，易于掌握，力求科学而又通俗地介绍中医药学的深奥内容，重点阐述国外常见而中医药颇具疗效的疾病的防治。

This Library encompasses a systematic summarization of the teaching experience accumulated in Nanjing University of TCM and Shanghai University of TCM that run the collaborating centers of traditional medicine and the international training centers on acupuncture and moxibustion set by WHO. I am sure that the publication of this Library will further promote the development of traditional Chinese med-

本套文库蕴含了南京中医药大学和上海中医药大学作为WHO传统医学合作中心、国际针灸培训中心多年留学生教学的实践经验和系统总结，更为全面、系统、准确地向世界传播中医药学。相信本书的出版将对中医更好地走向世界，让世界更好地了解中医产生更

icine abroad and enable the whole world to have a better understanding of traditional Chinese medicine.

Professor Zhu Qingsheng

Vice-Minister of Health Ministry of the People's Republic of China

Director of the State Administrative Bureau of TCM

December 14, 2000 Beijing

为积极的影响。

朱庆生教授

中华人民共和国卫生部副部长

国家中医药管理局局长

2000年12月14日于北京

Foreword Ⅱ

Before the existence of the modern medicine, human beings depended solely on herbal medicines and other therapeutic methods to treat diseases and preserve health. Such a practice gave rise to the establishment of various kinds of traditional medicine with unique theory and practice, such as traditional Chinese medicine, Indian medicine and Arabian medicine, etc. Among these traditional systems of medicine, traditional Chinese medicine is a most extraordinary one based on which traditional Korean medicine and Japanese medicine have evolved.

Even in the 21st century, traditional medicine is still of great vitality. In spite of the fast development of modern medicine, traditional medicine is still disseminated far and wide. In many developing countries, most of the people in the rural areas still depend on traditional medicine and traditional medical practitioners to meet the need for primary healthcare. Even in the countries with advanced modern medicine, more and more people have begun to accept traditional medicine and other therapeutic methods, such as homeopathy, osteopathy and naturopathy, etc.

With the change of the economy, culture and living style in various regions as well as the aging in the world population, the disease spectrum has changed. And such a change has paved the way for the new application of traditional medicine. Besides,

序　二

在现代医学形成之前，人类一直依赖草药和其他一些疗法治病强身，从而发展出许多有理论、有实践的传统医学，例如中医学、印度医学、阿拉伯医学等。中医学是世界林林总总的传统医学中的一支奇葩，在它的基础上还衍生出朝鲜传统医学和日本汉方医学。在跨入21世纪的今天，古老的传统医学依然焕发着活力，非但没有因现代医学的发展而式微，其影响还有增无减，人们对传统医学的价值也有了更深刻的体会和认识。在许多贫穷国家，大多数农村人口仍然依赖传统医学疗法和传统医务工作者来满足他们对初级卫生保健的需求。在现代医学占主导地位的许多国家，传统医学及其他一些“另类疗法”，诸如顺势疗法、整骨疗法、自然疗法等，也越来越被人们所接受。

伴随着世界各地经济、文化和生活的变革以及世界人口的老龄化，世界疾病谱也发生了变化。传统医学有了新的应用，而新疾病所引起的新需求以及现代医学的成

the new requirements initiated by the new diseases and the achievements and limitations of modern medicine have also created challenges for traditional medicine.

WHO sensed the importance of traditional medicine to human health early in the 1970s and have made great efforts to develop traditional medicine. At the 29th world health congress held in 1976, the item of traditional medicine was adopted in the working plan of WHO. In the following world health congresses, a series of resolutions were passed to demand the member countries to develop, utilize and study traditional medicine according to their specific conditions so as to reduce medical expenses for the realization of "health for all".

WHO has laid great stress on the scientific content, safe and effective application of traditional medicine. It has published and distributed a series of booklets on the scientific, safe and effective use of herbs and acupuncture and moxibustion. It has also made great contributions to the international standardization of traditional medical terms. The safe and effective application of traditional medicine has much to do with the skills of traditional medical practitioners. That is why WHO has made great efforts to train them. WHO has run 27 collaborating centers in the world which have made great contributions to the training of acupuncturists and traditional medical practitioners. Nanjing University of TCM and Shanghai University of TCM run the collaborating centers with WHO. In recent years it has, with the cooperation of WHO and other countries, trained about ten thousand international students from over

就与局限又向传统医学提出了挑战，推动它进一步发展。世界卫生组织早在20世纪70年代就意识到传统医学对人类健康的重要性，并为推动传统医学的发展做了努力。1976年举行的第二十九届世界卫生大会将传统医学项目纳入世界卫生组织的工作计划。其后的各届世界卫生大会又通过了一系列决议，要求各成员国根据本国的条件发展、使用和研究传统医学，以降低医疗费用，促进"人人享有初级卫生保健"这一目标的实现。

世界卫生组织历来重视传统医学的科学、安全和有效使用。它出版和发行了一系列有关科学、安全、有效使用草药和针灸的技术指南，并在专用术语的标准化方面做了许多工作。传统医学的使用是否做到安全和有效，是与使用传统疗法的医务工作者的水平密不可分的。因此，世界卫生组织也十分重视传统医学培训工作。它在全世界有27个传统医学合作中心，这些中心对培训合格的针灸师及使用传统疗法的其他医务工作者做出了积极的贡献。南京中医药大学、上海中医药大学是世界卫生组织传统医学合作中心之一，近年来与世界卫生组织和其他国家合作，培训了近万名来自90多个国

90 countries.

In order to further promote the dissemination of traditional Chinese medicine in the world, *A Newly Compiled Practical English-Chinese Library of Traditional Chinese Medicine*, compiled by Nanjing University of TCM with Professor Zuo Yanfu as the general compiler-in-chief and published by the Publishing House of Shanghai University of TCM, aims at systematic, accurate and concise expounding of traditional Chinese medical theory and introducing clinical therapeutic methods of traditional medicine according to modern medical nomenclature of diseases. Undoubtedly, this series of books will be the practical textbooks for the beginners with certain English level and the international enthusiasts with certain level of Chinese to study traditional Chinese medicine. Besides, this series of books can also serve as reference books for WHO to internationally standardize the nomenclature of acupuncture and moxibustion.

The scientific, safe and effective use of traditional medicine will certainly further promote the development of traditional medicine and traditional medicine will undoubtedly make more and more contributions to human health in the 21st century.

Zhang Xiaorui

WHO Coordination Officer

December, 2000

家和地区的留学生。

在南京中医药大学左言富教授主持下编纂的、由上海中医药大学出版社出版的《(英汉对照)新编实用中医文库》,旨在全面、系统、准确、简要地阐述中医基础理论,并结合西医病名介绍中医临床治疗方法。因此,这套文库可望成为具有一定英语水平的初学中医者和具有一定中文水平的外国中医爱好者学习基础中医学的系列教材。这套文库也可供世界卫生组织在编写国际针灸标准术语时参考。

传统医学的科学、安全、有效使用必将进一步推动传统医学的发展。传统医学一定会在21世纪为人类健康做出更大的贡献。

张小瑞

世界卫生组织传统医学协调官员

2000年12月

90 countries.

In order to further promote the dissemination of traditional Chinese medicine in the world, *A Newly Compiled Practical English-Chinese Library of Traditional Chinese Medicine* compiled by Nanjing University of TCM with Professor Zuo Yanfu as the general compiler-in-chief and published by the Publishing House of Shanghai University of TCM, aims at systematic, accurate and concise expounding of traditional Chinese medical theory and introducing clinical therapeutic methods of traditional medicine according to modern medical nomenclature of diseases. Undoubtedly, this series of books will be the practical textbooks for the beginners with certain English level and the international enthusiasts with certain level of Chinese to study traditional Chinese medicine. Besides, this series of books can also serve as reference books for WHO to internationally standardize the nomenclature of acupuncture and moxibustion.

The scientific, safe and effective use of traditional medicine will certainly further promote the development of traditional medicine and traditional medicine will undoubtedly make more and more contributions to human health in the 21st century.

Zhang Xiaorui

WHO Coordination Officer

December, 2000

Preface

The Publishing House of Shanghai University of TCM published *A Practical English-Chinese Library of Traditional Chinese Medicine* in 1990. The Library has been well-known in the world ever since and has made great contributions to the dissemination of traditional Chinese medicine in the world. In view of the fact that 10 years has passed since its publication and that there are certain errors in the explanation of traditional Chinese medicine in the Library, the Publishing House has invited Nanjing University of TCM and Shanghai University of TCM to organize experts to recompile and translate the Library.

Nanjing University of TCM and Shanghai University of TCM are well-known for their advantages in higher education of traditional Chinese medicine and compilation of traditional Chinese medical textbooks. The compilation of *A Newly Compiled Practical English-Chinese Library of Traditional Chinese Medicine* has absorbed the rich experience accumulated by Nanjing University of Traditional Chinese Medicine in training international students of traditional Chinese medicine. Compared with the previous Library, the Newly Compiled Library has made great improvements in many aspects, fully demonstrating the academic system of traditional Chinese medicine. The whole series of books has systematically introduced the basic theory and thera-

前　言

上海中医药大学出版社于1990年出版了一套《(英汉对照)实用中医文库》,发行10年来,在海内外产生了较大影响,对推动中医学走向世界起了积极作用。考虑到该套丛书发行已久,对中医学术体系的介绍还有一些欠妥之处,因此,上海中医药大学出版社特邀南京中医药大学主编、上海中医药大学主译,组织全国有关专家编译出版《(英汉对照)新编实用中医文库》。

《(英汉对照)新编实用中医文库》的编纂,充分发挥了南京中医药大学和上海中医药大学在高等中医药教育教学和教材编写方面的优势,吸收了作为WHO传统医学合作中心之一的两校,多年来从事中医药学国际培训和留学生学历教育的经验,对原《(英汉对照)实用中医文库》整体结构作了大幅度调整,以突出中医学术主体内容。全套丛书系统介绍了中医基础理论和中医辨证论治方法,讲解了中药学和方剂学的基本理论,详细介绍了236味中药、152首常用方剂和100种常用中成药;详述

peutic methods based on syndrome differentiation, expounding traditional Chinese pharmacy and prescriptions; explaining 236 herbs, 152 prescriptions and 100 commonly-used patent drugs; elucidating 264 methods for differentiating syndromes and treating commonly-encountered and frequently-encountered diseases in internal medicine, surgery, gynecology, pediatrics, traumatology and orthopedics, ophthalmology and otorhinolaryngology; introducing the basic methods and theory of acupuncture and moxibustion, massage (tuina), life cultivation and rehabilitation, including 70 kinds of diseases suitable for acupuncture and moxibustion, 38 kinds of diseases for massage, examples of life cultivation and over 20 kinds of commonly encountered diseases treated by rehabilitation therapies in traditional Chinese medicine. For better understanding of traditional Chinese medicine, the books are neatly illustrated. There are 296 line graphs and 30 colored pictures in the Library with necessary indexes, making it more comprehensive, accurate and systematic in disseminating traditional Chinese medicine in the countries and regions where English is the official language.

This Library is characterized by following features:

1. Scientific　Based on the development of TCM in education and research in the past 10 years, efforts have been made in the compilation to highlight the gist of TCM through accurate theoretical exposition and clinical practice, aiming at introducing authentic theory and practice to the world.

2. Systematic　This Library contains 14 sepa-

264 种临床内、外、妇、儿、骨伤、眼、耳鼻喉各科常见病与多发病的中医辨证论治方法；系统论述针灸、推拿、中医养生康复的基本理论和基本技能，介绍针灸治疗病种 70 种、推拿治疗病种 38 种、各类养生实例及 20 余种常见病证的中医康复实例。为了更加直观地介绍中医药学术，全书选用线图 296 幅、彩图 30 幅，并附有必要的索引，从而更加全面、系统、准确地向使用英语的国家和地区传播中医学术，推进中医学走向世界，造福全人类。

本丛书主要具有以下特色
(1) 科学性：在充分吸收近 10 余年来中医教学和科学研究最新进展的基础上，坚持突出中医学术精华，理论阐述准确，临床切合实用，向世界各国介绍“原汁原味”的中医药学术；(2) 系统性：本套丛书包括《中医基础理论》、《中医诊断学》、《中药学》、《方剂学》、《中医

rate fascicles, i.e. *Basic Theory of Traditional Chinese Medicine*, *Diagnostics of Traditional Chinese Medicine*, *Science of Chinese Materia Medica*, *Science of Prescriptions*, *Internal Medicine of Traditional Chinese Medicine*, *Surgery of Traditional Chinese Medicine*, *Gynecology of Traditional Chinese Medicine*, *Pediatrics of Traditional Chinese Medicine*, *Traumatology and Orthopedics of Traditional Chinese Medicine*, *Ophthalmology of Traditional Chinese Medicine*, *Otorhinolaryngology of Traditional Chinese Medicine*, *Chinese Acupuncture and Moxibustion*, *Chinese Tuina (Massage)*, *and Life Cultivation and Rehabilitation of Traditional Chinese Medicine*.

3. Practical Compared with the previous Library, the Newly Compiled Library has made great improvements and supplements, systematically introducing therapeutic methods for treating over 200 kinds of commonly and frequently encountered diseases, focusing on training basic clinical skills in acupuncture and moxibustion, tuina therapy, life cultivation and rehabilitation with clinical case reports.

4. Standard This Library is reasonable in structure, distinct in categorization, standard in terminology and accurate in translation with full consideration of habitual expressions used in countries and regions with English language as the mother tongue.

This series of books is not only practical for the beginners with certain competence of English to study TCM, but also can serve as authentic textbooks for international students in universities and colleges of TCM in China to study and practice TCM. For those from TCM field who are going to go

科学》、《中医外科学》、《中医妇科学》、《中医儿科学》、《中医骨伤科学》、《中医眼科学》、《中医耳鼻喉科学》、《中国针灸》、《中国推拿》、《中医养生康复学》14 个分册,系统反映了中医各学科建设与发展的最新成果;(3) 实用性:临床各科由原来的上下两册,根据学科的发展进行大幅度的调整和增补,比较详细地介绍了 200 多种各科常见病、多发病的中医治疗方法,重点突出了针灸、推拿、养生康复等临床基本技能训练,并附有部分临证实例;(4) 规范性:全书结构合理,层次清晰,对中医各学科名词术语表述规范,对中医英语翻译执行了更为严格的标准化方案,同时又充分考虑到使用英语国家和地区人们的语言习惯和表达方式。

本丛书不仅能满足具有一定英语水平的初学中医者系统学习中医之用,而且也为中医院校外国留学生教育及国内外开展中医双语教学提供了目前最具权威的系列教材,同时也是中医出国人员进

abroad to do academic exchange, this series of books will provide them with unexpected convenience.

Professor Xiang Ping, President of Nanjing University of TCM, is the director of the Compilation Board. Professor Zuo Yanfu from Nanjing University of TCM, General Compiler-in-Chief, is in charge of the compilation. Zhang Wenkang, Minister of Health Ministry, is invited to be the honorary director of the Editorial Board. Li Zhenji, Vice-Director of the State Administrative Bureau of TCM, is invited to be the director of the Approval Committee. Chen Keji, academician of China Academy, is invited to be the General Advisor. International advisors invited are Mr. M. S. Khan, Chairman of Ireland Acupuncture and Moxibustion Fund; Miss Alessandra Gulí, Chairman of "Nanjing Association" in Rome, Italy; Doctor Secondo Scarsella, Chief Editor of YI DAO ZA ZHI; President Raymond K. Carroll from Australian Oriental Touching Therapy College; Ms. Shulan Tang, Academic Executive of ATCM in Britain; Mr. Glovanni Maciocia from Britain; Mr. David, Chairman of American Association of TCM; Mr. Tzu Kuo Shih, director of Chinese Medical Technique Center in Connecticut, America; Mr. Helmut Ziegler, director of TCM Center in Germany; and Mr. Isigami Hiroshi from Japan. Chen Ken, official of WHO responsible for the Western Pacific Region, has greatly encouraged the compilers in compiling this series of books. After the accomplishment of the compilation, Professor Zhu Qingsheng, Vice-Minister of Health Ministry and Director of the State Administrative Bureau of TCM, has set a high value on the books in his fore-

行中医药国际交流的重要工具书。

全书由南京中医药大学校长项平教授担任编委会主任、左言富教授任总主编，主持全书的编写。中华人民共和国卫生部张文康部长担任本丛书编委会名誉主任，国家中医药管理局李振吉副局长担任审定委员会主任，陈可冀院士欣然担任本丛书总顾问指导全书的编纂。爱尔兰针灸基金会主席萨利姆先生、意大利罗马"南京协会"主席亚历山大·古丽女士、意大利《医道》杂志主编卡塞拉·塞肯多博士、澳大利亚东方触觉疗法学院雷蒙特·凯·卡罗院长、英国中医药学会学术部长汤淑兰女士、英国马万里先生、美国中医师公会主席大卫先生、美国康州中华医疗技术中心主任施祖谷先生、德国中医中心主任赫尔木特先生、日本石上博先生担任本丛书特邀外籍顾问。世界卫生组织西太平洋地区官员陈恳先生对本丛书的编写给予了热情鼓励。全书完成后，卫生部副部长兼国家中医药管理局局长朱庆生教授给予了高度评价，并欣然为本书作序；WHO 传统医学协调官员张小瑞对于本丛书的编写给予高度关注，百忙中也专为本书作序。我国驻外教育机构，特别是中国驻英国曼彻斯特领事张益群先生、中国驻美国休斯敦领事严美华

word for the Library. Zhang Xiaorui, an official from WHO's Traditional Medicine Program, has paid great attention to the compilation and written a foreword for the Library. The officials from the educational organizations of China in other countries have provided us with some useful materials in our compilation. They are Mr. Zhang Yiqun, China Consul to Manchester in Britain; Miss Yan Meihua, Consul to Houston in America; Mr. Wang Jiping, First Secretary in the Educational Department in the Embassy of China to France; and Mr. Gu Shengying, the Second Secretary in the Educational Department in the Embassy of China to Germany. We are grateful to them all.

The Compilers
December, 2000

女士、中国驻法国使馆教育处一秘王季平先生、中国驻德国使馆教育处二秘郭胜英先生在与我们工作联系中,间接提供了不少有益资料。在此一并致以衷心感谢!

编　者
2000年12月

Notes for compilation

The compilation of this book is marked by conciseness, diagrams and systematic introduction to the basic knowledge, theory and techniques of acupuncture and moxibustion as well as specific therapeutic methods for the treatment of various diseases for the benefit of the international readers in learning acupuncture and moxibustion. Therefore in the arrangement of contents and compilation, the following aspects are emphasized:

1. Systematic introduction to the knowledge of meridians and acupoints.

2. Emphasis is made on the relation between basic theory and clinical techniques. Apart from introduction to the location of acupoints, the ways to locate acupoints are also discussed. The discussion does not include topography and techniques for acupuncture and moxibustion. Comprehensive explanations of the anatomy and needling methods for various acupoints are given in the third chapter.

3. Seventy diseases clinically proved and applicable to the clinical application abroad are introduced in terms of the conception, syndrome differentiation, usage and needling methods.

In the compilation, introduction, Chapters 3, 4 and sections 8 - 10 in Chapter 5 are compiled by Zhao Jingsheng who is also responsible for drafting the compiling outline and polishing the whole book;

编写说明

为适合海外读者学习和运用中国针灸疗法的需要，本书的编写力争以简明准确的语言，配以图表，系统地介绍针灸学的基本知识、基本理论、基本技能和各科疾病的治疗方法，以使读者能对中医理论指导下的针灸理论和应用，有一个初步而又较完整的了解。为此，本书在内容和编排上有如下特点：

1. 系统介绍经络和腧穴知识。

2. 突出针灸学理论知识与临床技能之间的密切联系，便于掌握运用：腧穴部分除介绍位置外，还详述取穴法；各穴不单独设局部解剖和刺灸法项，重要部位的解剖和各部腧穴针刺方法等集中于第三章“各部常用腧穴的针刺方法”一节加以说明。

3. 精选临床上针灸疗效肯定、适合海外临床实际的病种 70 个，介绍其概念、辨证、用穴，详述针灸操作方法，使本书具有很强的临床实用性。

书中绪言、第三章、第四章及第五章的第八至第十节由赵京生编写，并负责制定编写大纲、全书中文稿的修订和统稿等工作；第一

Chapter 1, parts 1 - 6 in section 1 and section 2 in Chapter 2 and sections 1 - 7 in Chapter 5 are compiled by Liu Yueguang who is also responsible for drawing the diagrams; section 3 and parts 7 - 12 in section 1 in Chapter 2 as well as sections 11 - 14 in Chapter 5 are compiled by Hu Kui who is also responsible for drawing the diagrams.

章、第二章第一节的一至六和第二节、第五章的第一至第七节由刘跃光编写,并完成配图工作;第二章第一节的七至十二和第三节、第五章的第十一至第十四节由胡葵编写,并完成配图工作。

Contents

目　录

Introduction

Introduction to science of acupuncture and moxibustion

Acupuncture and moxibustion, one of the therapeutic nethods in traditional Chinese medicine (TCM) with a histoy of several thousand years, developed in the ancient times nd has contributed much to the healthcare and medical reatment for the Chinese people.

During their long clinical practice, people accumuated rich clinical experience and discovered a number of he therapeutic principles. The summarization of the linical experience and therapeutic principles has gradully paved the way to the establishment of the theory of icupuncture and moxibustion which has, in turn, pronoted the clinical practice and development of acupuncure and moxibustion, and eventually directing it to evolve into an independent clinical specialty—science of icupuncture and moxibustion.

Science of acupuncture and moxibustion develops under the guidance of TCM theory, its essential theory is the doctrine of meridians and collaterals which mainly includes meridians, collaterals and acupoints, directly guiding the clinical practice of acupuncture and moxibustion. Clinical treatment with acupuncture and moxibustion is done in light of syndrome differentiation, therapeutic principles and methods, by means of needling and moxibustion with certain manipulating

绪　言

一、针灸学简介

针灸疗法是古代中国人民创造的一种治病方法,其广泛使用的历史已有数千年之久,是中医治病的主要手段之一,对中国人民的医疗保健起着重大的作用。

在长期的应用过程中,人们积累起极为丰富的针灸临床经验,总结、发现了许多针灸治疗规律,逐渐形成了针灸理论,用以指导针灸临床实践,更加促进了针灸疗法的发展,至今已发展成为一门独立的临床学科——针灸学。

针灸学是中医学的一个组成部分,以中医理论为指导,其核心理论为经络学说。经络学说的主要内容是经络和腧穴理论,对针灸临床起着直接的理论指导作用。针灸临床治疗是在诊察辨证的基础上,按照治疗原则和治疗

methods to stimulate the selected acupoints for the prevention and treatment of disease.

方法，利用针刺、艾灸等手段，以一定的操作方式刺激相关的腧穴部位，以达到防病、治病的目的。

Acupuncture and moxibustion is an external therapy. By means of needling and moxibustion, it can stimulate the body and activate the regulating functions of the body to improve and rectify the disturbance and dysfunction of certain organs in the body. Such a therapy not only can treat disease, but also can prevent disease. It is noted for extensive application, significant curative effects and no side effects.

针灸疗法是一种外治方法，通过针刺、艾灸对机体的刺激，激发、调动其自身的调整功能，来改善、纠正紊乱的功能状态，使之趋于正常。不但能够治疗疾病，而且还能预防疾病。所以，针灸疗法具有广泛的适用范围，疗效明确，没有副作用。

It is just because of the characteristics mentioned above, the therapy of acupuncture and moxibustion is not only used in China, but also practised in over 100 countries in the world. It has gradually become a component in the world medicine and plays a certain role in the healthcare course for all human beings.

正是由于针灸疗法经过了千百年的长期临床实践检验，有完整的、能够指导临床实践的理论体系，适应证广，有效而较为安全，所以不但至今为中华民族所广泛使用，在中国的社会医疗保健事业中继续发挥着积极的作用，而且越来越受到世界医学界和各国人民的欢迎，前来中国学习针灸医学的人数不断增多，蔚然成风。目前世界上在使用和研究针灸的国家和地区已有 100 多个，针灸学已成为世界医学的组成部分，在人类医疗保健事业中发挥着越来越重要的作用。

2 Brief history

A brief introduction to the establishment and development of acupuncture and moxibustion is helpful for the study, practice and research of such a unique therapy.

In the ancient literature since the sixth century B.C., there was the record of "treatment of disease with stone needle". The earliest needle was made of stone. In *Huangdi Neijing* (*Huangdi's Canon on Medicine*) published over 2,000 years ago, silk medical books unearthed in the modern times and ancient Chinese classics, there was the description about how to treat disease with stone needle. In the 1960s, a stone needle was found in the ruins of new stone age in the north of China. With the development of metallurgy, needles were gradually made of bronze, iron, gold and silver. *Huangdi Neijing* (*Huangdi's Canon on Medicine*) mentions "Nine Needles", the relics of which were found in archaeology. The materials used for moxibustion were various in the early practice, gradually moxa was selected as the most suitable material for performing moxibustion.

In using acupuncture and moxibustion to treat disease, people discovered some therapeutic rules. Purposeful study of these rules led to theoretical cognition like the conception of meridians. In the silk medical books unearthed in the tomb of West Han Dynasty in

二、针灸学发展简史

了解针灸学的形成、发展过程，有助于对这门学科的学习、掌握和研究。

自公元前6世纪以来的中国古代文献中，就有“以砭石治病”和用艾治病的记载。针刺工具的前身是砭石。成书于2 000多年前的中医经典著作《黄帝内经》、近代考古发现的医学简帛书，以及中国文化典籍中，都有用称为“砭石”的石制针具治病的记载。20世纪60年代曾在中国北方的一个新石器时代遗址中出土一枚石针。冶金技术发明后，逐渐出现了铜针、铁针、金针和银针等金属针具。《黄帝内经》中记载有“九针”，其实物亦经考古发现。灸疗治病的材料，曾用过多种植物的枝叶，经过反复实践后选用艾叶作为灸治的主要材料。

在以针刺、艾灸治病的实践中，人们发现了某些治疗规律，并进而有意识地加以探索，逐渐形成一些理性认识，如经络的

1970s in Mawangdui, Changsha City, Hunan Province, there are the descriptions of eleven meridians named as "Eleven meridians of foot and arm for moxibustion" and "Eleven yin and yang meridians for moxibustion".

概念等。20 世纪 70 年代在湖南长沙马王堆西汉古墓中出土的医学帛书中,有两种记载十一条经脉的书,分别命名为"足臂十一脉灸经"、"阴阳十一脉灸经",反映了经络理论的早期面貌。

Huangdi Neijing (*Huangdi's Canon on Medicine*) compiled in the Han Dynasty contains rich knowledge of acupuncture and moxibustion, including meridians, acupoints, needling methods, indications and cautions as well as therapeutic principles, tenets, diagnosis and syndrome differentiation. *Huangdi Neijing* (*Huangdi's Canon on Medicine*) lays the foundation for the theory of acupuncture and moxibustion and guides the development of such a unique specialty.

成书于汉代的《黄帝内经》,对经络、腧穴、刺灸方法、适应病证、注意事项,针灸治疗思想、原则、原理,以及诊察和辨证方法等,有丰富而较为系统的论述,奠定了针灸理论的基础,在针灸学术的形成、发展中一直起着指导性的作用。

Zhenjiu Jiayijing (*A-B Classics on Acupuncture and Moxibustion*) compiled by Huangfu Mi in the Jin Dynasty is a collection of the related contents in *Huangdi Neijing* (*Huangdi's Canon on Medicine*) and *Mingtang Kongxue Zhenjiu Zhiyao* and described the locations, indications and needling methods of 349 acupoints as well as specific treatments for various diseases.

晋代医家皇甫谧所著的《针灸甲乙经》,将《黄帝内经》、《明堂孔穴针灸治要》等书的针灸内容汇集整理,确立了 349 个腧穴的位置、主治及操作等,还有大量常见病证的针灸治疗方法。对后世针灸学的发展有很大影响。

Sun Simiao, a great doctor in the Tang Dynasty, described Ashi Point and moxibustion methods for healthcare in *Qianjin Fang* (*Golden Prescriptions*) with colored illustrations of meridians. This book also contains many therapeutic methods for various diseases. In the book *Waitai Miyao* written by Wang Tao

唐代著名医家孙思邈在所著《千金方》中记载了阿是穴的取用方法,以及灸法强身防病的方法,并绘制了彩色经脉图;书中还大量记载了各种病证的

contains rich methods for performing moxibustion, which has promoted the development of moxibustion therapy. In the Imperial Medical Bureau, acupuncture and moxibustion became an independent specialty practised by doctors, assistants and acupuncturists who were also responsible for teaching.

针灸治法。王焘搜集大量灸法内容记于《外台秘要》中,其对灸疗的推崇在灸法发展过程中有一定促进作用。在唐代的太医署里,针灸已独立设科,配有针博士、针助教、针师等以进行针灸教学。

In the 11th century A.D., Wang Weiyi, an official in charge of medicine in the government in the Song Dynasty, rectified 354 acupoints and compiled *Tongren Shuxue Zhenjiu Tujing* (*Diagrams of Meridians and Acupoints on Bronze Figure*) which was published nationally. Two bronze figures, the normal size of man, were modelled for teaching and examination of acupuncture and moxibustion. Such an improvement promoted the unity in the location of acupoints and education of acupuncture and moxibustion.

公元 11 世纪,宋政府令医官王惟一对前人针灸文献进行整理,考订腧穴达 354 个,编撰《铜人腧穴针灸图经》并颁行全国;还首次铸造了两座成年男子大小的铜人腧穴模型,用于针灸教学和考试。这一举措有效地促进了腧穴定位的统一,对针灸教学的发展也有深远的影响。

In the Jin and Yuan Dynasties, there was further development in the theory of meridians, methods for selecting acupoints and needling techniques. Hua Boren, a celebrated doctor in the Yuan Dynasty, believed that the governor and conception vessels were as important as the twelve meridians. Therefore he called them fourteen meridians and described meridians and acupoints according to the fourteen meridians in his book *Shisijing Fahui* (*Elucidation of Fourteen Meridians*). Such an arrangement was helpful for understanding and using the theory of meridians and acupoints in the later generations. Famous doctors like He Ruoyu and Dou Hanqing thought highly of midnight-noon ebb-flow method for selecting acupoints and described such a

金元时期,在经络理论、用穴方法、刺法等方面都有进一步发展。元代名医滑伯仁,认为督脉、任脉与十二经脉同等重要而将其并称为十四经,在所著《十四经发挥》中按十四经排列腧穴。对后人理解、运用经脉腧穴理论很有启发。针灸名医何若愚、窦汉卿等,推崇子午流注取穴法,著书论述根据时间取用腧穴的方法,丰富了时间针灸的内容。窦汉卿

way to use acupoints in their books, and therefore enriching the content of time medicine. Dou Hanqing also developed the methods of needling by putting forward the methods of cold and heat reinforcing and reducing needling.

还丰富了针刺的操作术式，提出了寒热补泻的具体方法。

In the Ming Dynasty, acupuncture and moxibustion developed to its peak marked by publication of many monographs on acupuncture and moxibustion, active academic discussion and further development of needling methods, meridian theory and therapeutic methods. Yang Jizhou, a famous doctor then, compiled *Zhenjiu Dacheng* (*Compendium of Acupuncture and Moxibustion*) by summarizing the experience of his own and many others'. Xu Feng described many needling methods in his book *Zhenjiu Daquan* (*A Comprehensive Collection of Acupuncture and Moxibustion*) which further enriched the content of needling methods. Wang Ji studied many aspects of the theory and methods of acupuncture and moxibustion, which was beneficial to the normal development of acupuncture and moxibustion. In his book *Zhenjiu Juying*, Gao Wu collected various theoretical and therapeutic literature related to acupuncture and moxibustion with his personal ideas. Li Shizhen made thorough studies on extraordinary vessels and added new content to the doctrine of meridians in his book *Qijing Bamaikao* (*Textual Research on Extraordinary Meridians*).

明代是针灸学的兴盛时期，表现为针灸名家众多，有多部针灸著作问世，学术思想活跃，在针法、经脉理论、病证治法等方面又有所发展。针灸名医杨继洲将前人及自己的经验总结编著成《针灸大成》，内容丰富，在国内外都相当有影响。徐凤在其《针灸大全》中记载了大量针刺手法，使针法内容更为丰富。汪机则对许多针灸理论、方法进行探讨争鸣，有利于针灸学术的健康发展。高武的《针灸聚英》汇集多种针灸文献的理论和治疗经验，并有自己的见解与体会。李时珍的《奇经八脉考》，对奇经进行了专门的研究，丰富了经络学说。

Books on acupuncture and moxibustion published in the Qing Dynasty lacked innovative development. In the middle of the Qing Dynasty the specialty of acupuncture and moxibustion was banned in the Imperial Hospital. However, folk practice was still extensive.

清代的针灸著作少有新意，至中后期官方废除太医院的针灸科，从而阻碍了针灸学的进一步发展。但在民间，仍广泛使用着针灸疗法。

After the founding of the People's Republic of China and owing to the policy made by the government for developing traditional Chinese medicine, the academic studies of acupuncture and moxibustion have developed fast. The rapid development of acupuncture and moxibustion is marked by extensive application of acupuncture and moxibustion therapy, higher education, establishment of academic institutes, recompilation of ancient classics, publication of a great number of academic books and journals, thorough studies on the meridians, acupoints, needling and moxibusting methods and tenets of acupuncture and moxibustion therapy as well as development of various needling methods like acupuncture anesthesia and devices for performing acupuncture and moxibustion.

中华人民共和国成立后，由于中医政策的实施而使针灸学得到空前的发展。针灸疗法被广泛使用，发展针灸高等教育，建立针灸研究机构，整理针灸古籍，出版大量针灸著作、学术刊物；采用现代科学技术开展针灸临床研究，对经络、腧穴、刺灸方法、影响因素以及针灸作用原理等进行了深入的研究；发展、创造了多种针灸应用方法，如针刺麻醉等，研制各种刺灸器具和针灸治疗仪。所有这些极大地丰富了针灸医学的内容。

Acupuncture and moxibustion spread to the other countries even in the ancient times. In about 6th century A. D., *Zhenjiu Jiayijing* (*A-B Classics on Acupuncture and Moxibustion*) was spread to Korea and Japan. In 552 A. D., the Chinese Government then presented a set of *Zhenjing* (*Acupuncture Canon*) to Japanese Emperor. In the Tang Dynasty, *Qianjin Fang* (*Golden Prescriptions*) and *Waitai Miyao* were brought to Korea. Following the example of the Tang Dynasty, Japan also established acupuncture and moxibustion specialty and Korea appointed doctorate position for acupuncture. The textbooks used were *Zhenjing* (*Acupuncture Canon*) and *Zhenjiu Jiayijing* (*A-B Classics on Acupuncture and Moxibustion*). In the 17th century, acupuncture and moxibustion was spread to Europe. Since 1950s, many countries have sent

针灸医学很早就传到国外。约在公元 6 世纪，《针灸甲乙经》传到朝鲜、日本，公元 552 年中国赠送日本天皇一套《针经》。在唐代，《千金方》、《外台秘要》等书传至朝鲜；日本仿照唐制而设置针灸专科，朝鲜仿照唐制设针博士，皆以《针经》、《针灸甲乙经》等书为教材。17 世纪，针灸传到了欧洲。自 20 世纪 50 年代以来，有不少国家派医师来中国学习针灸技术。中国也不断派遣针灸专家小组到国外进

doctors to China to study acupuncture and moxibustion. Chinese government has sent acupuncture and moxibustion experts group abroad to offer clinical treatment. Since 1975, to meet the requirement of WHO, China has set up international training centers for acupuncture and moxibustion in Beijing, Shanghai and Nanjing to train acupuncture and moxibustion doctors for a number of countries. Currently acupuncture and moxibustion therapy has been used in about 100 countries and regions. A number of international academic organizations have been set up. In 1987, Federation of World Acupuncture and Moxibustion Society was established in China and many international conferences have been held since then. The science of acupuncture and moxibustion has developed smoothly in the whole world.

行临床治疗工作。自1975年以后,中国应联合国世界卫生组织(WHO)的要求,先后在北京、上海、南京等地成立国际针灸培训中心,为许多国家培训了针灸人才。目前世界上在使用和研究针灸的国家和地区已有100多个,多个国际性针灸学术组织相继建立,1987年世界针灸学会联合会在中国成立,针灸医学已在世界范围内得到发展。

1 General introduction to meridians and acupoints

第一章 经络腧穴总论

The theory of meridians and acupoints is the basic theory of acupuncture and moxibustion therapy. The science of meridians expounds the routes that connect different parts of the body based on the clinical application of acupoints; while the science of acupoints elucidates the relation between the viscera and the meridians in light of the theory of meridians.

经络、腧穴理论是针灸疗法的基本理论，其中，经络学主要是以腧穴的临床应用为依据，阐述人体各部之间的联系通路；腧穴学，又以经络理论为依据，阐明其与脏腑经络的关系，两者是一个不可分割的整体。

Meridians and acupoints are one of the essential parts demonstrating the organic wholeness in TCM. The theory of meridians, the theory of viscera and the theory of qi, blood and body fluids constitute the theoretic base of TCM and run through the physiology, pathology, diagnosis and treatment in TCM.

经络腧穴是中医学整体观念赖以构成的基础；经络理论与藏象理论、气血津液理论等共同构成中医学理论的基础，是中医基础理论的重要组成部分，贯串于中医学的生理、病理、诊断和治疗等各个方面。

1.1 General introduction to meridians

第一节 经络总论

Meridians refer to the routes that transport qi and blood, regulate yin and yang, connect the zang-organs with the fu-organs, associate the external with the internal as well as the upper with the lower.

经络是人体运行气血、协调阴阳、联络脏腑、沟通内外、贯串上下的通路。

Meridians include both meridians and collaterals. Meridians refer to the longitudinal trunk parts of the

经络是经脉和络脉的总称。经，有路径的意思，是指

meridian system, while collaterals refer to the branches of meridians. Collaterals can be further divided into subcollaterals. The shallow collaterals are called superficial collaterals which distribute all over the body. In this way meridians and collaterals form a network connecting all parts of the body, including the viscera, five sensory organs, nine orifices, four limbs and skeleton, into an organic whole.

经络系统中的直行主干部分；络，有网络的意思，是指由“经”分出的小的横行分支，络还可再分出更细小的分支称为“孙络”，其中浮现于体表的称为“浮络”，它们遍布全身，不计其数。这样就由经络构成了联系人体各部的网络结构系统，人体的五脏六腑、五官九窍、四肢百骸等，皆有赖于这些纵横交错贯穿其间的经络而联系成为一个有机的整体。

Meridians not only connect all parts of the body, but also coordinate their functions. By means of regulating their own conditions of qi and blood, the meridians influence the states of the viscera and regulate the physiological activities between the zang-organs, the zang and fu organs, the viscera and five sensory organs and nine orifices as well as the four limbs and skeleton to coordinate the functional activities of different parts of the body. Under morbid conditions, the meridians also influence various complicated pathological changes. The basic tenets of acupuncture and moxibustion in treating disease lie in their regulating functions through activating meridian qi to adjust the states of the viscera.

经络不仅对人体的脏腑、器官、组织起着结构上的联系，而且具有功能上的协调作用，它通过对自身气血的盛衰调节而影响脏腑的功能状态，并调节着脏与脏、脏与腑、腑与腑、脏腑与五官九窍、四肢百骸之间的复杂的生理活动，使机体各部分的功能活动得以保持协调；在疾病状态下，它也影响着多种复杂的病理变化过程。针灸治疗疾病的基本原理，就是通过激发经气的调整功能，来调节脏腑的功能状态。

1.1.1 Composition of meridian system

The system of meridians is mainly composed of the twelve regular meridians, twelve meridian branches, fifteen collaterals, twelve meridian tendons, twelve skin areas and eight extraordinary vessels (see Table 1-1).

一、经络系统的组成

经络系统主要是由十二经脉、十二经别、十五络脉、十二经筋、十二皮部和奇经八脉所组成(见表 1－1)。

Table 1 - 1 **System of meridians**

- Meridian System
  - Twelve regular meridians
    - Three yin meridians of hand
      - Lung meridian of hand-taiyin
      - Pericardium meridian of hand-jueyin
      - Heart meridian of hand-shaoyin
    - Three yang meridians of hand
      - Large intestine meridian of hand-yangming
      - Triple energizer meridian of hand-shaoyang
      - Small intestine meridian of hand-taiyang
    - Three yang meridians of foot
      - Stomach meridian of foot-yangming
      - Gallbladder meridian of foot-shaoyang
      - Bladder meridian of foot-taiyang
    - Three yin meridians of foot
      - Spleen meridian of foot-taiyin
      - Liver meridian of foot-jueyin
      - Kidney meridian of foot-shaoyin
  - (↑ to Twelve regular meridians)
    - Twelve meridian branches
    - Twelve meridian tendons
    - Twelve skin areas
    - Twelve collaterals
  - Fifteen major collaterals
    - Twelve collaterals
    - Large collateral of the spleen
    - CV collateral
    - GV collateral
  - Eight extraordinary vessels
    - Conception vessel ... CV collateral
    - Governor vessel ... GV collateral
    - Thoroughfare vessel
    - Belt vessel
    - Yin link vessel
    - Yang link vessel
    - Yin heel vessel
    - Yang heel vessel

表 1 - 1 **经络系统表**

- 经络系统
  - 十二经脉
    - 手三阴经
      - 手太阴肺经
      - 手厥阴心包经
      - 手少阴心经
    - 手三阳经
      - 手阳明大肠经
      - 手少阳三焦经
      - 手太阳小肠经
    - 足三阳经
      - 足阳明胃经
      - 足少阳胆经
      - 足太阳膀胱经
    - 足三阴经
      - 足太阴脾经
      - 足厥阴肝经
      - 足少阴肾经
  - （↑ 十二经脉）
    - 十二经别
    - 十二经筋
    - 十二皮部
    - 十二经络脉
  - 十五大络
    - 十二经络脉
    - 脾之大络
    - 任络
    - 督络
  - 奇经八脉
    - 任脉……任络
    - 督脉……督络
    - 冲脉
    - 带脉
    - 阴维脉
    - 阳维脉
    - 阴蹻脉
    - 阳蹻脉

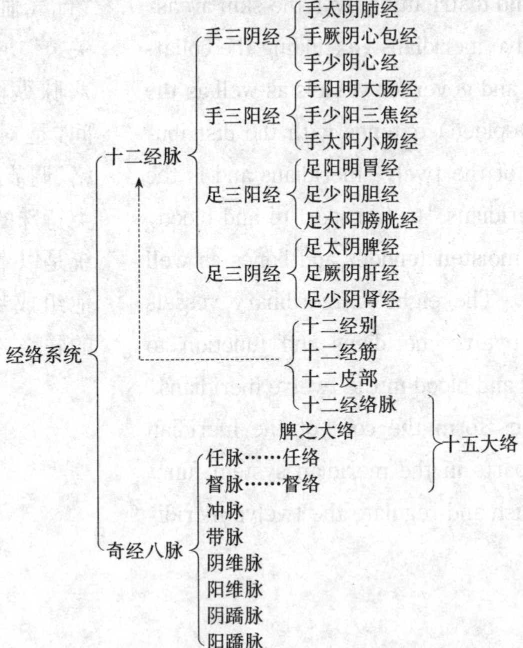

The twelve meridians are the trunk parts of the meridian system and "are connected with the viscera internally and limbs and skeleton externally" to transport qi and blood to the viscera, limbs and skeleton. The twelve meridian branches are the branches of the twelve meridians to reinforce the connection between the zang and fu organs externally and internally related and the meridians distributing over the head and face in external and internal relation. The fifteen collaterals stem from the twelve meridians and the conception and governor vessels as well as the spleen for reinforcement of the connection of the meridians with internal and external relationship on the four limbs as well as the association of the anterior, posterior and lateral parts of the trunk of the body. The twelve meridian tendons stem from the twelve meridians for nourishing and governing the musculature and joints as well as for reinforcing the connection with the three yin meridians and three yang meridians at the same side. The twelve skin areas refer to the collaterals stemming from the twelve meridians and distributing over the skin areas. The system of the twelve meridians (excluding the collaterals of the conception and governor vessels as well as the major collateral of the spleen) extends with the distribution of the trunk parts of the twelve meridians and is the base for the twelve meridians "to transport qi and blood, nourish yin and yang, moisten tendons and bones as well as smooth the joints". The eight extraordinary vessels distribute among the twelve meridians and function to connect and regulate qi and blood in the twelve meridians. So the twelve meridians form the core of the meridian system and the other parts in the meridian system function to connect, replenish and regulate the twelve meridians.

十二经脉是经络系统的主干,"内属于府藏,外络于肢节",将气血输布到人体的五脏六腑、四肢百骸。十二经别,是从十二经脉分出的支脉,以加强躯干部表里脏腑和头面表里经的联系。十五络脉,是从十二经以及任脉、督脉、脾脏分出的支脉,加强四肢部表里经和躯干前、后、侧三部的联系。十二经筋,是从十二经脉分出的濡养、支配筋肉关节的部分,并加强同侧三阴、三阳之间的联系。十二皮部,是十二经脉分出的络脉分布于皮肤的区域。上述十二经体系(任络 、督络、脾之大络除外),是围绕着十二经脉主干的支脉延伸,是十二经脉"行气血,营阴阳,濡筋骨,利关节"功能的结构基础。奇经八脉纵横交错于十二经脉之间,是对十二经脉起综合联络、调节经脉气血作用的另一类特殊的经脉。所以,经络系统是以十二经脉为核心的,其他组成部分都是对十二经脉的联络、补充和综合、调节。

1.1.2 Distribution of meridian system

1.1.2.1 The twelve meridians

The twelve meridians are the main part of the meridian system and are also known as "the twelve regular meridians" including three yin meridians of the hand, three yang meridians of the hand, three yin meridians of the foot and three yang meridians of the foot.

1.1.2.1.1 Distribution on the surface of the body

The twelve meridians distribute in symmetry on the face, head, trunk and limbs.

Four limbs: The yin meridians distribute along the inner side of the four limbs, yang meridians on the lateral side of the four limbs. According to yin and yang, taiyin and yangming meridians distribute along the anterior side, shaoyin and taiyang along the posterior side, and jueyin and shaoyang along the middle side. Among these meridians, only jueyin meridian of the foot turns and converges with others in distribution. It runs anterior to the taiyin meridian of the foot 8 cun down to the medial malleolus. From the region 8 cun above the medial malleolus, it converges with taiyin meridian and runs between the taiyin and shaoyin meridians.

Trunk: The six meridians of the foot distribute in the way mentioned above. The only difference is that they pertain to either yin or yang according to the inner side and lateral side of the trunk. The three yang meridians of the foot distribute the surface of the trunk, yangming on the front, taiyang on the back and shaoyang on the lateral side, while the three yin meridians of the foot run in the interior part corresponding to the yang meridians that they are internally and externally related to. Among the

二、经络系统的分布概貌

(一)十二经脉

十二经脉是经络系统的主体,故又称之为"十二正经";是手三阴经脉、手三阳经脉、足三阳经脉、足三阴经脉的总称。

1. 体表分布规律

十二经脉在体表左右对称地分布于头面、躯干、四肢。

(1) 四肢部:阴经分布于四肢的内侧,阳经分布于四肢的外侧;按三阴、三阳来分,则太阴、阳明在前,少阴、太阳在后,厥阴、少阳在中。其中只有足厥阴经有例外的曲折交叉,在足内踝上8寸以下循行于足太阴经之前,至内踝上8寸处与足太阴经交叉之后,行于太阴与少阴之间。

(2) 躯干部:足六经:仍按上述规律分布,所不同的是以躯干的内、外分阴阳,即足三阳经分布于躯干的表面:阳明在前,太阳在后,少阳在侧,而足三阴经则循行于与其相表里阳经的里面。

手六经:手三阳经都经过肩部上颈项;手三阴经则多由

six meridians of the hand, the three yang meridians all run over the shoulder to the neck while the three yin meridians all come out of the chest from the armpit.

胸内直接出于腋下。

Head and face: The six yang meridians of the hand and foot all reach the head and face to connect with the five sense organs. That is why it is said "the head is the convergence of all yang meridians". All the six yin meridians run deep in the head and neck to connect with the throat, tongue and eyes.

(3) 头面部:手足六阳经皆上头面联系五官,故有"头为诸阳之会"之说;六阴经多走在头、颈的深部,联系喉咙(颃颡)、舌、目系等器官。

1.1.2.1.2 Association of the twelve meridians with the viscera

2. 十二经脉与脏腑的联系

As to its rule, the association of the twelve meridians with the viscera is mainly demonstrated as "pertaining and connection". Yin meridians pertain to the zang organs and connect with the fu organs, while yang meridians pertain to the fu organs and connect with the zang organs. Besides the regular "pertaining and connection", the taiyang meridians of the hand and the foot in the six yang meridians also associate with the stomach and the brain; the six yin meridians usually associate with the other zang and fu organs. The following table is a thorough demonstration of such relations among the meridians.

十二经脉与脏腑的联系,就其规律性而言,主要表现为"属、络"关系,即:阴经属于脏而络于腑,阳经属于腑而络于脏。十二经脉除固定的"属络"脏腑外,六阳经中只有手、足太阳经还联系到胃和脑;六阴经则多联系其他脏腑,其详尽内容见表1-2。

Table 1-2 Association of the twelve meridians with the viscera

Meridians		Viscera pertaining to and connecting with	Other viscera
Three yin meridians of the hand	Hand-taiyin Hand-shaoyin Hand-jueyin	Lung, large intestine Heart, small intestine Pericardium, triple energizer	Stomach and middle energizer Lung
Three yin meridians of the foot	Foot-taiyin Foot-shaoyin Foot-jueyin	Spleen, stomach Kidney, bladder Liver, gallbladder	Heart Liver, lung, heart Lung, stomach
Three yang meridians of the hand	Hand-yangming Hand-taiyang Hand-shaoyang	Large intestine, lung Small intestine, heart Triple energizer, pericardium	Stomach
Three yang meridians of the foot	Foot-yangming Foot-taiyang Foot-shaoyang	Stomach, spleen Bladder, kidney Gallbladder, liver	Brain

表 1-2 十二经脉与脏腑联系表

经 脉		属络脏腑	其他脏腑
手 三 阴	手 太 阴	肺,大肠	胃,中焦
	手 少 阴	心,小肠	肺
	手 厥 阴	心包,三焦	
足 三 阴	足 太 阴	脾,胃	心
	足 少 阴	肾,膀胱	肝,肺,心
	足 厥 阴	肝,胆	肺,胃
手 三 阳	手 阳 明	大肠,肺	
	手 太 阳	小肠,心	胃
	手 少 阳	三焦,心包	
足 三 阳	足 阳 明	胃,脾	
	足 太 阳	膀胱,肾	脑
	足 少 阳	胆,肝	

1.1.2.1.3 Running direction, circulation and convergent principle of the twelve meridians

Running direction: Qi and blood in the twelve meridians flow in the same direction according to the distinction of three yin meridians of the hand and foot as well as three yang meridians of the hand and foot. Such a running direction is described in *Lingshu* (*Spiritual Pivot*) as "The three yin meridians of the hand run from the chest to the hand; the three yang meridians run from the hand to the head; the three yang meridians of the foot run from the head to the foot; the three yin meridians run from the foot to the abdomen."

Circulation: The twelve meridians form a cycle of qi and blood circulatory system with their regular and adverse circulatory directions. The circulatory order is demonstrated in the following table.

3. 十二经脉的循行走向、循环流注与交接规律

(1) 循行走向:十二经脉在人体的气血运行按手足三阴、三阳划分,其循行方向是一致的,这就是《灵枢·逆顺肥瘦》所说的:"手之三阴,从胸走手;手之三阳,从手走头;足之三阳,从头走足;足之三阴,从足走腹。"

(2) 循环流注:十二经脉循行走向有顺有逆,这就使得十二经脉连贯起来,构成"阴阳相贯,如环无端"的十二经脉整体气血循环系统。其流

注次序见表1-3。

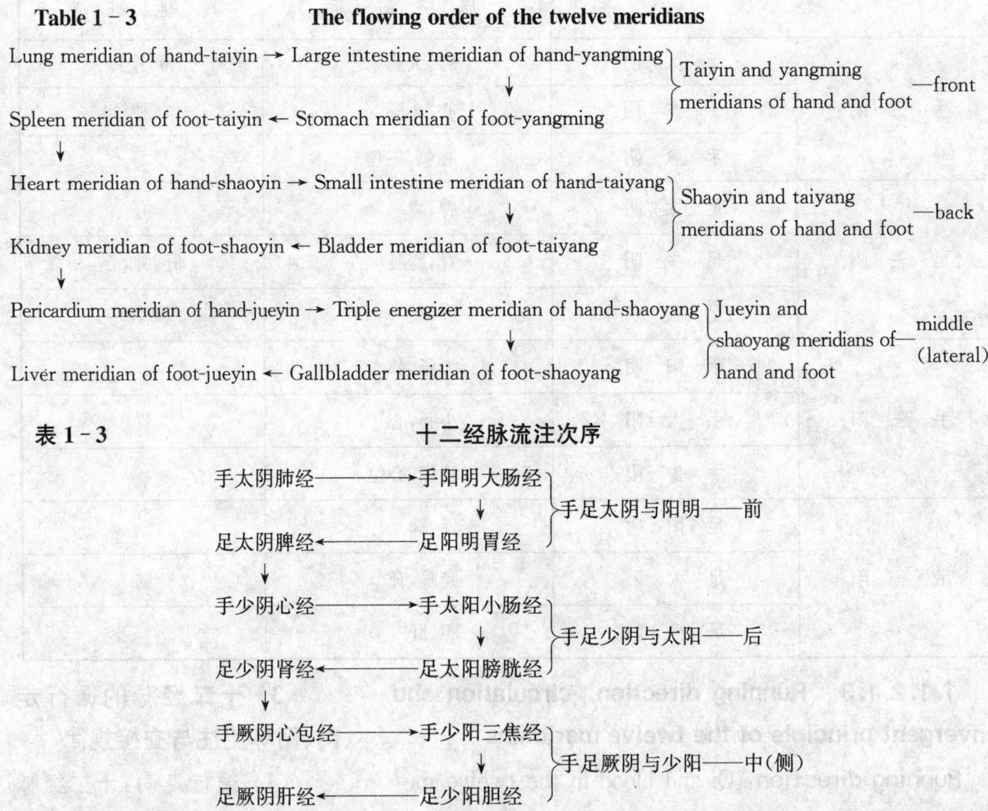

Convergent principle: The circulatory order shows that the first four meridians of taiyin and yangming of the hand and foot distribute along the anterior border of the body, the middle four meridians of shaoyin and taiyang of the hand and foot distribute along the posterior border of the body, the last four meridians of jueyin and shaoyang of the hand and foot distribute along the side or centre of the body. In this way qi and blood circulate in the twelve meridians for actually three cycles. The convergent way in each cycle follows the order of yin and yang meridians in external and internal relation as well as the yang meridians with the same name. According to such a convergent way and in light of the circulatory direction of the meridi-

(3) 交接规律：从上述十二经脉的流注次序可以看出，前四条经是手足太阴与阳明，分布于人体的前缘，中间四条经是手足少阴与太阳，分布于人体的后缘，后四条经是手足厥阴与少阳，分布于人体的侧面或中央，这样，气血沿着十二经脉完成一次循环流注，实际上在人体运行了三个回环；而在每个回环里，其连接的方式是按照表里阴阳经、同名阳经、表里阴阳经的顺序，再结

ns, it is obvious that the twelve meridians converge with he following principle: the yin and yang meridians in ex ernal and internal relationship converge over the end of the our limbs; the yang meridians with the same name con- erge over the head and face; the yin meridians and yang neridians (in a cycle-like connection) converge over the hest.

合经脉的循行走向，就不难得出十二经脉的交接规律：表里阴阳经在四肢末端交接；同名阳经在头面部交接；阴经与阴经(回环连接)在胸部交接。

The running direction, circulation and convergence re interrelated and reflect the circulatory order of qi and lood in the twelve meridians from different angles.

循行走向、流注次序、交接规律三者是相互决定的关系，它们都是从不同的角度对十二经脉的气血运行规律所作的归纳总结。

1.1.2.1.4 External and internal relation

4. 表里关系

External and internal relation, an important interre- tion among the twelve meridians similar to that of the elation between zang organs and fu organs, refers to the orrespondence of the three yin and three yang meridians. uch an external and internal relation among the twelve eridians, apart from the convergence of the yin and yang eridians in internal and external relation at the end of e four limbs as well as the regular "pertaining and con- ection" with the viscera over the trunk, further rengthens such a relation through meridian branches and ollaterals. The meridian branches reinforce the relation ith the organs in external and internal relation by means "entering" and reinforce the relation of the meridians external and internal relation on the head and face. The ollaterals of the twelve meridians intensify the relation of e meridians in external and internal relation on the four nbs by means of forking into the meridians in external d internal relation.

所谓经络的表里关系指的是手足三阴三阳的对应关系与脏腑表里的一致性，或称表里相合关系，它是十二经脉之间一种主要的相互关系。十二经脉的表里关系除了通过经脉本身在四肢末端表里阴阳经的交接和躯干部固定的脏腑互相"属、络"以外，还通过经别和络脉进一步加强这种联系，经别通过其"入"加强与表里脏腑的联系，通过其"合"加强头面部表里两经的联系，而十二经之络脉则通过别走表里，加强表里两经在四肢部的联系。

1.1.2.2 The meridian branches of the velve meridians

(二) 十二经别

The meridian branches of the twelve meridians stem

十二经别是指从十二经

from the twelve meridians, run deep into the trunk, associate with the viscera and the branches of the meridians in external and internal relation. The meridian branches are actually the regular meridians that run along other routes. As to the nature, the meridian branches stemming from the twelve meridians pertain to the aspect of the twelve meridians. In distribution, the meridian branches run deep into the body, associate with the meridians in external and internal relation, indicating that the distribution of the meridian branches is centripetal.

脉分出，别行深入躯干，联络脏腑器官，沟通表里两经的支脉，是别道而行的正经。即十二经别在属性上：是从十二经脉分出的支脉，是属于十二正经的范畴；在分布特点上：别行深入躯干，联络脏腑器官沟通表里两经，表明其分布呈向心性。

The running of the branches of the twelve meridians is marked by "stemming, entering, outthrusting and combination".

十二经别的循行，具有"离、入、出、合"的特点。

"Stemming" means that the meridian branches stem from the areas below the knees and elbows, usually the meridian branches run parallel to or together with the meridians in external and internal relation; "entering" means that the meridian branches enter the body and usually associate with the viscera in external and internal relation, the branches of the three yang meridians of the foot also associate with the heart; "outthrusting" means that the meridian branches come out to run in the superficial areas over the head and neck; "combination" means that the branches of the yin meridians combine with the yang meridians that they are in internal and external relation with, while the branches of the yang meridians combine with the meridians that they stem from.

"离"是指从肘膝关节以上本经别出，一般多表里经别并行或合而行走；"入"是指进入躯干，多联系表里脏腑，足三阳经别还联系到心；"出"是指浅出于头项部；"合"是指阴经经别合于相表里的阳经，阳经经别合于本经。

In this way, the three yin and three yang meridians of the hand and foot constitute "six combinations". By means of "stemming, entering, outthrusting and combination", the branches of the twelve meridians further strengthen the meridians in external and internal relation, especially the association of the meridians with the viscera in external and internal relation. With such activities, the

这样，手、足三阴三阳经别就汇合为六对，所以又称为"六合"。十二经别通过其离、入、出、合，进一步加强了经脉的表里联系，特别是加强了经脉与表里脏腑之间的联系；补充了经脉在循行分布上的

meridian branches also widen the distribution of the meridians, reinforces the association of the twelve meridians with the whole body, and enlarges the indication of the acupoints.

足,使十二经脉对人体各部分的联系更趋周密,扩大了经穴的主治范围。

1.1.2.3 The fifteen collaterals

(三)十五络脉

The fifteen collaterals is a collective term for the collaterals of the twelve meridians, the governor and conception vessels as well as the major collateral of the spleen.

十二经脉和任、督两脉各自别出一络,加上脾之大络,总为十五络脉。

The cyclical running of the twelve collaterals is composed of two parts: after stemming from the "Luo-Connecting" acupoints located below the knees and elbows, one part runs to the meridian that it is in internal and external relation with; the other part runs parallel to the meridian that it stems from and associates with certain viscera, organ and region. Collaterals are fine and numerous, making it difficult to locate and nominate. But the collaterals of the twelve meridians have definite location. They are connected with the meridians in external and internal relation on one hand, and run parallel to the meridians sharing both the properties of the meridians and collaterals on the other. That is why they are called "major collaterals". The three collaterals over the trunk of the body distribute on the front, back and side of the body.

十二经络脉的循行分为两部分:在从四肢肘膝关节以下的络穴别出后,一支走向其表里经;另一支并经而行联系一定的脏腑、器官和部位。络脉细小而不计其数,难以定位而无法命名(且亦无意义),十二经之络脉,有明确的别出部位,既有"支而横"络于表里之经者,又有纵向并经而行者,似具有经与络的双重属性,故另立一类称之为"大络",以示其不同于一般意义上的络脉。躯干部的三络,分布于身前、身后、身侧。

The major collaterals of the twelve meridians further strengthen the association of the meridians in external and internal relation below the knees and elbows. It is also marked by definite distribution, association with certain viscera and organs and improvement of the distribution of the twelve meridians. The three collaterals on the trunk of the body mainly function to infuse qi and blood in the front, back and side of the body.

十二经之大络,进一步加强了肘膝关节以下表里两经的联系;同时亦有一定的循行分布部位,特定地联系某些脏腑、器官,补充了经脉循行的不足;躯干三络主要是对身前、身后、身侧起渗灌气血的作用。

Both the meridian branches and collaterals function to strengthen the association of the meridians in external and

经别和络脉都是加强表里两经的联系,所不同的是:

internal relation. The difference is that the meridian branches mainly strengthen the association of the viscera in external and internal relation as well as the association of the meridians in external and internal relation on the head and face; while the collaterals mainly reinforce the association of the meridians in external and internal relation below the knees and elbows.

经别主内，主要是加强躯干部表里脏腑之间的联系和表里经脉在头面部的联系；而络脉主外，主要是加强肘膝关节以下表里两经之间的联系。

1.1.2.4 The tendons of the twelve meridians

（四）十二经筋

The tendons of the twelve meridians refer to the areas where qi from the twelve meridians accumulates and are the regions where the twelve meridians are connected with the musculature and joints.

十二经筋是十二经脉之气结聚散络于筋肉关节的体系，是十二经脉连属于筋肉关节的部分。

The distribution of the twelve meridian tendons agree with the projection of the meridians that they are connected with on the body surface, especially on the four limbs. The function of the meridian tendons is to nourish and govern the musculature and joints to maintain the normal activities of the body and strengthen the relation of the twelve meridians with the three yin and three yang meridians on the same side.

十二经筋的分布部位，与其所辖之经脉的体表投影基本一致，这种分布特点在四肢部尤为明显；经筋的作用主要是濡养和支配人体的筋肉关节，保持人体正常的运动功能；并加强十二经脉同侧三阴、三阳之间的联系。

1.1.2.5 The twelve skin areas

（五）十二皮部

The skin areas, the regions where the twelve meridians distribute on the skin, are the regions where the meridian qi effuse over the skin and the functional activities of the twelve meridians are reflected on the body surface.

皮部是十二经络脉在皮肤的分布区域，它是络脉之气在皮肤的散布所在，也是十二经功能活动反映于体表的部位。

The distribution of the skin areas follows the distribution of the twelve meridians on the body surface.

皮部的分布区域是以十二经脉在体表的分布范围为依据的。

The skin areas govern closure and opening and are the pivot responsible for the association of the body with the nature. The skin areas regulate the closing and opening states of the muscular interstices and the functions of the viscera in response to the outward stimulation so as to

皮部主司开合，是人体与自然接触交流的枢纽，它能随外界刺激的变化而相应地调整皮肤腠理的开合和内脏的功能状态，以使人体与自然相

enable the body to be in harmony with the nature. Such a function is closely related to the functions of defensive qi and the lung. That is why skin areas are regarded as the defensive screen of the body. Under path-ological conditions, the skin areas may act as the routes to transmit pathogenic factors inside and reflect the pathological conditions of the viscera and meridians. Clinical diagnosis and treatment of disease according to the examination of the external manifestations is actually done in light of the theory of skin areas.

适应，它的这一功能主要是与卫气和肺的功能密切相关，所以是机体的卫外屏障。在病理状态下，也可由浅入深成为传注病邪的途径和脏腑、经络病变时反映于体表的部位，临床上从外部的诊察和施治可推断和治疗内部的疾病，就是结合了皮部理论的运用。

1.1.2.6 The eight extraordinary vessels

（六）奇经八脉

The eight extraordinary vessels is a collective term for the governor vessel, conception vessel, thoroughfare vessel, belt vessel, yin link vessel, yang link vessel, yin heel vessel and yang heel vessel.

奇经八脉是督脉、任脉、冲脉、带脉、阴维脉、阳维脉、阴蹻脉、阳蹻脉的总称。

Compared with the twelve meridians, there is no external and internal relation among the eight extraordinary vessels. In terms of visceral association, the eight extraordinary vessels are in close relation with the extraordinary fu organs. In terms of the distribution, they do not have their own distributing routes and just run around among the twelve meridians except the governor and conception vessels. In terms of the acupoints, they do not have their own specific acupoints except the governor and conception vessels. In terms of the functions, they do not transport qi and blood like that of the twelve meridians, just accumulate and regulate qi and blood in the twelve regular meridians.

与十二正经相比较，奇经八脉没有表里属络关系，在脏腑联系上主要与奇恒之腑联系较密切；在循行分布上除督、任二脉外，它较少有属于自己的分布路线，纵横交错于十二经之间；在腧穴上除督、任二脉外，其他六条脉的穴位都寄附于十二经脉，没有专属于本经的穴位；在功能上也不像十二经脉那样运行气血，形成气血循环流注，而是对正经的气血起溢蓄和调节作用。

The functions of the eight extraordinary vessels are reflected in two aspects. One is to associate the twelve meridians to command qi and blood in certain meridians as well as to regulate yin and yang. The other is to accumulate, effuse and regulate qi and blood in the twelve meridians. "To accumulate" means that the extraordinary

奇经八脉的作用主要表现在两方面：一是沟通了十二经脉之间的联系，奇经八脉在其循行、分布过程中将功能相似的经脉联系起来，达到统摄有关经脉气血，协调阴阳的作用；

vessels can store up qi and blood in the twelve meridians when they are superabundant. "To effuse" means that the extraordinary vessels can provide qi and blood in case of need during the activity of the body or insufficiency of qi and blood in the twelve meridians to regulate the conditions of qi and blood as well as yin and yang related to the twelve meridians.

二是对十二经脉的气血有溢蓄调节作用,"蓄"是指当十二经脉和脏腑气血旺盛时,奇经能加以蓄积,"溢"是指在人体功能活动需要或正经气血不足时,奇经八脉又能渗灌供应,以调节正经气血阴阳的盛衰平衡。

1.2 General introduction to acupoints

第二节　腧穴总论

Acupoints are the spots where qi and blood from the viscera and meridians effuse and infuse in the body surface. The name of acupoints indicates that the basic characteristics: the spots where qi and blood from the viscera and meridians effuse and infuse; acupoints are usually located in the interstices in the thick muscles or between tendons and bones.

腧穴的"腧"与"输"义通,即有输注的含义;"穴"含有"孔"、"隙"的意思。腧穴是人体脏腑经络气血输注出入于体表的部位。腧穴的名称说明了腧穴的两个基本特征:其实质是脏腑经络之气的输注部位,其部位所在多为分肉筋骨之间的空隙之处。

The viscera, meridians and acupoints in the interior and exterior form an organic whole with close relation and harmonious unity. The meridians are connected with the viscera in the interior and with the acupoints in the exterior. The acupoints are the spots where qi from the viscera and meridians "effuse and infuse" as well as "run out and in". The viscera transform qi and blood, while the meridians and acupoints transport and infuse qi and blood. So the viscera form the base for the functional activities of the meridians and acupoints. Under pathological conditions, disorders of the viscera can be reflected on certain acupoints through the meridians. Stimulation of the acupoints with abnormal manifestations or related acupoints may regulate the functional activities of the corresponding viscera.

脏腑-经络-腧穴内外相应,是一个联系密切而又协调统一的整体。经脉内连于脏腑,外通于腧穴;腧穴是脏腑、经络之气"渗灌"和"游行出入"的部位;脏腑化生气血,经络腧穴运行、输注气血,因此脏腑是经络腧穴功能活动的基础。在病理状态下,脏腑疾患能通过经络在某些相应的腧穴出现异常反应,刺激这些异常反应点或相关腧穴,可以对相应脏腑的功能活动起到相对特异的调整作用。

1.2.1 Classification of acupoints

Acupoints can usually be classified into meridian acupoints, extraordinary acupoints and Ashi points according to the characteristics of acupoints.

1.2.1.1 Meridian acupoints

Meridian acupoints, also known as acupoints of the fourteen meridians, refer to the acupoints located on the twelve meridians as well as the governor and conception vessels. Meridian acupoints are the main part in acupoints and are the acupoints frequently used. Meridian acupoints are marked by pertaining to definite meridians, fixed names and location. Altogether there are 361 acupoints.

1.2.1.2 Extraordinary acupoints

Extraordinary acupoints refer to the acupoints not included in the acupoints of the fourteen meridians. These acupoints have definite location and names and are effective in treating certain diseases.

The extraordinary acupoints are marked by definite location, fixed names and no pertaining to any meridians. However, the extraordinary acupoints and meridian acupoints are closely related to each other. Firstly, some extraordinary acupoints include meridian acupoints. For example, in Xiyan (EX-LE 5), Waixiyan is actually Dubi (ST 35); Bafeng (EX-LE 10) includes Ying-Spring acupoint of the foot meridian. Secondly, some extraordinary acupoints are in fact formed by several meridian acupoints. For example, Siguan is a combination of Hegu (LI 4) and Taichong (LR 3), Sihua is a combination of Geshu

一、腧穴分类

根据腧穴的不同特点，通常可将其分为经穴、奇穴、阿是穴三大类。

（一）经穴

又称十四经穴，是指分布于十二经脉及任、督两脉上的腧穴。经穴是腧穴的主要组成部分，也是针灸主要的施术部位。经穴具有以下三个特点：有固定的归经，即所有的腧穴都分布在十四经脉上；有固定的名称，即每一腧穴都有其相对应的穴名；有固定的部位，就某一腧穴而言，其定位是固定不变的。经穴共有361个。

（二）奇穴

又称经外奇穴，是指十四经以外，有一定的位置和名称，对某些病证有专门的治疗作用的腧穴。

奇穴的特点是：有固定位置，就某一奇穴而言，其位置是固定不变的；有固定名称，即一个奇穴就有一个与其相对应的名称；无归经，奇穴既不归属于十二经脉，也不归属于奇经八脉。但奇穴与经穴之间关系还是相当密切的。首先，有些奇穴中就包含有经穴，如：膝眼穴中的外膝眼就是犊鼻穴，八风穴中就含有足

(BL 17) and Danshu (BL 19). Thirdly, the distri-bution and indication of some extraordinary acupoints are similar to those of the acupoints on certain meridians.

经的"荥"穴等;其次,有些奇穴直接就是几个经穴的组合,如四关穴就是合谷和太冲,四花穴为膈俞和胆俞等;另外,有些奇穴在分布和主治上与某些经脉的有穴通路和主治规律相符合,只是尚未归入经穴中而已。

1.2.1.3 Ashi points

Ashi points actually refer to tenderness spots. Such points are marked by no fixed location, no pertaining meridians and no names.

Ashi points have no fixed location. They are actually tender spots. They often change because the affected regions vary with diseases. Since they do not have fixed location, they have no names and no direct relationship with meridians.

(三)阿是穴

是指病痛局部或与病痛有关部位的压痛点,故近代又称其为"压痛点"。

阿是穴的特点是:无固定的位置,即以病痛局部的压痛点为穴,病痛部位不同,其腧穴部位也多随之发生改变;无穴位名称、无归经,由于阿是穴的部位不固定,自然就难以有相应的名称,也就不可能归入某条经脉。

1.2.2 Functions of acupoints

The functions of acupoints are marked by proximal curative effect, distal curative effect and special curative effect.

1.2.2.1 Proximal curative effect

Proximal curative effect is the common feature of all acupoints. That means that all acupoints can be needled to treat disorders to the regions, tissues and organs around them, especially the acupoints located on the head, face and trunk.

二、腧穴作用

腧穴具有近治作用、远治作用、特殊作用三大特点。

(一)近治作用

或称局部作用,这是所有腧穴都具有的共同特点。即所有腧穴均可以治疗所在部位及邻近组织、器官的病证,即所谓:"腧穴所在,主治所在。"头面、躯干部的腧穴以近治作用为主。

1.2.2.2 Distal curative effect

Distal curative effect is the feature of the acupoints on the fourteen meridians, especially the acupoints of the twelve meridians located below the knees and elbows which not only can be needled to treat disorders of the regional tissues, but also can be applied to treat the disorders of the viscera, tissues and organs associated with the meridians in their distribution. Some of the meridian acupoints even can be needled to treat the disorders of the whole body. That is what " the indication extends to where the meridian reaches" means. For example, Zusanli (ST 36), located on the shank, can be needled to treat flaccidity and pain of the lower limbs with its proximal curative effect on one hand, and on the other, treat disorders of the spleen and stomach which the stomach meridian (Zusanli (ST 36) is located) connects with or pertains to as well as disorders of the head and face where the meridian runs through. Besides, Zusanli (ST 36) can be used as a key acupoint for healthcare because it can be needled to supplement healthy qi for the body and reinforce the resistance of the body to exert distal curative effect.

(二)远治作用

这主要为十四经穴的主治规律。十四经穴,尤其是十二经脉位于肘膝关节以下的腧穴,不仅可以治疗所在局部组织的病证,而且还可以治疗经脉循行所联系的远隔部位的脏腑、组织、器官的病变,有些腧穴甚至具有影响全身的治疗作用。这也就是"经脉所通,主治所及。"如足三里穴,其位置在小腿部,它可以治疗下肢痿痹,这是其近治疗作用;此外,它还可治疗所属经脉属络的脾、胃两脏和经脉所过的头面病变;另外,它还作为强壮要穴,具有补益人体正气,提高机体抗病能力的影响全身的远治作用。

1.2.2.3 Special curative effect

Special curative effect of acupoints includes bi-directional and relative specific effect.

(三)特殊作用

包括双向性和相对特异性两个方面。

1.2.2.3.1 Bi-directional effect

Bi-directional effect, also known as favourable bi-directional regulating effect, refers to the needling of the same acupoints with different manipulating techniques to stimulate meridian qi to regulate different functional activities of the body bi-directionally. That means to balance the functions of the body when they become hyperactive with the inhibiting effect and to restore the normal functions of the body when they become hypoactive with the exciting effect. For example, when the heart is beating

1. 双向性

又称为良性双向调整作用,是指针刺相同的腧穴,施以不同的手法,激发经气,可以对机体的不同功能状态产生良性的双向调整作用,即当机体功能亢进时,针刺能使亢进的功能趋于正常,因而具有抑制作用;而当机体功能低下时,针刺则能使低下的功能恢

too fast, needling Neiguan (PC 6) can reduce heart rate; when the heart is beating too slow, needling Neiguan (PC 6) can increase the heart rate. Take Zusanli (ST 36) for another example, for stomach spasm, needling Zusanli (ST 36) can relieve spasm; but for gastrectasis, needling Zusanli (ST 36) can promote the peristalsis of the stomach.

复正常，因而具有兴奋作用。如在心动过速时针刺内关，可以减缓心率，而在心动过缓时，针刺内关则可以加速心率。再如胃痉挛的患者，针刺足三里，具有解痉止痛的作用；而当胃蠕动减缓而表现为胃扩张时，针刺足三里又具有促进胃蠕动的作用等等。

1.2.2.3.2 Relative specific effect

Relative specific effect means that some of the acupoints bear special or specific curative effect on certain diseases. For example, Dazhui (GV 14) abates fever and Zhiyin (BL 67) rectifies the position of fetus.

2. 相对特异性作用

是指某些腧穴对某些病证具有独特的或特殊的治疗作用。如大椎退热、至阴纠正胎位等。

1.2.3 Special acupoints

Special acupoints refer to the acupoints on the fourteen meridians with special curative effect. A majority of the acupoints bear special effect and are commonly used in clinical treatment.

There are ten types of special acupoints, including Five-Shu acupoints below the knees and elbows, Yuan-Source acupoints, Luo-Connecting acupoints, Lower He-Sea acupoints, Xi-Cleft acupoints and eight convergent acupoints; Back-Shu acupoints and Front-Mu acupoints located on the trunk; as well as eight confluent acupoints and crossing acupoints located on the whole body.

三、特定穴

特定穴是指十四经中，具有特殊治疗作用，并有特定称号的腧穴。特定穴在经穴中占有相当的比例，是临床最常用的腧穴。

特定穴共有十大类，包括分布于肘膝关节以下的五输穴、原穴、络穴、下合穴、郄穴、八脉交会穴；位于躯干部的背俞穴、募穴；遍布周身的八会穴、交会穴。

1.2.3.1 Five-Shu acupoints

Five-Shu acupoints refer to Jing-Well, Ying-Spring, Shu-Stream, Jing-River and He-Sea which are five acupoints located on the twelve meridians below the knees and elbows. They are situated in the above order from the distal extremities to the elbows or knees. These five

（一）五输穴

即井、荥、输、经、合穴，是十二经脉分布在肘、膝关节以下的五个特定腧穴，总称为“五输穴”。五输穴的分布，从四肢末端至肘、膝关节依次排

acupoints reflect the indication of the acupoints below the knees and elbows.

列。五输穴反映的是四肢肘膝关节以下的分部主治规律。

1.2.3.2 Yuan-Source acupoints

(二)原穴

Yuan-Source acupoints, the regions where the primary qi of the viscera flows by and retains, are usually located around the wrists and ankles, reflecting the pathological changes of the viscera. They are clinically used to diagnose and treat the disorders of the related viscera.

原穴是脏腑原气经过和留止的部位,多位于腕、踝关节附近,能反映脏腑的病变,故临床多用以诊治相关脏腑的病证。

1.2.3.3 Luo-Connecting acupoints

(三)络穴

Luo-Connecting acupoints refer to the points where the fifteen collaterals stem from the twelve meridians, the governor and conception vessels as well as the major collateral of the spleen. All the Luo-Connecting acupoints of the twelve meridians are located below the elbows and knees.

十五络脉在由经脉所别出部位各有一个腧穴,称为"络穴"。十二经脉的络穴都位于肘膝关节以下,加上位于躯干前、后、侧部的任脉络穴、督脉络穴和脾之大络,共十五络穴。

Luo-Connecting acupoints are used to treat the disorders of the regions that the meridians and collaterals run through as well as the disorders to the meridians in external and internal relation.

络穴除治疗本络循行所过处的病证外,还可用以治疗表里两经的病证。

1.2.3.4 Xi-Cleft acupoints

(四)郄穴

The Xi-Cleft acupoints are the sites where qi and blood from the meridians are deeply converged. Each of the twelve meridians and the four extraordinary vessels (Yin heel vessel, yang heel vessel, Yin link vessel and Yang link vessel) has a Xi-Cleft acupoint on the limbs, amounting to sixteen in all. All the Xi-Cleft acupoints, except Liangqiu (ST 34) on the stomach meridian, are all situated below the knees and elbows.

郄穴是经脉之气深聚的部位。十二经脉各有一个郄穴,加上奇经八脉中阴、阳维脉和阴、阳蹻脉各有一个郄穴,共计十六郄穴。郄穴中除足阳明胃经之梁丘,其余均位于肘膝关节以下。

Clinically Xi-Cleft acupoints are used to treat severe acute disorders of the meridians. The Xi-Cleft acupoints on the yin meridians are usually used to treat various blood syndromes and the Xi-Cleft acupoints on the yang meridians are often used to treat various pain syndromes.

在临床上郄穴多用于治疗各经的重证和急性病证,阴经的郄穴多用于治疗各经的血证,阳经的郄穴多用于治疗各经的痛证。

1.2.3.5 The eight convergent acupoints

（五）八脉交会穴

The eight convergent acupoints refer to the eight acupoints on the twelve meridians that are connected with the eight extraordinary vessels. These eight acupoints are all located below the knees and elbows and are used to treat disorders involving the face, head and trunk related to the eight extraordinary vessels.

八脉交会穴是十二经脉与奇经八脉脉气相通的八个腧穴，都位于肘膝关节以下。

八脉交会穴具有主治头面躯干相关奇经八脉的病证。

1.2.3.6 The lower He-Sea acupoints

（六）下合穴

The lower He-Sea acupoints refer to six acupoints on the three yang meridians of the foot where qi from the six fu organs converges and are the key acupoints for the treatment of the disorders of the six fu organs.

下合穴是指六腑之气下合于足三阳经的六个腧穴，是治疗六腑病证的主要穴位。

1.2.3.7 Back-Shu acupoints

（七）背俞穴

The Back-Shu acupoints are located on the back and waist along the first lateral line of the bladder meridian (1.5 cun lateral to the back middle line) and are the regions where qi of the viscera is infused. The distributing order of Back-Shu acupoints is similar to that of the location of the viscera.

背俞穴是脏腑之气输注于背腰部的腧穴。背俞穴都分布在足太阳膀胱经背腰部的第一侧线上，即后正中线旁开1.5寸的直线上，其排列的顺序与体内脏腑所处的位置大致相应。

Clinically these acupoints are used to treat the disorders of the related viscera, tissues and organs.

背俞穴临床多用于治疗相应脏腑及其相关组织、器官的病证。

1.2.3.8 Front-Mu acupoints

（八）募穴

Front-Mu acupoints are those located on the chest and abdomen where qi of the viscera is infused and converged. The location of the Front-Mu acupoints is similar to that of the related viscera. Among these acupoints, six on the conception vessel are unilateral acupoints, the rest are bilateral acupoints.

募穴是脏腑之气输注于胸腹部的腧穴。十二募穴在胸腹部位置，与相关脏腑在体内的位置大致对应。其中分布于任脉上的6个募穴为单穴，其余为双穴。

Front-Mu acupoints can be used to treat disorders of the related viscera, especially the disorders of the six fu organs. Front-Mu acupoints are usually needled with the combination of Back-Shu acupoints.

募穴可治疗相关脏腑病证，尤多用于治疗六腑病证，常与背俞穴配合使用。

1.2.3.9 Eight confluent acupoints

Eight confluent acupoints, located on the trunk and four limbs below the knees and elbows, are the regions where the essence of qi, blood, tendons, vessels, bones, marrow, zang organs and fu organs converges.

Apart from treating diseases of the meridian proper, these acupoints are frequently used to treat diseases of the corresponding tissues and organs.

1.2.3.10 Crossing acupoints

Crossing acupoints are those at the intersections of two or more meridians. Most of them are located on the head, face and trunk, except a few which are located on the lower limbs. Crossing acupoints are clinically used to treat diseases related to the meridian proper and the meridians crossed with the meridian proper.

Clinically these acupoints are used to treat the disorders of the crossing meridians.

1.2.4 Methods for locating acupoints

Accurate location of acupoints is prerequisite to the treatment of disease with acupuncture and moxibustion therapy. However, accurate location of acupoints depends on proper selection of acupoints.

The methods commonly used to locate acupoints are bone-length measurement, anatomical landmarks, finger measurement, simple location and searching acupoints.

1.2.4.1 Bone-length measurement

Bone-length measurement means to use the major bones in the human body as signifiers to measure the length and size of each region and change into proportional units as the criteria for locating acupoints (see Table 1-4 and Fig. 1).

（九）八会穴

八会穴是指人体气、血、筋、脉、骨、髓、脏、腑精气聚会的八个腧穴，分布于躯干和四肢肘、膝关节以下。

八会穴除治疗本经病证外，常用以治疗相应的组织、器官病证。

（十）交会穴

交会穴，是指两经或两经以上的经气交叉、会合部位的腧穴。除极少数分布于下肢外，交会穴大多位于头面、躯干部。临床上主要用于治疗本经和与之交会经脉的相关病变。

在临床上这类腧穴多有治疗所交会经脉病证的作用。

四、取穴方法

准确地定取腧穴是针灸治疗疾病的前提，而要快速准确地定取穴位，必须采用恰当的取穴方法。

常用的定位方法包括骨度分寸法、体表标志法、同身寸法、简便取穴法和揣穴法。

（一）骨度分寸法

骨度分寸法是以人体各部位主要的骨节为重要标志，测量周身各部的长短、大小，并按比例折算，作为定穴的标准(见表 1－4、图 1)。

Table 1-4 Standards for commonly-used bone-length measurement (cun)

Body parts	Starting and terminating points	Bone measurements	Indications	Notes
Head	● Anterior hairline → posterior hairline ● Yintang → anterior hairline ● Dazhui → posterior hairline	12cun 3cun 3cun	Vertical cun for the vertex Vertical cun for the forehead Vertical cun for the neck	Cun measurement from Yintang to Dazhui can be used if hairline is not clear.
	● Between two frontal angles along hairline ● Between the two mastoid processes	9cun 9cun	Transverse cun for front head Transverse cun for back head	
Chest and abdomen	● Sternocostal angle → umbilicus center ● Umbilicus center → upper margin of pubic symphysis	8cun 5cun	Vertical cun for the upper abdomen Vertical cun for the lower abdomen	Sternocostal symphysis is usually parallel to the fifth costal space.
	● Between two nipples ● Between two midlines of clavicles	8cun 8cun	Transverse cun for chest and abdomen Transverse cun for chest and abdomen	Usually used for women
Back and waist	First thoracic vertebra →fourth sacral vertebra	21 vertebrae		Vertical cun for the acupoints on the back and waist with the spinal process as the evidence for location
Upper limbs	● Anterior axillary fold → cubital transverse crease ● Cubital transverse crease → wrist transverse crease	9cun 12cun	Vertical cun for the upper arm Vertical cun for the forearm	

(Following table)

Body parts	Starting and terminating points	Bone measurements	Indications	Notes
Lower limbs	● Upper border of pubic symphysis → medial epicondyle of femur ● Lower margin of the medial condyle → tip of the medial ankle ● Tip of the medial ankle→sole	18cun 13cun 3cun	Vertical cun for lateral side of the thigh Vertical cun for the medial side of the shank Vertical cun for the medial side of foot	Bone measurement of the medial side of the lower limbs is applicable to the location of acupoints on the three yin meridians of foot.
	● Greater trochanter of femur → middle of knee ● Buttock crease →popliteal crease ● Middle of knee→tip of the lateral ankle ● tip of the lateral ankle →sole	19cun 14cun 16cun 3cun	Vertical cun for the lateral side of thigh Vertical cun for the back of thigh Vertical cun for the lateral side of shank Vertical cun for the lateral side of foot	Applicable to the location of acupoints on the three yang meridians of foot. The horizontal line in the knee is parallel anterioroly to the lower margin of the patella, posteriorly to the popliteal transverse crease and to the Dubi when the knee is bent.

表 1-4 **常用骨度分寸表**

部 位	起 止 点	骨度分寸	适 应 范 围	备 注
头部	前发际至后发际 印堂至前发际 大椎至后发际	12 寸 3 寸 3 寸	头顶部直寸 前额部直寸 项部直寸	前后发际不明显时,可用印堂至大椎间的骨度分寸
	两额角发际间 耳后两乳突之间	9 寸 9 寸	前头部横寸 后头部横寸	
胸腹部	胸剑联合至脐中 脐中至耻骨联合上缘	8 寸 5 寸	上腹部直寸 下腹部直寸	胸剑联合大多平第五肋间隙处
	两乳头之间 两锁骨中线间	8 寸 8 寸	胸腹部横寸 胸腹部横寸	多用于女性
背腰部	第一胸椎至第四骶椎	21 椎		背腰部腧穴的直寸,以脊椎棘突作定位的依据
上肢部	腋前皱襞至肘横纹 肘横纹至腕横纹	9 寸 12 寸	上臂部直寸 前臂部直寸	

（续表）

部位	起止点	骨度分寸	适应范围	备　注
下肢部	耻骨联合上缘至股骨内上髁 胫骨内侧髁下缘至内踝尖 内踝尖至足底	18 寸 13 寸 3 寸	大腿内侧面直寸 小腿内侧面直寸 足内侧直寸	下肢内侧面骨度分寸，适用于定取足三阴经腧穴
	股骨大转子至膝中 臀横纹至腘横纹 膝中至外踝尖 外踝尖至足底	19 寸 14 寸 16 寸 3 寸	大腿外侧直寸 大腿后侧直寸 小腿外侧直寸 足外侧直寸	适用于定取足三阳经腧穴。膝中水平线前平髌骨下缘，后平腘横纹，屈膝时平犊鼻穴

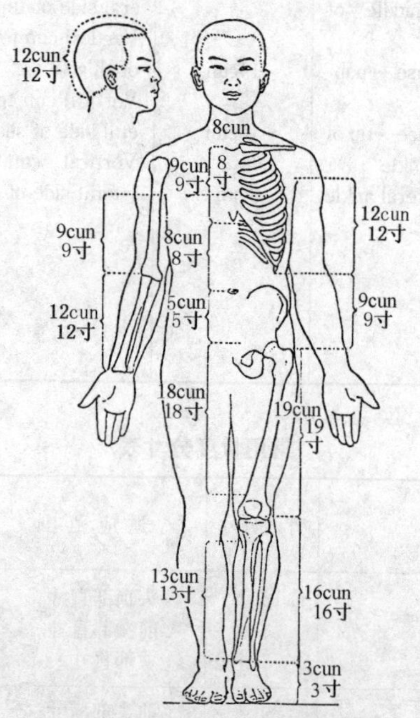

Fig. 1　Illustration of commonly-used bone-length measurement

图 1　常用骨度分寸示意图

Since the acupoints on the chest and side of the chest are mainly located in the costal interstices or parallel to the costal interstices, the costal interstices are used as signifiers to locate these acupoints.

由于胸部和侧胸部的腧穴多分布在肋间隙中或平肋间隙，在定取这些腧穴时，应以肋间隙为标志。

1.2.4.2　Anatomical landmarks

（二）体表标志法

Anatomical landmarks include fixed landmarks and

体表标志定取穴位包括

moving landmarks.

体表固定标志法和体表活动标志法两种。

1.2.4.2.1 Fixed anatomical landmarks

Fixed anatomical landmarks are those that would not change with body movement and visible or palpable on the body surface. They include the five sensory organs, hair, nails, nipple, umbilicus, and prominence and depression of the bones as well as texture of the muscles. With the aid of these landmarks, acupoints can be located directly. Examples are Suliao (CV 25) on the tip of the nose, Yuyao (EX-HN4) on the central point of the eyebrows and Shenque (CV 8) on the umbilicus.

1. 体表固定标志法

所谓的固定标志，是指不须借助活动，直接在体表能看到或能触及到的，如五官、毛发、指(趾)甲、乳头、脐、部分骨节凸起或凹陷、肌肉纹理等，利用这些标志可直接定取腧穴。如鼻尖高点取素髎、眉毛的中央取鱼腰、脐中取神阙等。

1.2.4.2.2 Moving anatomical landmarks

Moving landmarks refer to those that will appear only when a part of the body keeps in a specific position. Such anatomical landmarks can be used to locate some acupoints. For instance, the prominence on the masseter in chewing is Jiache (ST 6).

2. 体表活动标志法

所谓的活动标志，是指进行一定的活动使组织、器官处于特定的位置后，在体表看到或触及的标志，而利用这些标志定取腧穴的方法称为活动标志法。如进行咀嚼动作时，在咬肌隆起的高点处可取颊车穴等。

1.2.4.3 Finger measurement

Finger measurement means to take the length and width of the patient's finger(s) as a standard for locating acupoints because the fingers and the other parts of the body are in proportion. The following three methods are commonly used in clinical treatment.

(三) 指寸定位法

指寸定位法又名手指比量法、手指同身寸法，因人的手指与身体其他部分有一定的比例关系，因而先确定手指一定部位的长度，再在骨度分寸的基础上，用手指比量取穴的方法称为指寸定位法。"指寸"是患者自身(同身)手指的尺寸。它包括三种：

1.2.4.3.1 Middle finger measurement

When the patient's middle finger is flexed, the distance between the two medial ends of the creases of the

1. 中指同身寸

中指屈曲时，以中指中节桡侧两端纹头之间的距离作

interphalangeal joints is taken as one cun, this method is used to measure the vertical distance to locate acupoints on the limbs and to measure the horizontal distance to locate the acupoints on the back. (see Fig. 2)

为1寸。本法适用于四肢取穴的直寸及脊背取穴的横寸。(见图2)

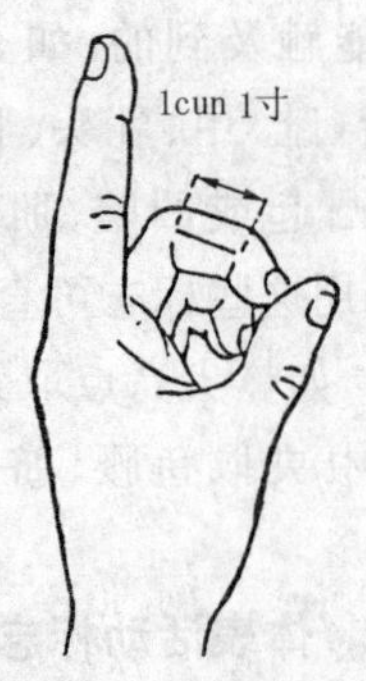
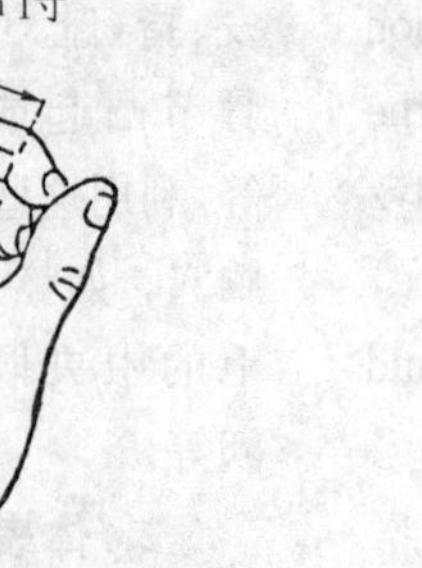

Fig. 2　Middle finger measurement
图2　中指同身寸法

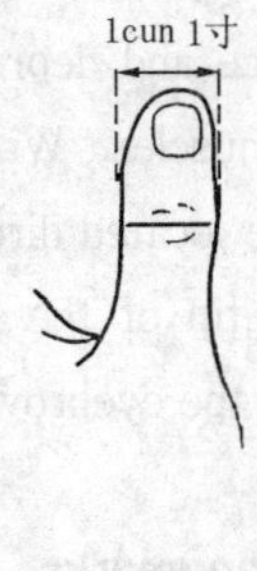

Fig. 3　Thumb measurement
图3　拇指同身寸法

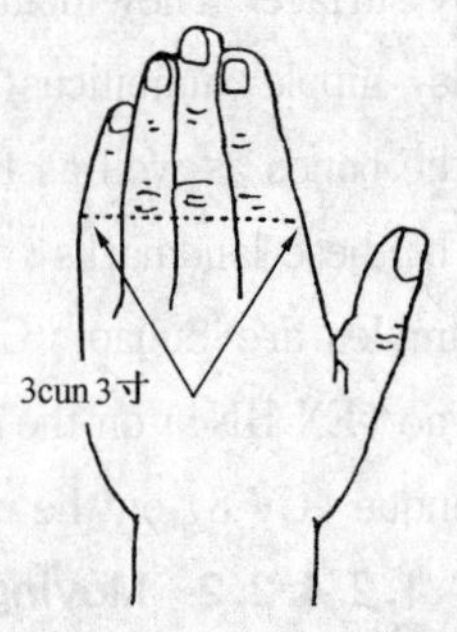

Fig. 4　Four-finger measurement
图4　横指同身寸法

1.2.4.3.2　Thumb measurement

The width of the interphalangeal joint of the patient's thumb is taken as one cun. This method is used for measuring the vertical distance to locate the acupoints on the limbs. (see Fig. 3)

1.2.4.3.3　Four-finger measurement

The width of the four fingers (index, middle, ring and little fingers) close together at the level of the dorsal skin crease of the proximal interphalangeal joint of the middle finger is taken as three cun. This method is used to locate the acupoints on the lower limbs, lower abdomen and the back. (see Fig. 4)

Each finger measurement method has its own range of application and one cannot replace the others. Finger measurement should be done on the basis of bone-length measurement. If finger measurement and bone-length measurement cannot agree with each other, the latter should be taken as the standard.

2. 拇指同身寸

拇指伸直时，以拇指指关节横纹的宽度作为1寸。本法适用于度量四肢部腧穴的直寸。(见图3)

3. 横指同身寸

是将食指、中指、无名指小拇指四指并拢，以过中指近端指关节横纹处四指的宽度作为3寸。本法多用于下肢下腹部的直寸和背部的横寸(见图4)

运用指寸定位法时，应注意不同的指寸有其不同的适用范围，不能以一种指寸遍用于周身。其次，必须在骨度分寸法的基础上运用指寸法，当两者出现抵触时，应以骨度分寸法为准。

1.2.4.4 Simple location

Simple location was developed by the ancient doctors according to their clinical experience. Fox example, the crossing point of the vertical line from the ear tip and the middle line from the front and back of the head is Baihui (GV 20); when the thumb webs are crossed, Lieque (LU 7) can be located; the point that the middle finger touches when the hand is put down naturally is Fengshi (GB 31).

(四) 简便取穴法

这是古今医家在多年的临床实践中总结出的简便、快捷的取穴方法，如两耳尖直上与头部前后正中线的交点取百会；两手虎口交叉取列缺；两手自然下垂于大腿外侧，当中指尖抵达处取风市等。

1.2.4.5 Searching acupoints

Searching acupoints means that the doctor presses around the acupoint to decide its exact location. The acupoints are usually located in the bone spaces, muscular interstices and depression, pressing around is helpful for finding such spaces and interstices. Acupoints usually reflect pathological changes. Under pathological conditions, searching such tenderness points for needling is often satisfactorily effective.

Searching acupoints is the method used to find the exact location of acupoints after the application of other methods. For example, Lanwei (EX-LE7) is the tenderness point 2 cun below Zusanli (ST 36) and Dannang (EX-LE 6) is the tenderness point 1 - 2 cun directly below Yanglingquan (GB 34).

(五) 揣穴

揣，为揣度、揣摸、寻找的意思。揣穴法是医者用手指在穴位部位上下左右按压，以揣摸腧穴的方法。腧穴大多位于骨缝、肌肉间隙及一些凹陷中，定取腧穴时，就要在相应的部位揣摸，以找到骨缝、间隙等；腧穴具有反应病候的功能，在人体发生病变时，寻找这些反应点进行针灸治疗，往往能取得满意的疗效。

揣穴法是在运用其他取穴法后，进一步精确定取穴位的方法。如取“阑尾”穴，在足三里穴下 2 寸处寻找压痛点；取“胆囊”穴，在阳陵泉穴直下 1～2 寸处找压痛点等。

1.3 Application of the theory of meridians and acupoints

第三节 经络腧穴理论的运用

3.1 Theoretical elucidation

一、用于理论说明

1.3.1.1 Elucidation of the pathological changes

The occurrence and changes of disease are closely

(一) 说明病理变化

疾病的发生和传变与经

related to the meridians. When the body is attacked by pathogenic factors, the pathogenic factors can be transmitted to the viscera through meridians. Due to the association of the viscera by meridians, the pathogenic factors are transmitted from one viscus to another. "Transmission through the six meridians" in febrile disease in the *Shanghan Lun* (*Treatise on Seasonal Febrile Disease*) is summarized according to the interrelation between the three yang meridians and three yin meridians as well as the meridians and the viscera. "Defensive qi, qi, nutrient qi and blood" in seasonal febrile disease school used to analyze the conditions of febrile diseases were also developed on the basis of the physiological functions of the meridians in transporting nutrient qi, defensive qi, qi and blood. Syndrome differentiation is used to explain viscera, interaction between two zang (or fu) organs or more organs and their pathological changes (such as attack by pathogenic cold followed by sudden abdominal pain and diarrhea due to "direct invasion into taiyin", liver disease involving the spleen and stomach as well as simultaneous onset of lung and kidney diseases) are exclusively caused by "the association of the meridians with the viscera in the interior and the limbs and joints in the exterior".

络有着密切的关系。当机体遇到病邪侵袭时，可以通过经络而传入内脏，由于内脏之间的经络连贯，病邪可从一个脏腑传入另一脏腑。《伤寒论》一书所总结的热性病的“六经传变”规律，就是基于三阳经和三阴经、经络和脏腑之间的联系；温病学派运用“卫、气、营、血”概念来分析热性病过程中的浅深关系，是以经络运行营卫气血的生理功能为基础；脏腑辨证中用以解释两脏（腑）或两脏（腑）以上病理方面的互相影响及其病理改变，例如人体感受寒邪以后突发腹痛、腹泻的“直中太阴”以及肝病影响脾胃和肺肾同病等都是因为“内属于府藏，外络于肢节”的经络的循行联系。

1.3.1.2 Elucidation of the treatment

The treatment of diseases with acupuncture and moxibustion is accomplished by the transmitting activities of the meridians in regulating meridian qi to restore the normal functions of the viscera and meridians. Such a function of the meridians lies in their physiological activities in transporting qi and blood as well as in harmonizing yin and yang. The meridians are closely related to the viscera, tissues and organs. Under pathological conditions the harmony between qi and blood is broken and the states of yin

（二）说明治疗作用

针灸防治疾病是通过经络的传导功能，通调经气，达到恢复脏腑、经络功能的的。经络的这一作用是建在其生理上运行气血、协调阳的基础上的。经络与人的脏腑组织器官有着密切内在联系，当疾病情况下出气血不和及阴阳偏盛偏衰

d yang may turn hyperactive or hypoactive, acupuncre and moxibustion therapy may stimulate the functions the meridians to treat meridian and visceral disorders enabling viscera and meridian qi and blood to infuse inthe acupoints "to regulate qi" and "to harmonize vital tivities". In acupuncture therapy, it is emphasized that rrival of qi ensures curative effect". The arrival of qi tually means the transmission of meridian qi. The exnples are clinical "obtaining qi" (appearance of needling nsation) and "transmission of qi".

虚实状态时，通过针灸脏腑、经络气血输注于体表的腧穴以"调气"、"治神"，激发经络本身的功能，治疗有关的经络、脏腑病证。针灸治疗疾病强调"气至而有效"，而气至的实质就是经气的传导感应，临床上的"得气"和"行气"现象就是经络传导感应的具体表现。

3.2 Guiding diagnosis and treatment

二、指导诊断治疗

1.3.2.1 Guiding the examination of acupoints

（一）指导经穴诊察

Under pathological conditions, meridians become the utes to transmit pathogenic factors. Pathological chans of the viscera and meridians can be revealed by abnoral reactions along the routes along which the meridians n. So meridians are also helpful for diagnosing diseases, hich is recorded in the chapter of *Back-Shu acupoints Lingshu* (*Spiritual Pivot*). Currently, diagnosis is ade by examining whether there appear tenderness, bcutaneous nodules, prominence and depression along e meridian routes or by pressing Shu-Stream, Frontu, Yuan-Source, Luo-Connecting and Xi-Cleft acuints.

在病理状态下，经络成为病邪传变的途径，经络、脏腑正常功能活动发生了病理的变化，就可以在经络循行路线和有关穴位上通过望、切等方法发现各种异常的反应，以此可以帮助诊断相关的脏腑疾病，这在《灵枢・背俞》中早有记载，现代则多采用按压俞、募、原、络、郄等特定穴或切循经络循行路线上有无压痛、皮下结节、隆起、凹陷等现象，以推断病变所在，在诊断上具有重要价值。

1.3.2.2 Guiding clinical syndrome differenation

（二）指导临床辨证

Clinically accurate diagnosis can be made in light of e symptoms and signs as well as the regions covered in clical flowing and the viscera connected with. In the Chap- of *Tendons of the Meridians in Lingshu* (*Spiritual*

在临床上，可根据疾病出现的症状及其性质，结合经络循行部位与其所联系的脏腑器官，作出正确的临床辨证定

Pivot), the syndromes of the twelve meridians, fifteen collaterals and twelve tendons were recorded. The twelve meridians, the core of the meridian system, were summarized in terms of the disorders of the regions covered in their cyclical flowing and the diseases of the viscera associated with them. Such a record is known as "diseases caused by morbid changes of the meridians" and "the diseases included in the indication of the meridians", which can be used as the principle for syndrome differentiation. Besides, the distribution of the meridians is also helpful for syndrome differentiation of the viscera. Examples are stomachache and vomiting due to disharmony between the liver and stomach; cough due to invasion of liver fire into the lung; hernia due to cold retention in the liver meridian; red eyes due to hyperactivity of liver fire; and dizziness and headache due to hyperactivity of liver yang. These symptoms are all caused through the meridians and may appear simultaneously or one after another. Syndrome differentiation with the eight principles, syndrome differentiation with the six meridians as well as syndrome differentiation of defensive qi, qi nutrient qi, and blood are all related to the doctrine of meridians in terms of their origin.

1.3.2.3 Guiding therapeutic methods

The doctrine of meridians is extensively applied to the treatment in all clinical specialties, especially to the clinical treatment with acupuncture and moxibustion. Such a guidance is well reflected in the location of acupoints which is done according to syndrome differentiation and the pertaining meridians as well as the distribution and cyclical flowing of the meridians. That is what "locating acupoints along the meridians" means. "Locating

位。应用经络对症状体征行分类，最早见于《黄帝经》，其中在《灵枢·经脉·筋》中集中叙述了十二经脉十五络脉和十二经筋的病候特别是作为经络系统核心、干的十二经脉，在《灵枢·脉》中高度概括了各经络循所过部位的外经病和有关腑病，即"是动则病"和"是某所生病"，临床可直接作辨证归经的依据。其次，经的循行分布也是脏腑辨证主要依据，如肝胃不和的痛、呕吐；肝火犯肺的咳嗽；凝肝脉的疝气；肝火上炎所目赤；肝阳上亢所致头晕、眩、头痛等等，都是因为经上的联系，上述诸症往往会时并见或先后出现，组成了病的证候。此外，中医学中八纲辨证、六经辨证、卫气血辨证，就其形成的来源，不与经络学说有着不可分的关系。

（三）指导治疗方法

经络学说的理论被广地运用于临床各科的治疗，别是对针灸的临床治疗更有重要的指导意义。这种导意义体现在取穴上，就是按照经络学说进行辨证归的基础上，再根据经络的循分布路线和联系范围来选

acupoints along the meridians" does not simply mean the cyclical flowing routes of the fourteen meridians. The meridian branches, collaterals and skin areas strengthen the relation between the meridians in external and internal relation as well as the three yin and three yang meridians with the same name and on the same side. Their distributing regions are larger than those of the twelve meridians. On the other hand, the eight extraordinary vessels run across the twelve meridians. Attention should also be paid to the crossing acupoints which are connected with several meridians. So the indication of a certain acupoint is complicated and multiple and should be analyzed according to various relations. Only when the theory of meridians is thoroughly understood can accurate location of acupoints be ensured. The guiding significance of the doctrine of meridians is also reflected in the application of needling and moxibusting techniques. According to the idea of "interrelation between man and the nature", the ancient doctors established "midnight-noon ebb-flow" and "eight magic turtle methods" by associating the circulation of qi and blood in the meridians "with the nature". Besides, the idea of "guiding herbs" developed by attributing medicinal herbs to the meridians is significant in understanding the indication and action of the medicinal herbs.

穴位，即"循经取穴"。对"循经取穴"的理解不能只是单纯地局限于十四经的循行路线上，由于经别、络脉、经筋、皮部加强了十二经脉的表里、同名、同侧三阴三阳经的联系，其循行分布的范围又较十二经脉广泛，奇经八脉纵横交错于十二经脉之间，加之交会穴，一穴通多经，某经的经穴主治是复杂、多层次的，因此应当从这种多重关系上去全面理解，只有系统深刻地理解经络学说的理论，才能在临床上做到取穴精当。经络学说对针灸治疗的指导意义还体现在刺法、灸法的运用上。后世医家根据"天人相应"的观点，将经络气血运行"与天地相参"、"与日月相应"，创立的"子午流注"和"灵龟八法"，则是经络腧穴理论在针灸临床运用的进一步发展。此外，中药归经学说以及根据药物归经理论创立"引经报使"学说，对掌握药物的主治、性能都具有十分重要的意义。

2 Specific discussions of the meridians and acupoints

2.1 The twelve meridians

2.1.1 Lung meridian of hand-taiyin

2.1.1.1 Cyclical flowing and distribution

The lung meridian of hand-taiyin originates from the middle energizer, running downward to connect with the large intestine. Winding back, it goes along the upper orifice of the stomach, passes through the diaphragm, and enters the lung, its pertaining organ. From the lung system, which refers to the portion of the lung communicating with the throat, it comes out transversely. Descending along the medial aspect of the upper arm, it goes continuously downward along the anterior border of the radial side in the medial aspect of the forearm and enters cunkou. Passing the thenar eminence, it goes along its radial border, ending at the medial side of the tip of the thumb.

The branch proximal to the wrist emerges and runs directly to the radial side of the tip of the index finger and ends at the medial side of the tip of the index finger where it links with the large intestine meridian. (see Fig. 5)

Associated viscera: Lung, large intestine, stomach and middle energizer.

Associated organs: Trachea and throat.

第二章 经络腧穴各论

第一节 十二经脉

一、手太阴肺经

(一)经脉循行

起始于中焦,向下联络大肠,回过来沿着胃上口,穿过膈肌,连属于肺脏,从气管、喉咙部横出腋下,沿着上肢内侧前缘,进入寸口,经过大鱼际部,沿其边际,出大指的末端。

其支脉:从腕后走向食指桡侧,出其末端,接手阳明大肠经。(见图5)

联系脏腑:肺、大肠、胃、中焦。

联系器官:气管、喉咙。

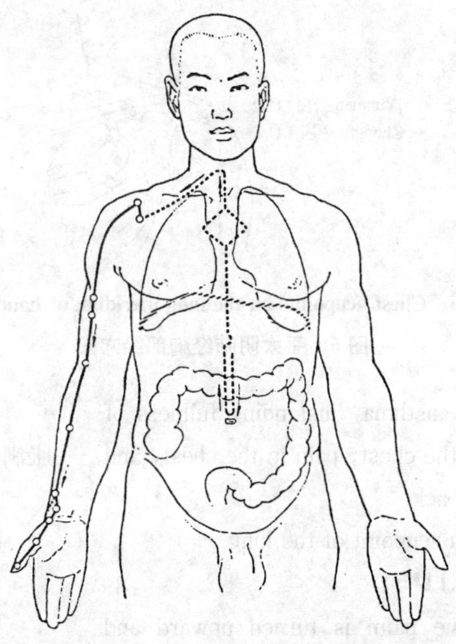

Fig. 5 Flowing route of the lung meridian of hand-taiyin
图 5 手太阴肺经循行示意图

2.1.1.2 Indications

Disorders of the chest, lung, throat and the regions the meridian running by.

2.1.1.3 Commonly used acupoints

2.1.1.3.1 Zhongfu (LU 1)

Location: Laterosuperior to the sternum at the lateral side of the first intercostals space, 1 cun below Yunmen (LU 2), parallel to the first costal interstice and 6 cun lateral to the median line (see Fig. 6). The patient sits straight or lies in supination for locating this acupoint. Yunmen (LU 2) is located in the depression between the acromion and the humerus when the hands are put against the waist. Directly below Yunmen (LU 2) in the first costal interstice is Zhongfu (LU 1).

(二)主治要点

本经腧穴主治胸、肺、喉病,以及经脉循行部位的其他病证。

(三)常用腧穴

1. 中府 LU1

【位置与取法】 正坐或仰卧,在胸部的外上方,云门穴下 1 寸,平第一肋间隙,距前正中线 6 寸处(见图 6)。以手叉腰,在锁骨肩峰端与肱骨之间凹陷中取云门穴,云门穴直下,第一肋间隙中为中府穴。

Yunmen 云门 LU 2
Zhongfu 中府 LU 1

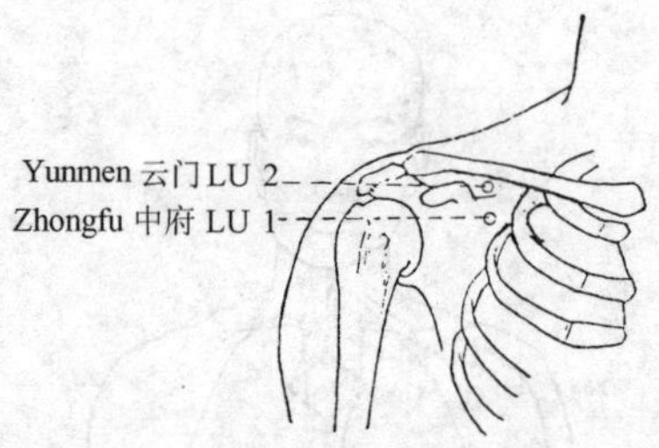

Fig. 6　Chest acupoints on the lung meridian of hand-taiyin

图 6　手太阴肺经胸部经穴图

Indications: Cough, asthma, distending fullness of the lung, suppression in the chest, pain in the chest, and pain in the shoulder and back.

【主治】 咳嗽，气喘，肺胀满；胸闷，胸痛；肩背痛。

Note: The Front-Mu acupoint of the lung.

【备注】 肺之"募"穴。

2.1.1.3.2　Chize (LU 5)

2. 尺泽　LU5

Location: When the palm is turned upward and slightly bent, this acupoint is located on the cubital crease and on the radial side of the tendon of m. biceps brachii (see Fig. 7 and 8).

【位置与取法】 仰掌，微屈肘，在肘横纹中，肱二头肌腱桡侧凹陷中(见图 7、图 8)。

3cun 3寸
Tianfu 天府 LU3
Xiabai 侠白 LU4
6 cun 6寸
Chize 尺泽 LU5

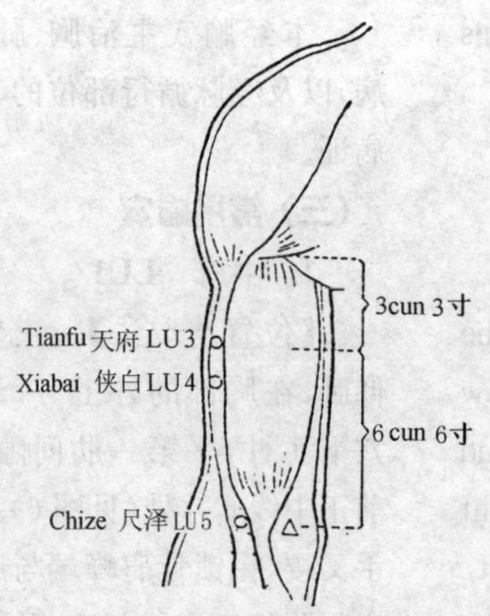

Fig. 7　Upper arm acupoints on the lung meridian of hand-taiyin

图 7　手太阴肺经上臂部经穴图

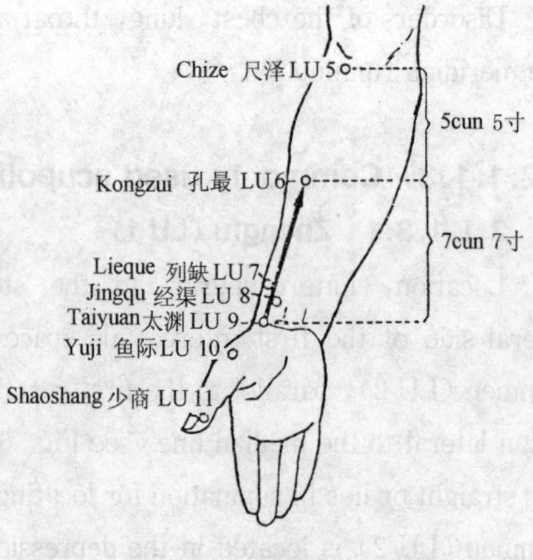

Chize 尺泽 LU 5
5cun 5寸
Kongzui 孔最 LU6
7cun 7寸
Lieque 列缺 LU 7
Jingqu 经渠 LU 8
Taiyuan 太渊 LU 9
Yuji 鱼际 LU 10
Shaoshang 少商 LU 11

Fig. 8　Forearm acupoints on the lung meridian of hand-taiyin

图 8　手太阴肺经前臂部经穴图

Indications: Cough, dyspnea, hemoptysis, afternoon

【主治】 咳嗽，气喘，咯

fever, sore throat, dryness of the tongue, fullness in the chest, spasmodic pain of the elbow and arm, vomiting and infantile convulsion.

Note: He-Sea acupoint of the lung meridian of hand-taiyin.

2.1.1.3.3 Kongzui (LU 6)

Location: When the elbow is slightly bent and the palms turn to face each other, or when the forearm is stretched and the palm turns over, this acupoint is located on the palmar aspect of the forearm on the line joining taiyuan (LU 9) and Chize (LU 5) and 7 cun above the transverse crease of the wrist (see Fig. 8).

Indications: Hemoptysis, cough, dyspnea, sore throat, aphonia, hemorrhoids, spasmodic pain of the elbow and arm, no sweating in febrile disease and headache.

Note: The Xi-Cleft acupoint of the lung meridian of hand-taiyin.

2.1.1.3.4 Lieque (LU 7)

Location: The elbow is bent slightly and the palms turn to face each other. This acupoint is superior to the styloid process of the radius, 1.5 cun above the transverse crease of the wrist (see Fig. 8). When the index finger and the thumbs of both hands are crossed with the index finger of one hand placed on the styloid process of the radius of the other, the depression right under the tip of the index finger is the acupoint (see Fig. 9).

血,潮热;咽喉肿痛;舌干;胸部胀满;肘臂挛痛;吐泻,小儿惊风。

【备注】 手太阴经之“合”穴。

3. 孔最 LU6

【位置与取法】 微屈肘,掌心相对,或伸前臂仰掌,在前臂掌面桡侧,当尺泽穴与太渊穴连线上,腕横纹上7寸(见图8)。或伸臂仰掌,于尺泽穴与太渊穴连线的中点向上1寸,桡骨内缘处是穴。

【主治】 咯血,咳嗽,气喘;咽喉肿痛,失音;痔疮;肘臂挛痛;热病无汗,头痛。

【备注】 手太阴经之“郄”穴。

4. 列缺 LU7

【位置与取法】 微屈肘,侧腕掌心相对,在前臂桡侧缘,桡骨茎突正上方,腕横纹上1.5寸。当肱桡肌腱与拇长展肌腱之间(见图8)。两手虎口交叉,一手食指按在另一手的桡骨茎突上,当食指尖下是穴(见图9)。

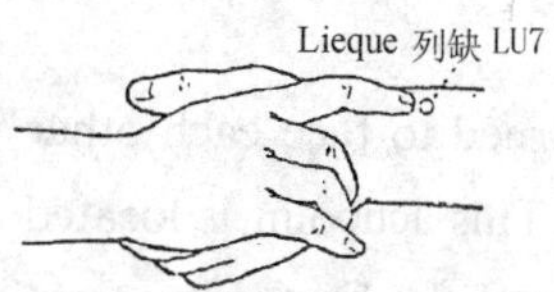

Fig. 9 Simple way to locate Lieque (LU 7) on the lung meridian of hand-taiyin

图9 手太阴肺经列缺简便取穴图

Indications: Cough, asthma, hemoptysis, migraine, stiff neck, sore throat, toothache, distorted face, hematuria, feverish urination, pain in the penis and feverish sensation in the palms.

Note: The Luo-Connecting acuponit of the lung meridian of hand-taiyin and one of the eight convergent acupoints "associating with the conception vessel".

【主治】 咳嗽，气喘，咯血；偏正头痛，项强；咽喉肿痛；齿痛；口眼㖞斜；尿血，小便热，阴茎痛；掌中热。

【备注】 手太阴经之"络"穴，八脉交会穴之一，通于任脉。

2.1.1.3.5 Jingqu (LU 8)

Location: The arm is stretched and the palm is turned over. This acupoint is located 1 cun above the transverse crease of the wrist in the depression on the lateral side of the radial artery (see Fig. 8). Or the point touched by the middle finger of the doctor in feeling pulse is this acupoint.

Indications: Cough, asthma, sore throat, pain in the chest and back as well as the wrist.

Note: Jing-River acupoint of the lung meridian of hand-taiyin.

5. 经渠　LU8

【位置与取法】 伸臂仰掌，在前臂掌面桡侧，桡骨茎突与桡动脉之间凹陷处，腕横纹上 1 寸(见图 8)。或医者按脉时中指所着处。

【主治】 咳嗽，气喘；喉痹；胸背痛；手腕痛。

【备注】 手太阴经之"经"穴。

2.1.1.3.6 Taiyuan (LU 9)

Location: The arm is stretched and the palm is turned over. This acupoint is located at the radial end of the transverse crease of the wrist and in the depression on the lateral side of the radial artery (see Fig. 8).

Indications: Cough, asthma, sorc throat, pain in the chest and back, feverish sensation in the palms, weakness and pain of the wrist and pulseless disease.

Note: The Shu-Stream and Yuan-Source acupoints of the lung meridian of hand-taiyin, and also the "vessel-confluent acupoint" of the eight confluent acupoints.

6. 太渊　LU9

【位置与取法】 伸臂仰掌，在腕掌侧横纹桡侧，桡动脉搏动处(见图 8)。

【主治】 咳嗽，气喘，咯血；喉痹；胸背痛；掌中热，手腕无力疼痛；无脉症。

【备注】 手太阴经之"输"穴、"原"穴，八会穴之"脉会"。

2.1.1.3.7 Yuji (LU 10)

Location: The palms are turned to face each other and the hands clench naturally. This acupoint is located at the radial side of the midpoint of the first metacarpal bone and the junction of the red and white skin, in the

7. 鱼际　LU10

【位置与取法】 侧腕掌心相对，自然半握拳，在手拇指本节后凹陷处，约当第一掌骨中点桡侧，赤白肉际处(见

depression proximal to the first metacarpophalangeal joint (see Fig. 8).

图8)。

Indications: Cough, hemoptysis, aphonia, sore throat, feverish sensation in the palms and febrile disease.

【主治】 咳嗽,咳血;失音,喉痹;掌心热;热病。

Note: Ying-Spring acupoint of the lung meridian of hand-taiyin.

【备注】 手太阴经之“荥”穴。

2.1.1.3.8 Shaoshang (LU 11)

8. 少商 LU11

Location: The thumb is stretched. The acupoint is located on the radial side of the thumb, about 0.1 cun lateroposterior to the corner of the nail (see Fig. 8).

【位置与取法】 伸拇指,在拇指末节桡侧,距指甲角0.1寸(见图8)。

Indications: Cough, asthma, sore throat, epistaxis, abdominal fullness, mania and febrile disease.

【主治】 咳嗽,气喘;咽喉肿痛;鼻衄;心下满,昏迷,癫狂;热病。

Note: Jing-Well acupoint of the lung meridian of hand-taiyin.

【备注】 手太阴经之“井”穴。

2.1.2 Pericardium meridian of hand-jueyin

二、手厥阴心包经

2.1.2.1 Cyclical flowing and distribution

(一)经脉循行

The pericardium meridian originates from the chest. Emerging, it enters its pertaining organ, the pericardium. Then, it descends through the diaphragm to the abdomen, connecting successively with the upper, middle and lower energizers.

从胸中开始,出来连属于心包,通过膈肌,历络于上、中、下三焦。

A branch arising from the chest runs inside the chest, emerges from the costal region at a point 3 cun below the anterior axillary fold and ascends to the axilla. It further runs downward to the forearm between the two tendons and reaches the palm where it passes along the middle finger right down to its tip.

分支一:从胸中出胁部(当腋下3寸处),向上到腋下,沿上肢内侧中央,走两筋之间,进入掌中,沿中指桡侧出于末端。

Another branch arises from the palm and runs along the ring finger to its tip and links with the triple energizer meridian. (see Fig. 10)

分支二:从掌中分出,沿无名指出其末端,接手少阳三焦经。(见图10)

Associated viscera: Pericardium and triple energizer.

联系脏腑:心包、三焦。

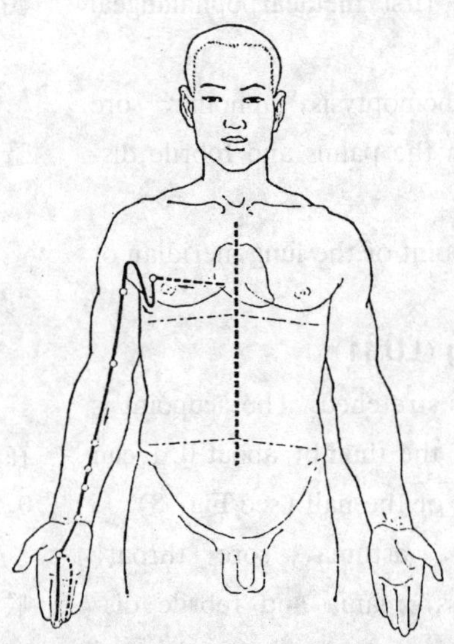

Fig. 10　Flowing route of the pericardium meridian of hand-jueyin
图 10　手厥阴心包经循行示意图

2.1.2.2　Indications

Disorders of the heart, chest, stomach and mind as well as diseases involving the regions covered by the cyclical flowing of the meridian.

2.1.2.3　Commonly used acupoints

2.1.2.3.1　Tianchi (PC 1)

Location: It is located in the fourth intercostal space, 1 cun lateral to the nipple and 5 cun lateral to the front median line (see Fig. 11).

(二) 主治要点

本经腧穴主治心、胸、胃、神志病以及经脉循行部位的其他病证。

(三) 常用腧穴

1. 天池　PC1

【位置与取法】　在胸部，当第四肋间隙，乳头外 1 寸，前正中线旁开 5 寸(见图 11)。

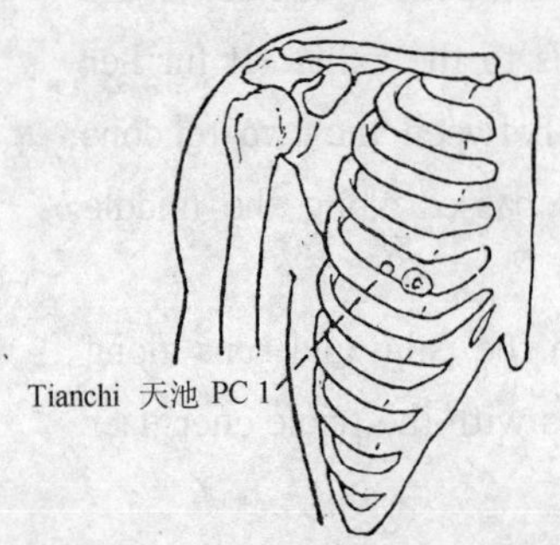

Fig. 11　Chest acupoints on the pericardium meridian of hand-jueyin
图 11　手厥阴心包经胸部经穴图

Indications: Dysphoria, angina pectoris, suppression in the chest, intercostal pain, breast abscess, cough, profuse sputum, asthma and scrofula.

【主治】 心烦,心痛;胸闷,胁肋疼痛;乳痈;咳嗽,痰多,气喘;瘰疬。

2.1.2.3.2 Quze (PC 3)

2. 曲泽 PC3

Location: It is located on the medial side of the forearm, on the transverse cubital crease and at the ulnar side of the tendon of m. biceps brachii (see Fig. 12 and 13).

【位置与取法】 在臂内侧,在肘横纹中,当肱二头肌腱的尺侧缘(见图12、图13)。

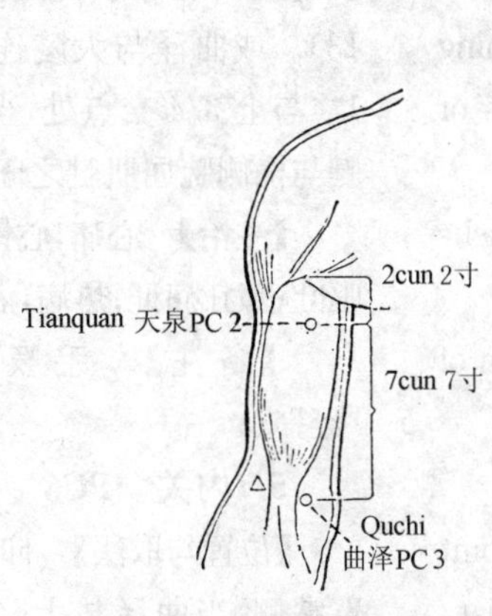

Fig. 12 Upper arm acupoints on the pericardium meridian of hand-jueyin

图 12 手厥阴心包经上臂部经穴图

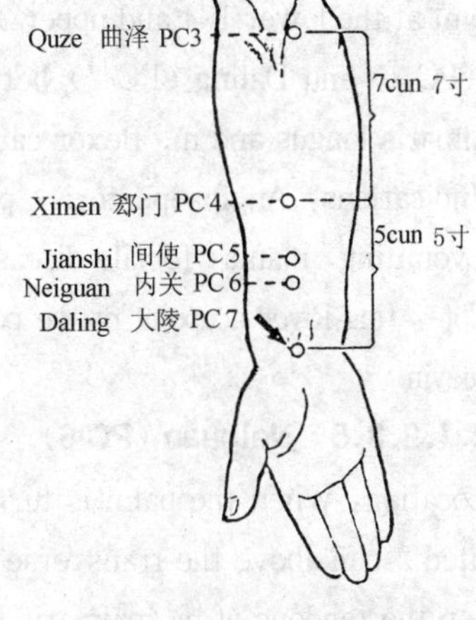

Fig. 13 Forearm acupoints on the pericardium meridian of hand-jueyin

图 13 手厥阴心包经前臂部经穴图

Indications: Angina pectoris, palpitation, stomachache, vomiting, spasmodic pain of the elbow and forearm, diarrhea and febrile disease.

【主治】 心痛,心悸;胃痛,呕吐;肘臂挛痛;泄泻;热病。

Note: He-Sea acupoint of the pericardium meridian of hand-jueyin.

【备注】 手厥阴经之"合"穴。

2.1.2.3.3 Ximen (PC 4)

3. 郄门 PC4

Location: The palm is turned up. The acupoint is located 5 cun above the transverse crease of the wrist, on the line connecting Quze (PC 3) and Daling (PC 7), between the tendons of m. palmaris longus and m. flexor carpi radialis (see Fig. 13).

【位置与取法】 仰掌,在前臂掌侧,当曲泽与大陵的连线上,腕横纹上5寸,掌长肌腱与桡侧腕屈肌腱之间(见图13)。

Indications: Angina pectoris, palpitation, hemoptysis,

【主治】 心痛,心悸;咳

hematemesis, epistaxis, epilepsy, chest pain and rooted furuncle.

Note: Xi-Cleft acupoint of the pericardium meridian of hand-jueyin.

2.1.2.3.4 Jianshi (PC 5)

Location: The palm is turned up. The acupoint is located 3 cun above the transverse crease of the wrist, between the tendons of m. palmaris longus and m. flexor carpi radialis (see Fig. 13). Or it is located on the crossing point at the lower 1/4 and upper 3/4 of the line joining Quze (PC 3) and Daling (PC 7) between the tendons of m. palmaris longus and m. flexor carpi radialis.

Indications: Angina pectoris, palpitation, stomachache, vomiting, mania, febrile disease and malaria.

Note: Jing-River acupoint of the pericardium meridian of hand-jueyin.

2.1.2.3.5 Neiguan (PC 6)

Location: When the palm is turned up, the acupoint is located 2 cun above the transverse crease of the wrist, between the tendons of m. palmaris longus and m. flexor radialis (see Fig. 13).

Indications: Angina pectoris, palpitation, stomachache, vomiting, hiccup, insomnia, dizziness, epilepsy, puerperal vertigo due to loss of blood, chest distress, spasmodic pain of elbow and forearm, migraine and febrile disease.

Note: Luo-Connecting acupoint of the pericardium meridian and one of the eight convergent acuponits "associating with yin link vessel".

2.1.2.3.6 Daling (PC 7)

Location: When the palm is turned up, the acupoint is located in the middle of the transverse crease of the wrist, between the tendons of the m. palmaris longus and m. flexor carpi radialis (see Fig. 13).

Indications: Angina pectoris, palpitaiton, stomachache,

血,呕血,衄血;癫痫;胸痛;疔疮。

【备注】 手厥阴经之"郄"穴。

4. 间使 PC5

【位置与取法】 仰掌,在前臂掌侧,当曲泽与大陵的连线上,腕横纹上 3 寸,掌长肌腱与桡侧腕屈肌腱之间(见图 13)。或曲泽与大陵连线的下 1/4与上 3/4 交点处,当掌长肌腱与桡侧腕屈肌腱之间取穴。

【主治】 心痛,心悸;胃痛,呕吐;癫狂痫证;热病,疟疾。

【备注】 手厥阴经之"经"穴。

5. 内关 PC6

【位置与取法】 仰掌,在前臂掌侧,当曲泽与大陵的连线上,腕横纹上 2 寸,掌长肌腱与桡侧腕屈肌腱之间(见图 13)。

【主治】 心痛,心悸;胃痛,呕吐,呃逆;失眠,眩晕,癫痫,产后血晕;胸闷;肘臂挛痛;偏头痛;热病。

【备注】 手厥阴经之"络"穴,八脉交会穴之一,通于阴维脉。

6. 大陵 PC7

【位置与取法】 仰掌,在腕横纹的中点处,当掌长肌腱与桡侧腕屈肌腱之间(见图 13)。

【主治】 心痛,心悸;胃

vomiting, mania, hypochondriac pain and ulcer.

Note: Shu-Stream and Yuan-Source acupoints of the pericardium meridian of hand-jueyin.

痛,呕吐;癫狂;胸胁痛;疮疡。

【备注】 手厥阴经之"输"穴、"原"穴。

2.1.2.3.7 Laogong (PC 8)

Location: When the palm is turned up, the acupoint is located on the transverse crease of the palm, between the second and third metacarpal bones (see Fig. 14). When the fist is clenched, the point is just below the tip of the middle finger.

7. 劳宫 PC8

【位置与取法】 仰掌,在手掌心横纹中,当第二三掌骨之间偏于第三掌骨处(见图14)。屈指握拳,当中指尖下是穴。

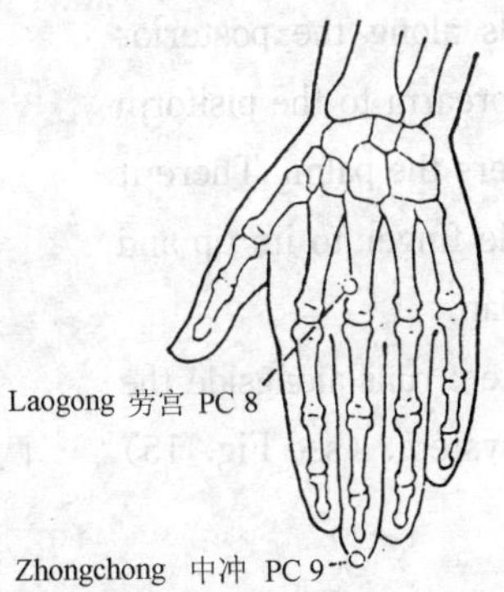

Fig. 14 Hand acupoints on the pericardium meridian of hand-jueyin

图 14 手厥阴心包经手部经穴图

Indications: Angina pectoris, palpitation, vomiting, foul breath, oral ulcer, coma due to apoplexy, sunstroke, mania, epilepsy and toothache.

Note: Ying-Spring acupoint of the pericardium meridian of hand-jueyin.

【主治】 心痛,心悸;呕吐,口疮,口臭;中风昏迷,中暑,癫狂痫证;牙痛。

【备注】 手厥阴经之"荥"穴。

2.1.2.3.8 Zhongchong (PC 9)

Location: The acupoint is located in the center of the tip of the middle finger (see Fig. 14).

Indications: Angina pectoris, coma, sunstroke apoplexy, infantile convulsion, stiffness and swelling of the tongue and febrile disease.

Note: Jing-Well acupoint of the pericardium meridian of hand-jueyin.

8. 中冲 PC9

【位置与取法】 在手中指末节尖端中央(见图14)。

【主治】 心痛;昏迷,中暑,中风,小儿惊风;舌强肿痛,热病。

【备注】 手厥阴经之"井"穴。

2.1.3 Heart meridian of hand-shaoyin

2.1.3.1 Cyclical flowing and distribution

The heart meridian orginates from the heart. It emerges and spreads over the heart system. It passes through the diaphragm to connect with the small intestine. The exteriorly running part runs from the heart system to the lung. Then it turns downward and emerges from the axilla. From there it goes along the posterior border of the medial aspect of the upper arm and down to the cubital fossa. Then it descends along the posterior border of the medial aspect of the forearm to the pisiform region proximal to the palm and enters the palm. There it follows the medial aspect of the little finger to its tip and links with the small intestine meridian.

The branch from the heart system runs alongside the esophagus to connect with the eye system. (see Fig. 15)

三、手少阴心经

(一)经脉循行

从心中开始,出经心系,下过膈肌,联络小肠。其外行主干:从心系上至肺,向下出于腋下,沿上肢内侧后缘,抵达掌后豌豆骨部,进入掌内后缘,沿小指的桡侧出其末端,接手太阳小肠经。

其支脉:从心系向上挟食管两旁,联系到目系。(见图 15)

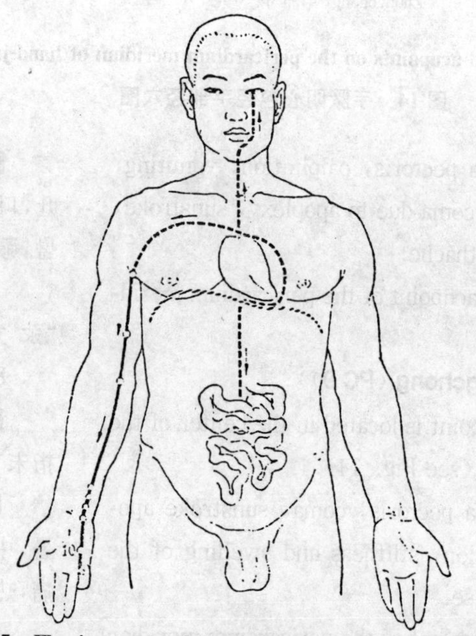

Fig. 15 Flowing route of the heart meridian of hand-shaoyin

图 15 手少阴心经循行示意图

Associated viscera: Heart, small intestine and lung.

Associated organs: Eye system, tongue, throat and larynx.

联系脏腑：心、小肠、肺。

联系器官：目系、舌、咽、喉咙。

2.1.3.2 Indications

Disorders of the heart and chest and mental problems as well as diseases involving the regions covered by the meridian in cyclical flowing.

(二) 主治要点

本经腧穴主治心、胸、神志病以及经脉循行部位的其他病证。

2.1.3.3 Commonly used acupoints

(三) 常用腧穴

2.1.3.3.1 Jiquan (HT 1)

Location: The patient sits down or lies in supination with the arm stretched out. The acupoint is located in the center of the axilla, on the pulsation point of the axillary artery (see Fig. 16).

1. 极泉 HT1

【位置与取法】 正坐或仰卧位，上臂外展，在腋窝顶点，腋动脉搏动处(见图 16)。

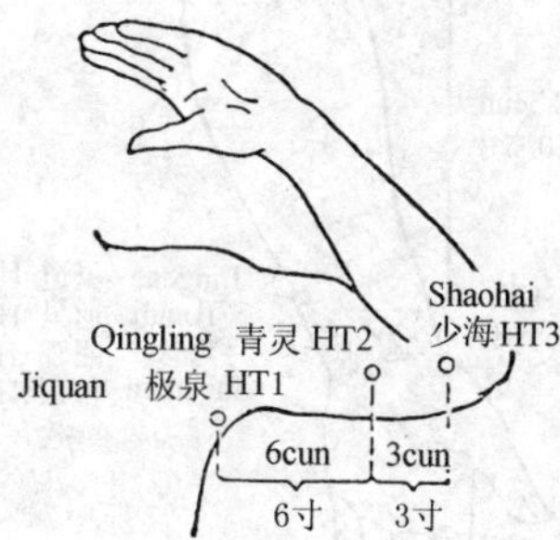

Fig. 16 Upper arm acupoints on the heart meridian of hand-shaoyin

图 16 手少阴心经上臂部经穴图

Indications: Angina pectoris, chest distress, hypochondriac and costal pain, dry mouth, terrible thirst, yellowish eyes, cold pain in the arm and scrofula.

【主治】 心痛，心悸；胸闷，胁肋疼痛；咽干烦渴，目黄；手臂冷痛；瘰疬。

2.1.3.3.2 Shaohai (HT 3)

Location: When the elbow is bent, the acupoint is in the depression between the medial end of the transverse and cubital crease and the medial epicondyle of the humerus (see Fig. 16). Or when the elbow is flexed as close as possible, the acupoint is located at the medial end of the transverse crease of the elbow.

2. 少海 HT3

【位置与取法】 屈肘，在肘横纹内侧端与肱骨内上髁连线的中点处(见图 16)。或尽量曲肘，在肘横纹内侧纹头处。

Indications: Angina pectoris, amnesia, susceptibility

【主治】 心痛；健忘，善

to laugh, mania, epilepsy, spasmodic pain of the elbow and arm, numbness of arm, tremor of hand, scrofula, headache, dizziness, toothache and pain in the axilla.

Note: He-Sea acupoint of the heart meridian of hand-shaoyin.

笑，癫狂，痫证；肘臂挛痛，臂麻，手颤；瘰疬；头痛，目眩；齿痛；腋胁痛。

【备注】 手少阴经之“合”穴。

2.1.3.3.3 Lingdao (HT 4)

Location: When the palm is turned up, the acupoint is on the radial side of the tendon of the m. flexor carpi ulnaris, 1.5 cun above the transverse crease of the wrist (see Fig. 17).

3. 灵道　HT4

【位置与取法】 仰掌，在前臂掌侧，当尺侧腕屈肌腱的桡侧缘，腕横纹上 1.5 寸(见图 17)。

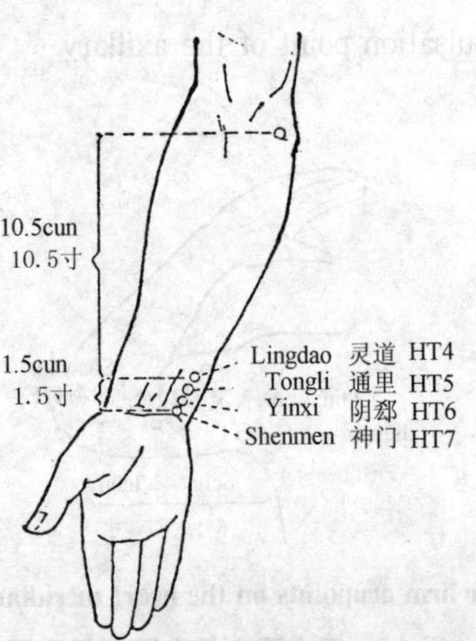

Fig. 17　Forearm acupoints on the heart meridian of hand-shaoyin

图 17　手少阴心经前臂部经穴图

Indications: Angina pectoris, palpitation, susceptibility to laugh, sorrow and fright, sudden aphonia, aphasia due to stiff tongue and spasmodic pain of the elbow and arm.

【主治】 心痛，心悸，怔忡；善笑，悲恐；暴喑，舌强不语；肘臂挛痛。

2.1.3.3.4 Tongli (HT 5)

Location: When the palm is turned upward, the acupoint is on the radial side of the tendon of m. flexor carpi ulnaris, 1 cun above the transverse crease of the wrist (see Fig. 17).

Indications: Palpitation, severe palpitation, sudden aphonia, aphasia due to stiff tongue, pain in the wrist and arm.

4. 通里　HT5

【位置与取法】 仰掌，在前臂掌侧，当尺侧腕屈肌腱的桡侧缘，腕横纹上 1 寸(见图 17)。

【主治】 心悸，怔忡；暴喑，舌强不语；腕臂痛。

Note: Luo-Connecting acupoint of the heart meridian of hand-shaoyin.

【备注】 手少阴经之"络"穴。

2.1.3.3.5 Yinxi (HT 6)

5. 阴郄 HT6

Location: When the palm is turned upward, the acupoint is on the radial side of the tendon of m. flexor carpi ulnaris, 0.5 cun above the transverse crease of the wrist (see Fig. 17).

【位置与取法】 仰掌,在前臂掌侧,当尺侧腕屈肌腱的桡侧缘,腕横纹上 0.5 寸(见图 17)。

Indications: Angina pectoris, palpitation due to fright, hematemesis, epistaxis, sudden loss of voice, bone-steaming and night sweating.

【主治】 心痛,惊悸;吐血,衄血;暴喑失语;骨蒸盗汗。

Note: Xi-Cleft acupoint of the heart meridian of hand-shaoyin.

【备注】 手少阴经之"郄"穴。

2.1.3.3.6 Shenmen (HT 7)

6. 神门 HT7

Location: When the palm is turned upward, the acupoint is at the ulnar end of the transverse crease of the wrist, in the depression on the radial side of the tendon of m. flexor carpi ulnaris (see Fig. 17).

【位置与取法】 仰掌,腕横纹尺侧端,尺侧腕屈肌腱的桡侧凹陷处(见图 17)。

Indications: Angina pectoris, dysphoria, palpitation, severe palpitations, amnesia, insomnia, mania, epilepsy, hypochondriac pain, wrist pain and finger numbness.

【主治】 心痛,心烦,惊悸,怔忡;健忘,失眠,癫狂痫证;胸胁痛;腕痛,指麻。

Note: Shu-Stream and Yuan-Source acupoints of the heart meridian of hand-shaoyin.

【备注】 手少阴经之"输"穴、"原"穴。

2.1.3.3.7 Shaofu (HT 8)

7. 少府 HT8

Location: When the palm is turns upward, the acupoint is located between the fourth and fifth metacarpal bones (see Fig. 18). When a fist is formed, this acupoint is where the tip of the little finger touches.

【位置与取法】 在手掌面,第四五掌骨之间,当掌骨头后缘凹陷中(见图 18)。手指曲向掌心横纹,当小指尖下是穴。

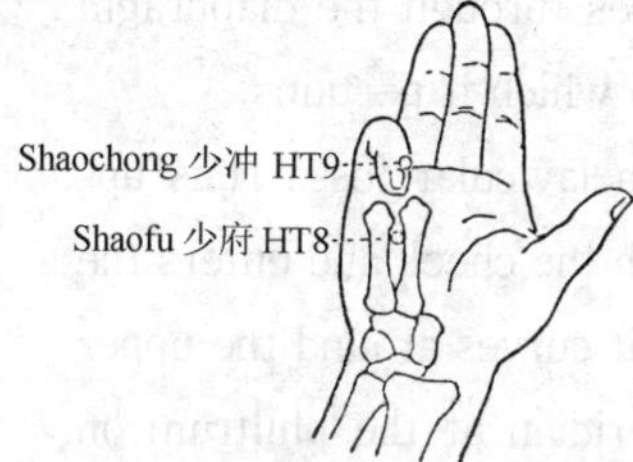

Fig. 18 Hand acupoints on the heart meridian of hand-shaoyin
图 18 手少阴心经手部经穴图

Indications: Palpitation, chest pain, spasmodic pain of the little finger, furuncle, ulcer, pruritus of the external genitalia, pudendal pain, dysuria and enuresis.

【主治】 心悸;胸痛;手小指拘挛;痈疡;阴痒,阴痛,小便不利,遗尿。

Note: Ying-Spring acupoint of the heart meridian of hand-shaoyin.

【备注】 手少阴经之"荥"穴。

2.1.3.3.8 Shaochong (HT 9)

8. 少冲 HT9

Location: The acupoint is on the radial side of the little finger, about 0.1 cun latero-posterior to the corner of the nail (see Fig. 18).

【位置与取法】 在手小指末节桡侧,距指甲角 0.1 寸(见图 18)。

Indications: Palpitation, angina pectoris, mania, coma, hypochondriac pain and febrile disease.

【主治】 心悸,心痛;癫狂,昏迷;胸胁痛;热病。

Note: Jing-Well acupoint of the heart meridian of hand-shaoyin.

【备注】 手少阴经之"井"穴。

2.1.4 Large intestine meridian of hand-yangming

四、手阳明大肠经

2.1.4.1 Cyclical flowing and distribution

(一) 经脉循行

The large intestine meridian starts from the tip of the index finger. It runs upward along the radial side of the index finger and passes through the interstice of the first and second metacarpal bones, dipping into the depression between the tendons of m. extensor pollicis longus and brevis. Following the lateral anterior aspect of the forearm, it reaches the lateral side of the elbow where it ascends along the lateral anterior aspect of the upper arm to the highest point of the shoulder. Along the anterior border of the acromion, it goes up to the seventh cervical vertebra and descends to the supraclavicular fossa to connect with the lung. It then passes through the diaphragm and enters the large intestine to which it pertains.

起于食指末端,沿食指桡侧缘向上,循经手背第一二掌骨间,向上经腕关节桡侧拇长与拇短伸肌腱之间,沿上臂外侧前缘上行,上肩,出肩峰前缘,向上出于柱骨之会上,向下由缺盆部入内,联络肺脏,穿过膈部,连属大肠。

The branch from the supraclavicular fossa runs upward to the neck, passes through the cheek and enters the gums of the lower teeth. Then it curves around the upper lip and crosses the opposite meridian at the philtrum on the governor vessel and upward to both sides of the nose

其支脉:从缺盆处分出经过颈部,穿过面颊,进入下牙中,并返出挟口角,左右经脉交会于督脉的人中穴而循行至对侧,挟行于鼻之两旁,与足阳明

to connect with the stomach meridian. (see Fig. 19)

经相交接。(见图 19)

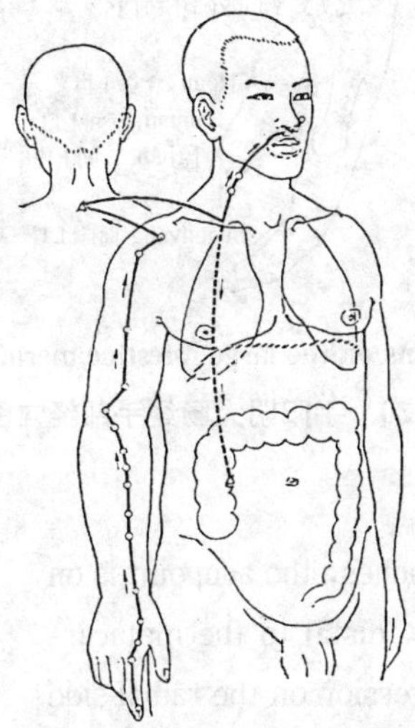

Fig. 19 Flowing route of the large intestine meridian of hand-yangming

图 19 手阳明大肠经循行示意图

Associated viscera: Large intestine and lung.

Associated organs: Mouth, lower teeth and nose.

联系脏腑:大肠、肺。

联系器官:口、下齿、鼻。

2.1.4.2 Indications

(二)主治要点

Disorders of the mouth, teeth, nose and throat as well as diseases involving the lateral border of the upper limbs, anterior part of the shoulder and neck.

本经腧穴主治口、齿、鼻等头面器官病、咽喉病,及经脉循行所过的上肢外侧前缘、肩前、颈部的病变。

2.1.4.3 Commonly used acupoints

(三)常用腧穴

2.1.4.3.1 Shangyang (LI 1)

1. 商阳 LI1

Location: The acupoint is located on the radial side of the index finger, about 0.1 cun latero-posterior to the corner of the nail (see Fig. 20).

Indications: Apoplexy, coma, toothache, deafness, numbness of fingers and high fever.

Note: Jing-Well acupoint of the large intestine meridian of hand-yangming.

【位置与取法】 在食指桡侧,距指甲角 0.1 寸(见图 20)。

【主治】 中风,昏迷;齿痛,耳聋;手指麻木;高热。

【备注】 手阳明经之“井”穴。

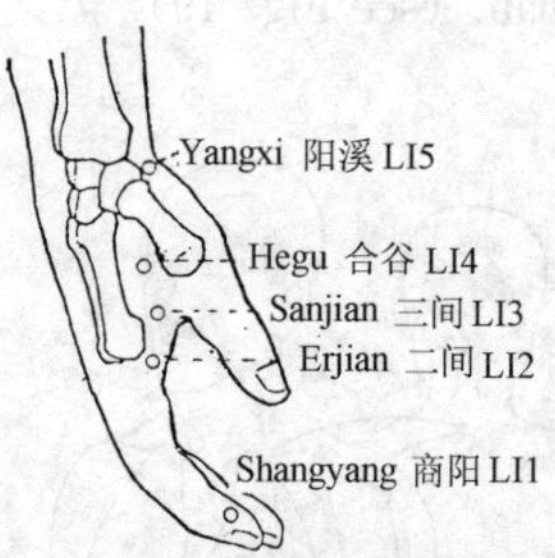

Fig. 20 Hand acupoints on the large intestine meridian of hand-yangming

图 20 手阳明大肠经手部经穴图

2.1.4.3.2 Erjian (LI 2)

Location: When the hand clenches, the acupoint is on the radial side of the index finger, distal to the metacarpal-phalangeal joint and in the depression on the radial side (see Fig. 20).

Indications: Toothache, facial paralysis, dry mouth, sore throat, numbness of fingers and febrile disease.

Note: Ying-Spring acupoint of the large intestine meridian of hand-yangming.

2. 二间 LI2

【位置与取法】 微握拳，在手第二掌指关节前，桡侧凹陷中(见图 20)。

【主治】 齿痛，面瘫，口干，咽喉肿痛；手指麻木；热病。

【备注】 手阳明经之"荥"穴。

2.1.4.3.3 Sanjian (LI 3)

Location: When the hand slightly clenches, the acupoint is on the radial side of the index finger, in the depression behind the second metacarpophalangeal joint (see Fig. 20).

Indications: Toothache, epistaxis, sore throat, swelling and pain of the dorsum of hand, numbness of fingers and somnolence.

Note: Shu-Stream acupoint of the large intestine meridian of hand-yangming.

3. 三间 LI3

【位置与取法】 微握拳，在手第二掌指关节后，桡侧凹陷中(见图 20)。

【主治】 齿痛，鼽衄，咽喉肿痛；手背肿痛，手指麻木；嗜睡。

【备注】 手阳明经之"输"穴。

2.1.4.3.4 Hegu (LI 4)

Location: The acupoint is located on the dorsum of the hand, between the first and second metacarpal bones, approximately in the middle of the second metacarpal bone on the radial side (see Fig. 20). When the transverse

4. 合谷 LI4

【位置与取法】 位于手背，第一二掌骨间，平第二掌骨桡侧的中点处(见图 20)。拇、食二指张开，以一手拇指

crease of the interphalangeal joint of the thumb is placed in coincident position with the margin of the web between the thumb and the index finger of the other hand, the acupoint is where the tip of the thumb touches (see Fig. 21). When the thumb and index finger join together, the prominence of the muscle is the location of the acupoint. When the thumb and the index finger open, the middle point on the line from the web between the thumb and index finger to the line connecting the first and second metacarpal bones is the location of the acupoint.

指关节横纹放在另一手的虎蹼缘上，当拇指尖下是穴（见图21）。也可拇、食二指并拢，在肌肉隆起的最高处。还可拇、食二指张开，虎口与第一二掌骨结合部连线的中点处。

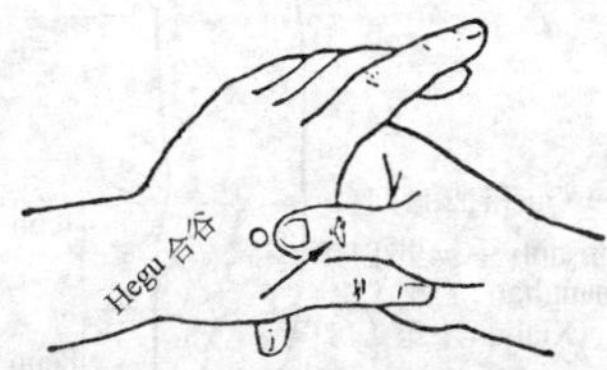

Fig. 21 Simple way to locate Hegu (LI 4) on the large intestine meridian of hand-yangming

图21 手阳明大肠经合谷穴简便取穴图

Indications: Redness, swelling and pain of eyes, facial paralysis, epistaxis, toothache, swelling pain of the throat, abdominal pain, diarrhea, constipation, dysentery, common cold, cough, no sweating, profuse sweating, delayed labour, irregular menstruation, obstruction syndrome in apoplexy, infantile convulsion, paralysis and spasm of fingers.

【主治】 目赤肿痛，面瘫，齿痛，鼻衄，咽喉肿痛；腹痛，泄泻，便秘，痢疾；感冒，咳嗽，无汗，多汗；滞产，月经不调；中风闭证，小儿惊风；半身不遂，指挛。

Note: Yuan-Source acupoint of the large intestine meridian of hand-yangming.

【备注】手阳明经之"原"穴。

2.1.4.3.5 Yangxi (LI 5)

5. 阳溪 LI5

Location: The acupoint is located on the radial side of the wrist. When the thumb is tilted upward, it is in the depression between the tendons of m. extensor pollicis longus and brevis (see Fig. 20).

【位置与取法】 位于腕背横纹桡侧端，大拇指向上翘起时，当拇短伸肌腱与拇长伸肌腱之间的凹陷中（见图20）。

Indications: Headache, toothache, tinnitus, deafness, mania, epilepsy, and spasmodic pain in the wrist.

【主治】 头痛，齿痛，耳鸣，耳聋；癫证，狂证，痫证；手腕挛痛。

Note: Jing-River acupoint of the large intestine meridian of hand-yangming.

【备注】 手阳明经之"经"穴。

2.1.4.3.6 Pianli (LI 6)

6. 偏历　LI6

Location: When the elbow is flexed, the acupoint is located at the radial side of the forearm, on the line joining Yangxi (LI 5) and Quchi (LI 11), 3 cun above the transverse crease on the wrist (see Fig. 22). Or it is located on the crossing point at the lower 1/4 and upper 3/4 of the line joining Yangxi (LI 5) and Quchi (LI 11).

【位置与取法】 侧掌屈肘,在前臂背面桡侧,当阳溪与曲池连线上,腕横纹上 3 寸(见图 22)。或于阳溪与曲池连线的下 1/4 与上 3/4 的交点处取穴。

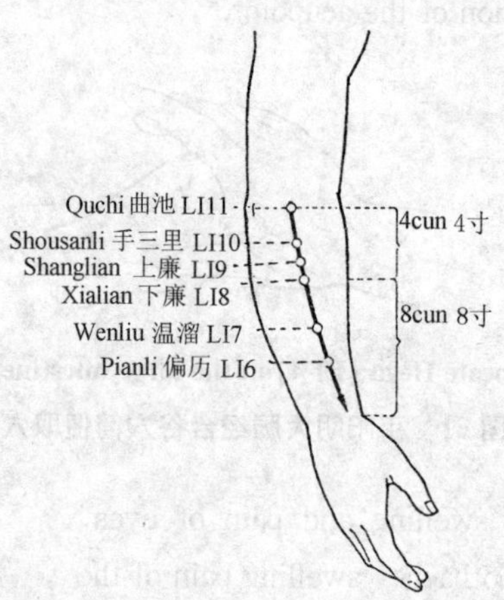

Fig. 22　Forearm acupoints on the large intestine meridian of hand-yangming

图 22　手阳明大肠经前臂部经穴图

Indications: Tinnitus, deafness, toothache, facial paralysis and spasmodic pain in the forearm.

【主治】 耳鸣,耳聋,齿痛,面瘫;前臂挛痛。

Note: Luo-Connecting acupoint of the large intestine meridian of hand-yangming.

【备注】 手阳明经之"络"穴。

2.1.4.3.7 Wenliu (LI 7)

7. 温溜　LI7

Location: When the elbow is flexed, the acupoint is located at the radial side of the forearm, on the line joining Yangxi (LI 5) and Quchi (LI 11), and 5 cun above the transverse crease on the wrist (see Fig. 22). Or it is 1 cun below the middle point on the line joining Yangxi (LI 5) and Quchi (LI 11).

【位置与取法】 屈肘,在前臂背面桡侧,当阳溪与曲池连线上,腕横纹上 5 寸(见图 22)。或于阳溪与曲池连线的中点下 1 寸处。

Indications: Headache, epistaxis, sore throat,

【主治】 头痛,鼻衄,咽

borborygmus, abdominal pain and aching pain in the shoulder and arm.

喉肿痛;肠鸣腹痛;肩臂酸痛。

Note: Xi-Cleft acupoint of the large intestine meridian of hand-yangming.

【备注】 手阳明经之"郄"穴。

2.1.4.3.8 Shousanli (LI 10)

8. 手三里 LI10

Location: It is located on the line joining Yangxi (LI 5) and Quchi (LI 11), 2 cun below the transverse crease on the elbow (see Fig. 22).

【位置与取法】 当阳溪与曲池连线上,肘横纹下 2 寸(见图 22)。

Indications: Toothache, swelling of cheeks, borborygmus, abdominal pain, diarrhea and paralysis of the upper limbs.

【主治】 齿痛颊肿;肠鸣腹痛,腹泻;上肢不遂。

2.1.4.3.9 Quchi (LI 11)

9. 曲池 LI11

Location: When the elbow is flexed 90°, the acupoint is located on the middle point on the line joining Chize (LU 5) and the external epicondyle of the humerus (see Fig. 22 and 23). When the elbow is flexed as close as possible, the end of the transverse crease of the elbow at the radial side is the location of the acupoint.

【位置与取法】 屈肘 90°,当尺泽与肱骨外上髁连线中点处(见图 22、图 23)。尽量屈肘,肘横纹桡侧端纹头尽处是穴。

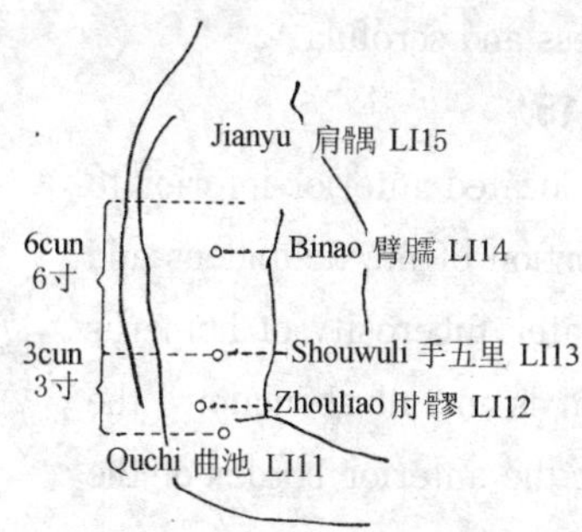

Fig. 23 Upper arm acupoints on the large intestine meridian of hand-yangming

图 23 手阳明大肠经上臂部经穴图

Indications: Toothache, redness, swelling and pain of eyes, sore throat, abdominal pain, diarrhea, paralysis of the upper limbs, spasmodic pain of the elbow and arm, febrile disease, hypertension and urticaria.

【主治】 齿痛,目赤肿痛,咽喉肿痛;腹痛,腹胀,腹泻;上肢不遂,肘臂挛痛;热病,高血压病,瘾疹。

Note: He-Sea acupoint of the large intestine meridian

【备注】 手阳明经之

of hand-yangming.

“合”穴。

2.1.4.3.10　Zhouliao (LI 12)

10. 肘髎　LI12

Location: When the elbow is flexed, the acupoint is located about 1 cun superolateral to Quchi (LI 11) and on the lateral border of the humerus (see Fig. 23).

【位置与取法】 屈肘，曲池上方1寸，当肱骨边缘处(见图23)。

Indications: Spasmodic pain in the elbow and arm, numbness of the upper limbs.

【主治】 肘臂挛痛，上肢麻木。

2.1.4.3.11　Shouwuli (LI 13)

11. 手五里　LI13

Location: It is located on the line joining Quchi (LI 11) and Jianyu (LI 15) and 3 cun above Quchi (LI 11) (see Fig. 23).

【位置与取法】 位于曲池与肩髃的连线上，曲池穴上3寸处(见图23)。

Indications: Spasmodic pain in the elbow and arm, scrofula and somnolence.

【主治】 肘臂挛痛；瘰疬；嗜卧。

2.1.4.3.12　Binao (LI 14)

12. 臂臑　LI14

Location: It is located on the line joining Quchi (LI 11) and Jianyu (LI 15), 7 cun above Quchi (LI 11) (see Fig. 23). Or it is superior to the lower end of m. deltoideus.

【位置与取法】 当曲池与肩髃连线上，曲池上7寸(见图23)。或于三角肌止点稍前上方处取穴。

Indications: Pain in the shoulder and arm, stiff neck, shortsightedness, night blindness and scrofula.

【主治】 肩臂痛，项强；近视，雀目；瘰疬。

2.1.4.3.13　Jianyu (LI 15)

13. 肩髃　LI15

Location: The acupoint is located anterior-inferior to the acromion, on the upper portion of m. deltoideus and between the acromion and greater tuberosity of humerus (see Fig. 23). When the arm is in full abduction, the acupoint is in the depression at the anterior border of the acromioclavicular joint.

【位置与取法】 肩峰端下缘，当肩峰与肱骨大结节之间，三角肌上部中央(见图23)。上臂外展平举时，肩前呈现的凹陷中是穴。

Indications: Pain in the shoulder and arm, flaccidity of the upper limbs, urticaria and scrofula.

【主治】 肩臂疼痛，上肢痿痹；瘾疹；瘰疬。

2.1.4.3.14　Futu (LI 18)

14. 扶突　LI18

Location: The acupoint is located on the lateral side of the laryngeal protuberance and between the sternal head and clavicular head of m. sternocleidomastoideus (see Fig. 24).

【位置与取法】 喉结旁开3寸，当胸锁乳突肌胸骨头与锁骨头之间(见图24)。

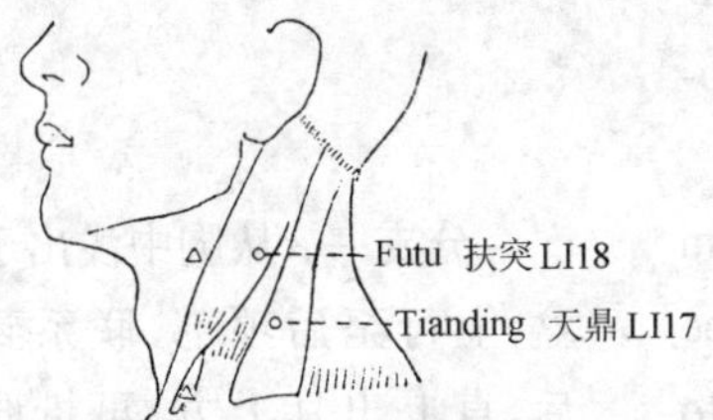

Fig. 24 Neck acupoints on the large intestine meridian of hand-yangming

图 24 手阳明大肠经颈部经穴图

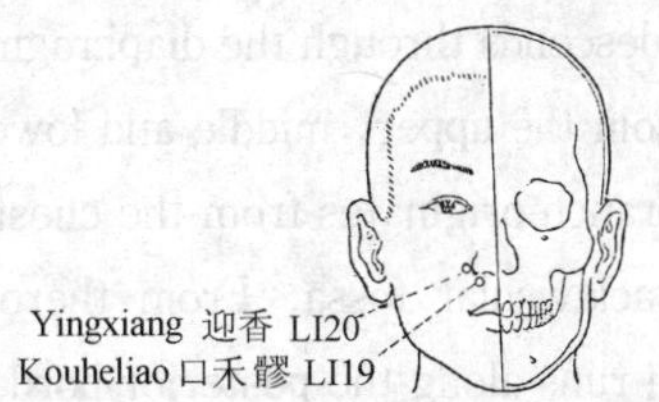

Fig. 25 Head and face acupoints on the large intestine meridian of hand-yangming

图 25 手阳明大肠经头面部经穴图

Indications: Cough, asthma, sore throat, scrofula and goiter.

【主治】 咳嗽,气喘;咽喉肿痛;瘰疬,瘿气。

2.1.4.3.15 Kouheliao (LI 19)

Location: The acupoint is located right below the lateral margin of the nostril and parallel to Shuigou (GV 26) (see Fig. 25).

Indications: Toothache, facial paralysis and nose disorders.

15. 口禾髎 LI19

【位置与取法】 在上唇部,鼻孔外缘直下,平水沟穴(见图 25)。

【主治】 齿痛,面瘫,鼻病。

2.1.4.3.16 Yingxiang (LI 20)

Location: The acupoint is located in the nasolabial groove and at the level of the midpoint of the lateral border of the nose (see Fig. 25).

Indications: Nasal obstruction, nasosinusitis, epistaxis, facial paralysis and syncope due to ascariasis.

16. 迎香 LI20

【位置与取法】 鼻翼外缘中点旁开,鼻唇沟中取穴(见图 25)。

【主治】 鼻塞,鼻渊,鼻衄;面瘫;蛔厥。

2. 1. 5 Triple energizer meridian of hand-shaoyang

2.1.5.1 Cyclical flowing and distribution

The triple energizer meridian originates from the tip of the ring finger and runs upward between the fourth and fifth metacarpal bones along the dorsal aspect of the wrist to the lateral aspect of the forearm between the radius and ulna. Then it passes through the olecranon along the lateral aspect of the upper arm and reaches the shoulder region. It moves forward into the supraclavicular fossa

五、手少阳三焦经

(一)循行分布

起于无名指末端,向上出于四五掌指关节之间,沿手背、腕关节,沿上臂外侧中央向上到达肩部,向前下进入缺盆,分布于胸中,散络心包,向下通过膈部,依次连属于上、中、下三焦。

and spreads in the chest to connect with the pericardium. Then it descends through the diaphragm down to the abdomen to join the upper, middle and lower energizers.

A branch originates from the chest and emerges from the supraclavicular fossa. From there it ascends to the neck and runs along the posterior border of the ear and to the corner of the anterior hairline. Then it turns downward to join the other branch at the cheek and terminates in the infraorbital region.

分支一：从胸中浅出于缺盆，上行至后项部，联系到耳后，直上出耳上方，再折向下行至面颊，抵达目下颧骨部。

The other branch arises from the retroauricular region and enters the ear. Then it emerges in front of the ear, crosses the previous branch at the cheek and reaches the outer canthus to link with the gallbladder meridian. (see Fig. 26)

分支二：从耳后进入耳中，出行到耳前，经上关，与前一支脉交于面颊，抵达目外眦，和足少阳胆经相交接。(见图 26)

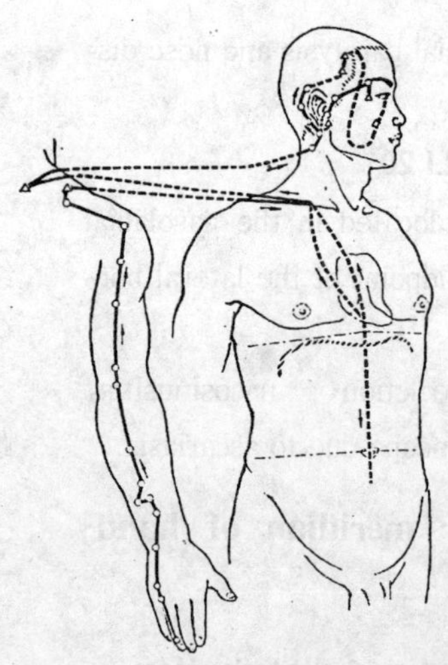

Fig. 26　Flowing route of the triple energizer meridian of hand-shaoyang

图 26　手少阳三焦经循行示意图

Associated viscera: Triple energizer and pericardium.

联系脏腑：三焦、心包。

Associated organs: Eyes and ears.

联系器官：目、耳。

2.1.5.2　Indications

（二）主治要点

Disorders of the side of the head, ears, eyes and throat as well as diseases involving the regions through

本经腧穴主要治疗侧头病，耳、目、咽喉病，以及经脉

which the meridian runs.

循行所过部位的其他病证。

2.1.5.3 Commonly used acupoints

（三）常用腧穴

2.1.5.3.1 Guanchong（TE 1）

1. 关冲 TE1

Location：The acupoint is located on the lateral side of the ring finger，about 0.1 cun latero-posterior to the corner of the nail (see Fig. 27).

【位置与取法】 在手无名指末节尺侧，距指甲角 0.1 寸（见图 27）。

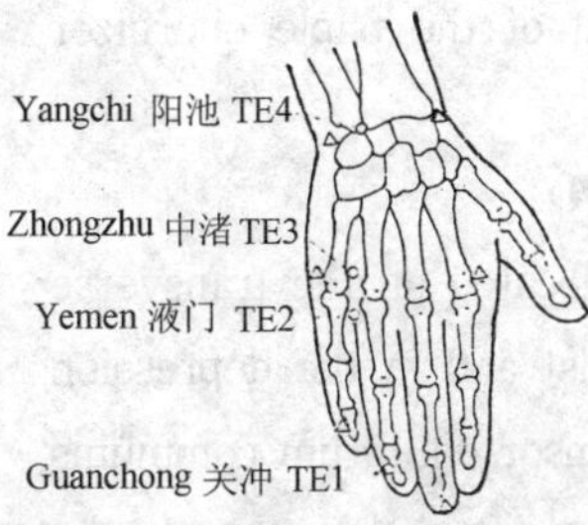

Fig. 27 Hand acupoints on the triple energizer meridian of hand-shaoyang

图 27 手少阳三焦经手部经穴图

Indications：Apoplexy，coma，headache，redness，swelling and pain of eyes，tinnitus，deafness，sore throat and high fever.

【主治】 中风，昏迷；头痛；目赤肿痛；耳鸣，耳聋；咽喉肿痛；高热。

Note：Jing-Well acupoint of the triple energizer meridian of hand-shaoyang.

【备注】 手少阳经之“井”穴。

2.1.5.3.2 Yemen（TE 2）

2. 液门 TE2

Location：The acupoint is located on the dorsum of the hand between the fourth and fifth fingers and in the depression proximal to the margin of the web between the ring and small fingers (see Fig. 27).

【位置与取法】 在手背部，当第四五指间，指蹼缘后方赤白肉际处（见图 27）。

Indications：Headache，redness and swelling pain of eyes，tinnitus，deafness，sore throat，numbness of fingers，swelling and pain of the dorsum of hand and febrile disease.

【主治】 头痛；目赤肿痛；耳鸣，耳聋；咽喉肿痛；手指麻木，手背肿痛；热病。

Note：Ying-Spring acupoint of the triple energizer meridian of hand-shaoyang.

【备注】 手少阳经之“荥”穴。

2.1.5.3.3 Zhongzhu（TE 3）

3. 中渚 TE3

Location：The acupoint is located on the dorsum of

【位置与取法】 手背部，

the hand, posterior to the metacarpophalangeal joint of the fourth finger and in the depression between the fourth and fifth metacarpophalangeal joints (see Fig. 27).

当无名指掌指关节的后方,第四五掌骨间的凹陷处(见图27)。

Indications: Headache, dizziness, redness and pain of the eyes, tinnitus, deafness, sore throat, aching pain in the shoulder, back, elbow and arm as well as spasmodic pain of the fingers.

【主治】 头痛;目眩,目赤肿痛;耳鸣,耳聋;咽喉肿痛;肩背肘臂酸痛,手指挛痛。

Note: Shu-Stream acupoint of the triple energizer meridian of hand-shaoyang.

【备注】 手少阳经之"输"穴。

2.1.5.3.4 Yangchi (TE 4)

4. 阳池 TE4

Location: The acupoint is located on the transverse crease of the dorsum of the wrist and in the depression lateral to the tendon of m. extensor digitorum communis (see Fig. 27). Or when the palm is turned upward, the acupoint is in the depression at the point on the transverse crease of the wrist dorsum crossed with the vertical interstice between the third and fourth metacarpal bones.

【位置与取法】 在腕背横纹中,当指总伸肌腱的尺侧缘凹陷处(见图27)。或俯掌,于第三四掌骨间直上与腕背横纹交点处的凹陷中取穴。

Indications: Tinnitus, deafness, sore throat, pain of the wrist joint, flaccidity and Bi-syndrome of the upper limbs and diabetes.

【主治】 耳鸣,耳聋;咽喉肿痛;腕关节疼痛,上肢痿痹;消渴。

Note: Yuan-Source acupoint of the triple energizer meridian of hand-shaoyang.

【备注】 手少阳经之"原"穴。

2.1.5.3.5 Waiguan (TE 5)

5. 外关 TE5

Location: The acupoint is located 2 cun above the transverse crease on the wrist, between the radius and ulna, on the line joining Yangchi (TE 4) and elbow tip.

【位置与取法】 在前臂背侧,当阳池与肘尖的连线上,腕横纹上2寸,尺骨与桡骨之间(见图28)。

Indications: Migraine, facial paralysis, tinnitus, deafness, redness, swelling and pain of eyes, hypochondriac pain, spasmodic pain in the elbow and arm, common cold and febrile disease.

【主治】 偏头痛;面瘫;耳鸣,耳聋;目赤肿痛;胁痛,肘臂挛痛;感冒,热病。

Note: Luo-Connecting acupoint of the triple energizer meridian of hand-shaoyang and one of the eight convergent acupoints "associating with yang link vessel".

【备注】 手少阳经之"络"穴,八脉交会穴之一,通于阳维脉。

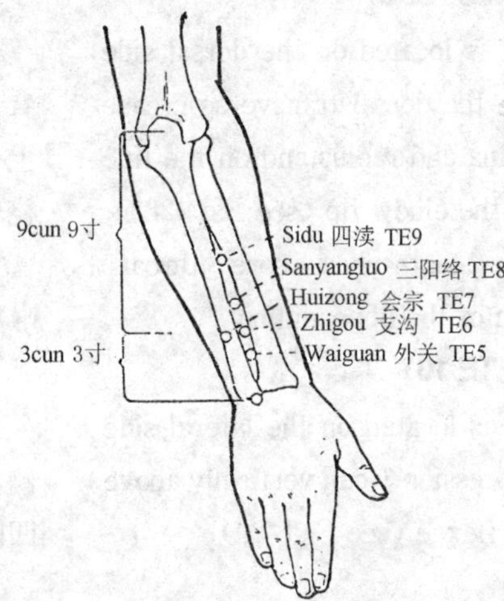

Fig. 28 Forearm acupoints on the triple energizer meridian of hand-shaoyang

图 28 手少阳三焦经前臂部经穴图

2.1.5.3.6 Zhigou (TE 6)

Location: The acupoint is located on the dorsal side of the forearm, 3 cun above the dorsal transverse crease of the wrist and between the ulna and radius (see Fig. 28).

Indications: Sudden loss of voice, tinnitus, deafness, hypochondriac pain, aching pain in the shoulder and back, constipation and febrile disease.

Note: Jing-River acupoint of the triple energizer meridian of hand-shaoyang.

2.1.5.3.7 Huizong (TE 7)

Location: The acupoint is located on the dorsal side of the forearm, 3 cun above the dorsal transverse crease of the wrist and at the ulnar border of Zhigou (TE 6) and radial border of the ulna (see Fig. 28).

Indications: Deafness and obstructive pain in the upper limbs.

Note: Xi-Cleft acupoint of the triple energizer meridian of hand-shaoyang.

6. 支沟 TE6

【位置与取法】 在前臂背侧,当腕背横纹上 3 寸,尺骨与桡骨之间(见图 28)。

【主治】 暴喑;耳鸣,耳聋;胁痛,肩背酸痛;便秘;热病。

【备注】 手少阳经之"经"穴。

7. 会宗 TE7

【位置与取法】 在前臂背侧,当腕背横纹上 3 寸。支沟尺侧,尺骨的桡侧缘。(见图 28)

【主治】 耳聋;上肢痹痛。

【备注】 手少阳经之"郄"穴。

2.1.5.3.8 Sanyangluo (TE 8)

Location: The acupoint is located on the dorsal side of the forearm, 4 cun above the dorsal transverse crease of the wrist, between the ulna and radius and on the line joining Yangchi (TE 4) and the elbow tip (see Fig. 28).

Indications: Deafness, toothache, sore throat, sudden loss of voice and pain of the upper limbs.

8. 三阳络 TE8

【位置与取法】 在前臂背侧，当阳池与肘尖的连线上，腕背横纹上 4 寸，尺骨与桡骨之间(见图 28)。

【主治】 耳聋，牙痛，咽喉肿痛，暴喑；上肢痹痛。

2.1.5.3.9 Tianjing (TE 10)

Location: The acupoint is located on the lateral side of the forearm and in the depression 1 cun vertically above elbow tip when the elbow is flexed (see Fig. 29).

9. 天井 TE10

【位置与取法】 在臂外侧，屈肘时，当肘尖直上 1 寸凹陷处(见图 29)。

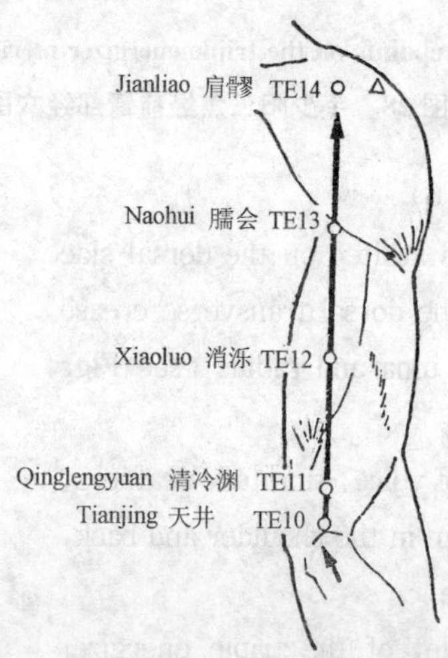

Fig. 29 Upper arm acupoints on the triple energizer meridian of hand-shaoyang

图 29 手少阳三焦经上臂部经穴图

Indications: Deafness, migraine, hypochondriac pain, spasmodic pain in the elbow and arm and epilepsy.

Note: He-Sea acupoint of the triple energizer meridian of hand-shaoyang.

【主治】 耳聋；偏头痛，胁痛，肘臂挛痛；癫痫。

【备注】 手少阳经之“合”穴。

2.1.5.3.10 Naohui (TE 13)

Location: The acupoint is located on the lateral side of the forearm, on the line joining the elbow tip and Jianliao (TE 14), 3 cun below Jianliao (TE 14) and on the

10. 臑会 TE13

【位置与取法】 在臂外侧，当肘尖与肩髎连线上，肩髎下 3 寸，三角肌的后下缘

posterior border of m. deltoideus (see Fig. 29).

（见图 29）。

Indications: Pain in the shoulder and arm, scrofula and goiter.

【主治】 肩臂痛；瘰疬，瘿气。

2.1.5.3.11 Jianliao (TE 14)

11. 肩髎 TE14

Location: The acupoint is located on the shoulder, in the depression posterior to the acromion when the arm is abducted (see Fig. 29).

【位置与取法】 在肩部，肩峰后下方之凹陷中(见图29)。上臂外展平举，肩关节部于肩峰后下方呈现的凹陷处。

Indications: Pain in the shoulder and arm and inflexibility of the shoulder joint.

【主治】 肩臂痛，肩关节活动不利。

2.1.5.3.12 Yifeng (TE 17)

12. 翳风 TE17

Location: The acupoint is located posterior to the lobule of the ear, in the depression between the mandible and mastoid process (see Fig. 30).

【位置与取法】 在耳垂后方，当乳突与下颌角之间的凹陷处(见图 30)。

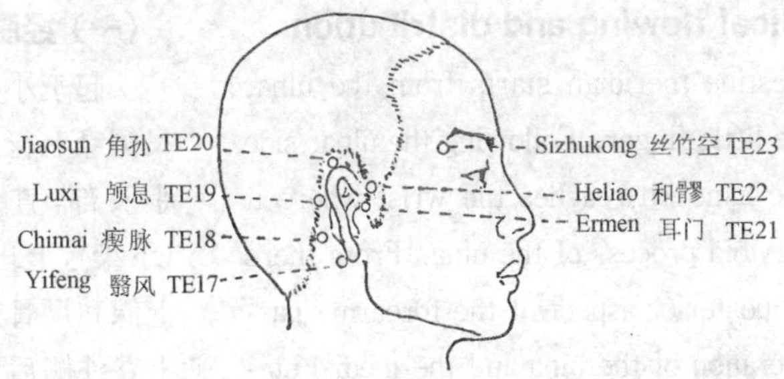

Fig. 30 Head and face acupoints on the triple energizer meridian of hand-shaoyang

图 30 手少阳三焦经头面部经穴图

Indications: Facial paralysis, tinnitus, deafness, swelling of cheeks, toothache and hiccup.

【主治】 面瘫；耳鸣，耳聋；颊肿；牙痛；呃逆。

2.1.5.3.13 Jiaosun (TE 20)

13. 角孙 TE20

Location: The acupoint is located directly above the ear apex, within the hair line (see Fig. 30).

【位置与取法】 在头部，当耳尖直上入发际处(见图 30)。

Indications: Migraine, swelling of cheeks, tinnitus, deafness, cataract and toothache.

【主治】 偏头痛，颊肿；耳鸣，耳聋；目翳；牙痛。

2.1.5.3.14 Ermen (TE 21)

Location: The acupoint is located on the face and in the depression anterior to the supratragic notch and slightly superior to the condyloid process of the mandible when the mouth is open (see Fig. 30).

Indications: Tinnitus, deafness, otorrhea, toothache and swelling of cheeks.

14. 耳门　TE21

【位置与取法】 在面部，当耳屏上切迹的前方，下颌骨髁状突后缘，张口有凹陷处(见图30)。

【主治】 耳鸣，耳聋，聤耳；牙痛；颊肿。

2.1.5.3.15 Sizhukong (TE 23)

Location: The acupont is located in the depression at the lateral end of the eyebrow (see Fig. 30).

Indications: Headache, dizziness, redness and swelling pain of the eyes, twitching of the eyelid, toothache and epilepsy.

15. 丝竹空　TE23

【位置与取法】 在面部，当眉梢凹陷处(见图30)。

【主治】 头痛；目眩，目赤肿痛，眼睑瞤动；牙痛；癫痫。

2. 1. 6 Small intestine meridian of hand-taiyang

六、手太阳小肠经

2.1.6.1 Cyclical flowing and distribution

The small intestine meridian starts from the ulnar side of the tip of the little finger. Following the ulnar side of the dorsum of the hand, it reaches the wrist where it emerges from the styloid process of the ulna. From there it ascends along the posterior aspect of the forearm, passes between the olecranon of the ulna and the medial epicondyle of the humerus, and runs along the posterior border of the lateral aspect of the upper arm to the shoulder joint. Circling around the scapular region, it converges over the shoulder and then turns downward to the supraclavicular fossa to connect with the heart. From there it descends along the esophagus, passes through the diaphragm, reaches the stomach, and finally enters the small intestine.

The branch from the supraclavicular fossa ascends to the neck, and further to the cheek. Then it reaches the outer canthus and enters the ear.

(一)经脉循行

起于小指外侧端，沿手掌尺侧缘上行到腕部，出于尺骨小头部，直上沿尺骨尺侧缘(下缘)，上出于肘内侧肱骨内上髁和尺骨鹰嘴之间，向上沿上臂外侧后缘，上出于肩后关节缝部，绕行肩胛，交会到肩上，向前下由缺盆入内，联络于心，沿食管向下穿过膈，抵达胃部，连属于小肠。

分支一：从缺盆向上沿颈部，上行到面颊，抵目外眦，再向后进入耳中。

The other branch from the cheeks runs upward to the infraorbital region and further to the lateral side of the nose and inner canthus to connect with the bladder meridian. (see Fig. 31)

分支二：从面颊部分出，上行到眼眶的下方，抵达鼻到目内眦，交足太阳膀胱经。(见图 31)

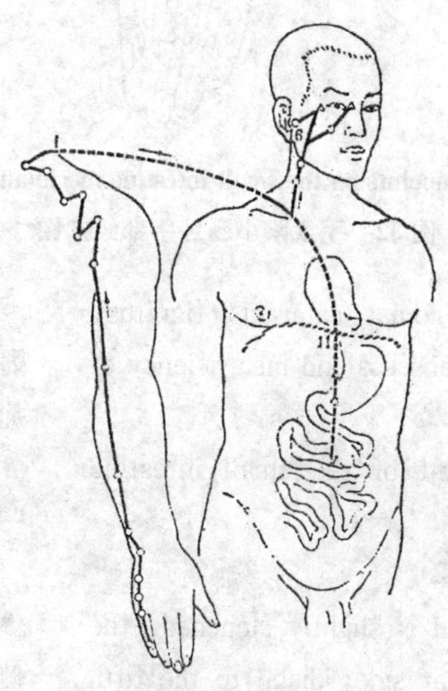

Fig. 31 Flowing route of the small intestine meridian of hand-taiyang

图 31 手太阳小肠经循行示意图

Associated viscera: Small intestine, heart and stomach.

联系脏腑：小肠、心、胃。

Associated organs: Throat, ears, nose and eyes.

联系器官：咽、耳、鼻、目。

2.1.6.2 Indications

(二) 主治要点

Disorders of the organs on the face and throat, febrile disease and pathological changes of the lateral side of the upper limbs, scapula and neck.

本经腧穴主治头面器官病、咽喉病、热病及经脉循行所过的上肢外侧后缘、肩胛部、颈项部、面部病变。

2.1.6.3 Commonly used acupoints

(三) 常用腧穴

2.1.6.3.1 Shaoze (SI 1)

1. 少泽 SI1

Location: The acupoint is located on the ulnar side of the little finger, about 0.1 cun latero-posterior to the corner of the nail (see Fig. 32).

【位置与取法】 在手小指末节尺侧，距指甲角 0.1 寸(见图 32)。

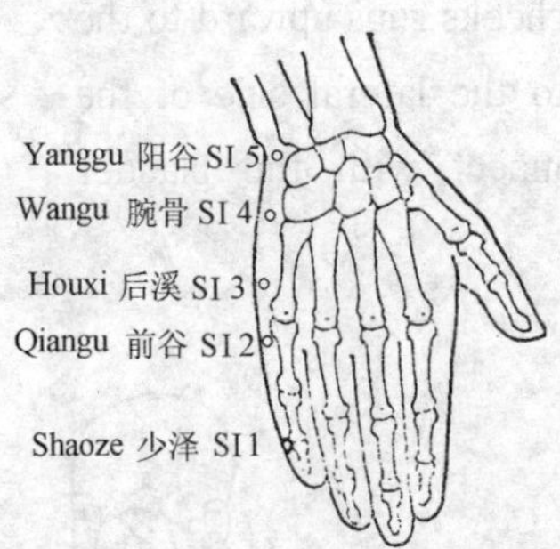

Fig. 32　Hand acupoints on the small intestine meridian of hand-taiyang

图 32　手太阳小肠经手部经穴图

Indications: Apoplexy, coma, cataract, tinnitus, deafness, sore throat, breast abscess and insufficiency of lactation.

【主治】 中风，昏迷；目翳，耳鸣，耳聋，咽喉肿痛；乳痛，乳少。

Note: Jing-Well acupoint of the small intestine meridian of hand-taiyang.

【备注】 手太阳经之"井"穴。

2.1.6.3.2 Qiangu (SI 2)

2. 前谷 SI2

Location: When the hand is slightly clenched, the acupoint is located on the ulnar side, distal to the fifth metacarpophalangeal joint, at the junction of the red and white skin (see Fig. 32).

【位置与取法】 在手尺侧，微握拳，当第五掌指关节前的掌指横纹头赤白肉际处（见图 32）。

Indications: Headache, redness, swelling and pain of eyes, tinnitus, deafness, insufficiency of lactation and numbness of fingers.

【主治】 头痛；目赤肿痛；耳鸣，耳聋；乳少；手指麻木。

Note: Ying-Spring acupoint of the small intestine meridian of hand-taiyang.

【备注】 手太阳经之"荥"穴。

2.1.6.3.3 Houxi (SI 3)

3. 后溪 SI3

Location: When the hand is slightly clenched, the acupoint is located on the ulnar side, proximal to the fifth metacarpophalangeal joint, at the end of the transverse crease and the junction of the red and white skin (see Fig. 32).

【位置与取法】 在手掌尺侧，微握拳，当第五掌指关节后的远侧掌横纹头赤白肉际（见图 32）。

Indications: Redness, swelling and pain of the eyes, sore throat, mania, epilepsy, stiff neck, acute lumbar muscle sprain, spasmodic pain in the elbow and arm,

【主治】 目赤肿痛；耳聋；咽喉肿痛；癫、狂、痫证；落枕，急性腰扭伤；肘臂挛痛，手

numbness of fingers, malaria and febrile disease.

Note: Shu-Stream acupoint of the small intestine meridian of hand-taiyang and one of the eight convergent acupoints "associating with the governor vessel".

指麻木;疟疾,热病。

【备注】 手太阳经之"输"穴、八脉交会穴之一,通于督脉。

2.1.6.3.4 Wangu (SI 4)

4. 腕骨 SI4

Location: The acupoint is located on the ulnar side of the palm, in the depression between the base of the fifth metacarpal bone and the triquetral bone (see Fig. 32).

【位置与取法】 在手掌尺侧,当第五掌骨基底与三角骨之间的凹陷处赤白肉际(见图 32)。

Indications: Stiffness and pain of neck and head, cataract, tinnitus, deafness, abdominal distension and pain, pain in the wrist, numbness of fingers, febrile disease, malaria and jaundice.

【主治】 头项强痛;目翳;耳鸣,耳聋;腹胀腹痛;腕关节疼痛,手指麻木;热病,疟疾,黄疸。

Note: Yuan-Source acupoint of the small intestine meridian of hand-taiyang.

【备注】 手太阳经之"原"穴。

2.1.6.3.5 Yanggu (SI 5)

5. 阳谷 SI5

Location: The acupoint is located on the ulnar end of the transverse crease on the dorsal aspect of the wrist, in the depression between the styloid process of the ulna and the triquetral bone (see Fig. 32).

【位置与取法】 在手腕尺侧,当尺骨茎突与三角骨之间的凹陷处(见图 32)。

Indications: Headache, redness, swelling and pain of the eyes, tinnitus, deafness, mania, epilepsy, spasmodic pain in the elbow, arm and wrist joint as well as exogenous febrile disease.

【主治】 头痛;齿痛;目赤肿痛;耳鸣,耳聋;癫、狂、痫证;肘臂挛痛,腕关节疼痛;外感热病。

Note: Jing-River acupoint of the small intestine meridian of hand-taiyang.

【备注】 手太阳经之"经"穴。

2.1.6.3.6 Yanglao (SI 6)

6. 养老 SI6

Location: The acupoint is located at the dorsal and ulnar side of the arm and in the depression at the radial side proximal to ulnar head (see Fig. 33). The palm turns downward, and the fingers of the other hand press on the prominent point of the ulnar head. Then the palm faces the chest, the point is in the bony cleft on the styloid process of the ulna.

【位置与取法】 在手臂背面尺侧,当尺骨小头近端桡侧凹陷中(见图 33)。掌心向下,用另一手指按捺在尺骨小头的最高点上;然后掌心转向胸部,当手指滑入的骨缝中是穴。

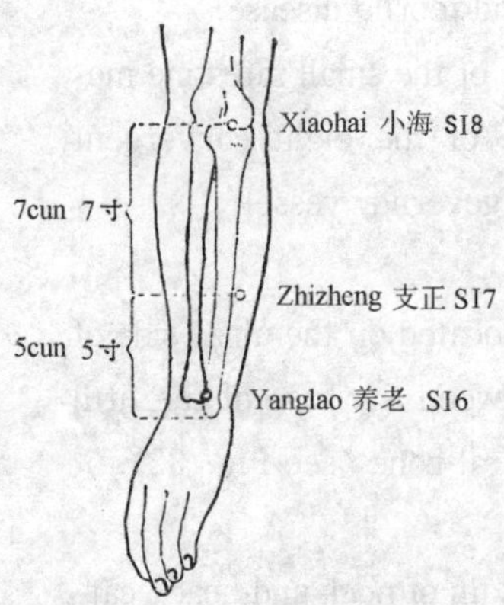

Fig. 33　Forearm acupoints on the small intestine meridian of hand-taiyang

图 33　手太阳小肠经前臂部经穴图

Indications: Blurred vision and aching pain in the shoulder, back, elbow and arm.

【主治】　目视不明；肩、背、肘、臂酸痛。

Note: Xi-Cleft acupoint of the small intestine meridian of hand-taiyang.

【备注】　手太阳经之"郄"穴。

2.1.6.3.7　Zhizheng (SI 7)

7. 支正　SI7

Location: The acupoint is located on the line joining Yanggu (SI 5) and Xiaohai (SI 8), 5 cun above the dorsal transverse crease of the wrist (see Fig. 33).

【位置与取法】　在前臂背面尺侧，当阳谷与小海的连线上，腕背横纹上 5 寸(见图 33)。

Indications: Headache, dizziness, depressive psychosis, manic psychosis, stiff neck and spasmodic pain in the elbow and arm.

【主治】　头痛，目眩；癫证，狂证；项强，肘臂挛痛。

Note: Luo-Connecting acupoint of the small intestine meridian of hand-taiyang.

【备注】　手太阳经之"络"穴。

2.1.6.3.8　Xiaohai (SI 8)

8. 小海　SI8

Location: The acupoint is located in the depression between the olecranon of the ulna and the medial epicondyle of the humerus when the elbow is flexed (see Fig. 33).

【位置与取法】　在肘内侧，当尺骨鹰嘴与肱骨内上髁之间凹陷处(见图 33)。

Indications: Headache, dizziness, tinnitus, deafness, epilepsy, spasmodic pain in the elbow and arm.

【主治】　头痛目眩，耳鸣耳聋；癫痫；肘臂挛痛。

Note: He-Sea acupoint of the small intestine meridian

【备注】　手太阳经

of hand-taiyang.

“合”穴。

2.1.6.3.9 Jianzhen (SI 9)

Location: The acupoint is posterior and inferior to the shoulder joint. When the arm is adducted, the acupoint is located 1 cun above the posterior end of the axillary fold (see Fig. 34).

9. 肩贞 SI9

【位置与取法】 在肩关节后下方，臂内收时，腋后纹头上1寸(见图34)。

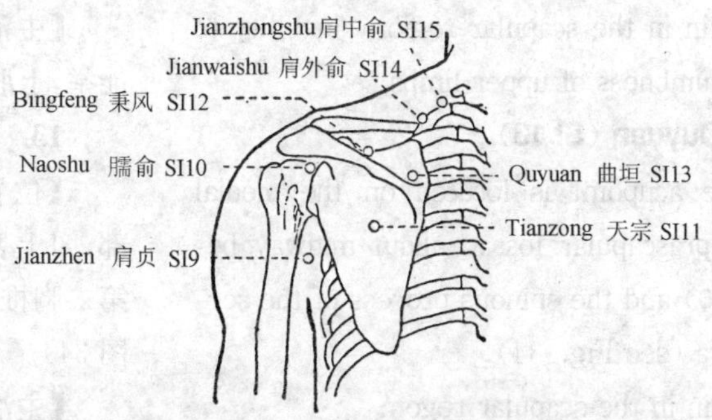

Fig. 34 Shoulder and back acupoints on the small intestine meridian of hand-taiyang

图34 手太阳小肠经肩背部经穴图

Indications: Pain in the scapular region, inability to raise shoulder, numbness of the upper limbs, tinnitus and deafness.

【主治】 肩关节疼痛，肩不能举，上肢麻木；耳鸣，耳聋。

2.1.6.3.10 Naoshu (SI 10)

Location: The acupoint is located on the shoulder and in the depression vertically above the posterior crease of the axilla and below the lower border of the spine of scapula (see Fig. 34).

Indications: Pain in the shoulder and scrofula.

10. 臑俞 SI10

【位置与取法】 在肩部，当腋后纹头直上，肩胛冈下缘凹陷中(见图34)。

【主治】 肩臂疼痛；瘰疬。

2.1.6.3.11 Tianzong (SI 11)

Location: The acupoint is in the infrascapular fossa, at the junction of the upper 1/3 and middle 1/3 of the distance between the lower border of the scapular spine and the inferior angle of the scapula (see Fig. 34).

11. 天宗 SI11

【位置与取法】 在肩胛部，当冈下窝中央凹陷处，与第四胸椎相平(见图34)。在肩胛冈下缘与肩胛骨下角等分线上，当上、中1/3交点处。与臑俞、肩贞约成三角形。

Indications: Pain in the scapular region, cough, asthma, and breast abscess.

2.1.6.3.12 Bingfeng (SI 12)

Location: The acupoint is located in the center of the suprascapular fossa, directly above Tianzong (SI 11). When the arm is raised, the acupoint is at the site of the depression.

Indications: Pain in the scapular region, inability to raise shoulder and numbness of upper limbs.

2.1.6.3.13 Quyuan (SI 13)

Location: The acupoint is located on the medial extremity of the suprascapular fossa, about midway between Naoshu (SI 10) and the spinous process of the second thoracic vertebra (see Fig. 34).

Indications: Pain in the scapular regon.

2.1.6.3.14 Jianwaishu (SI 14)

Location: The acupoint is located on the back, and 3 cun lateral to the lower border of the spinous process of the frist thoracic vertebra (see Fig. 34).

Indications: Aching pain in the shoulder and back, stiffness and pain of neck, cough and asthma.

2.1.6.3.15 Jianzhongshu (SI 15)

Location: The acupoint is located on the back and 2 cun lateral to the spinous process of the seventh cervical vertebra (see Fig. 34).

Indications: Aching pain in the shoulder and back, headache and stiff neck as well as cough and asthma.

2.1.6.3.16 Tianrong (SI 17)

Location: The acupoint is located in the lateral aspect of the neck and in the depression on the anterior border of m. sternocleidomastoideus and posterior to the angle of mandible (see Fig. 35).

Indications: Tinnitus, deafness, sore throat, swelling and pain of the neck.

【主治】 肩胛疼痛；咳嗽气喘；乳痈。

12. 秉风　SI12

【位置与取法】 在肩胛部，冈上窝中央，天宗直上，举臂有凹陷处（见图34）。

【主治】 肩胛疼痛，肩不能举，上肢麻木。

13. 曲垣　SI13

【位置与取法】 在肩胛部，冈上窝内侧端，当臑俞与第二胸椎棘突连线中点处（见图34）。

【主治】 肩胛疼痛。

14. 肩外俞　SI14

【位置与取法】 在背部，当第一胸椎棘突下，旁开3寸（见图34）。

【主治】 肩背酸痛，颈项强痛；咳嗽，气喘。

15. 肩中俞　SI15

【位置与取法】 在背部，当第七颈椎棘突下，旁开2寸（见图34）。

【主治】 肩背酸痛，头痛项强；咳嗽，气喘。

16. 天容　SI17

【位置与取法】 在颈外侧部，当下颌角的后方，胸锁乳突肌前缘凹陷中（见图35）。

【主治】 耳鸣，耳聋；咽喉肿痛；颈项肿痛。

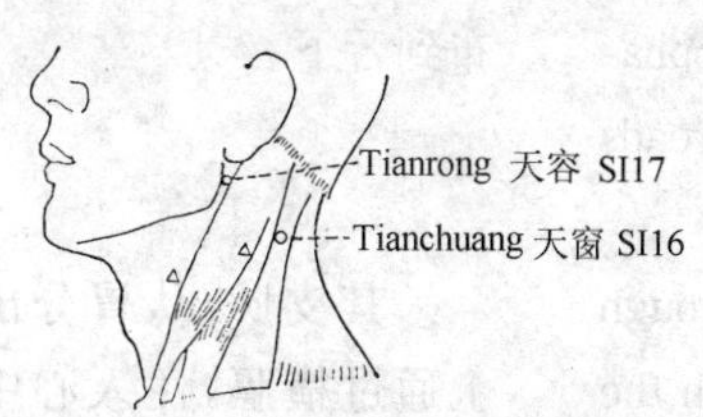

Fig. 35 Neck acupoints on the small intestine meridian of hand-taiyang

图 35 手太阳小肠经颈部经穴图

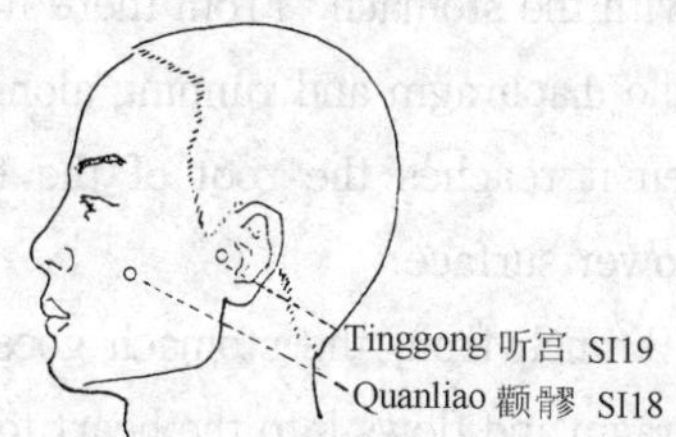

Fig. 36 Head and face acupoints on the small intestine meridian of hand-taiyang

图 36 手太阳小肠经头面部经穴图

2.1.6.3.17 Quanliao (SI 18)

Location: The acupoint is located directly below the outer canthus, in the depression on the lower border of zygoma (see Fig. 36).

Indications: Facial paralysis, twitching of eyelids, toothache and swelling of cheeks.

17. 颧髎 SI18

【位置与取法】 在面部，当目外眦直下，颧骨下缘凹陷处(见图 36)。

【主治】 面瘫；眼睑瞤动；齿痛；颊肿。

2.1.6.3.18 Tinggong (SI 19)

Location: The acupoint is located anterior to the tragus and posterior to the condyloid process of the mandible and in the depression formed when the mouth is open (see Fig 36).

Indications: Tinnitus, deafness, otorrhea, toothache depressive psychosis, manic psychosis, and epilepsy.

18. 听宫 SI19

【位置与取法】 在面部，耳屏前，下颌骨髁状突的后方，张口时呈凹陷处(见图 36)。

【主治】 耳鸣，耳聋，聤耳；齿痛；癫狂痫。

2.1.7 Spleen meridian of foot-taiyin

2.1.7.1 Cyclical flowing and distribution

The spleen meridian starts from the tip of the great toe. From there it runs along the medial aspect of the foot at the junction of the red and white skin. Then it ascends in front of the medial malleolus up to the medial aspect of the leg (an area 8 cun above the medial malleolus). Following the posterior aspect of the tibia, it crosses and goes in front of the liver meridian. Passing through the anterior medial aspect of the knee and thigh, it enters the abdomen and then the spleen to which it pertains and

七、足太阴脾经

(一) 循行分布

起于大趾末端，沿大趾内侧赤白肉际，经过第一跖趾关节、第一跖骨基底部前上向内踝前缘，经小腿内侧，沿胫骨内侧后缘(在内踝上 8 寸处)交出足厥阴肝经之前，而行于足厥阴和足少阴肾经之前，沿膝、大腿内侧前缘，进入腹内，连属于脾脏，络于胃腑，通过

connect with the stomach. From there it ascends, passing through the diaphragm and running alongside the esophagus. When it reaches the root of the tongue it spreads over its lower surface.

横膈,挟食道上行,连舌根,散布到舌下。

The branch from the stomach goes upward through the diaphragm and flows into the heart to connect with the heart meridian. (see Fig. 37)

其支脉:从胃分出来,向上通过横膈,注入心中,交手少阴心经。(见图 37)

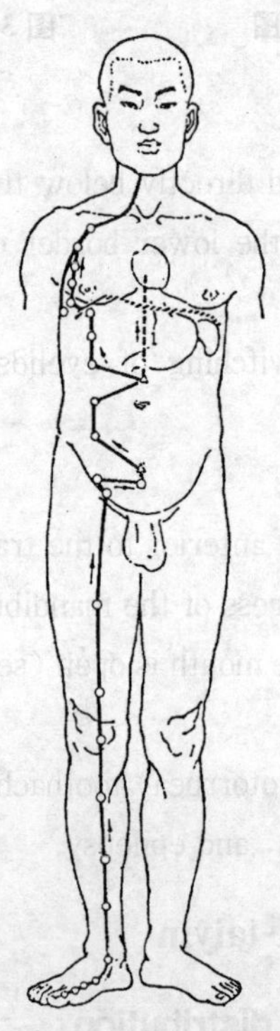

Fig. 37　Flowing route of the spleen meridian of foot-taiyin

图 37　足太阴脾经循行示意图

Associated viscera: Spleen, stomach and heart.

联系脏腑:脾、胃、心。

Associated organs: Throat and tongue.

联系器官:咽、舌。

2.1.7.2　Indications

(二)主治要点

Disorders of the spleen and stomach, gynecological diseases, genital problems and diseases involving the areas through which the meridian flows.

本经腧穴主治脾胃病,妇科、前阴病及经脉循行部位的其他病证。

2.1.7.3 Commonly used acupoints

2.1.7.3.1 Yinbai (SP 1)

Location: The acupoint is located on the medial side of the great toe, 0.1 cun latero-posterior to the corner of the nail (see Fig. 38).

(三)常用腧穴

1. 隐白 SP1

【位置与取法】 在足大趾末节内侧,距趾甲角0.1寸(见图38)。

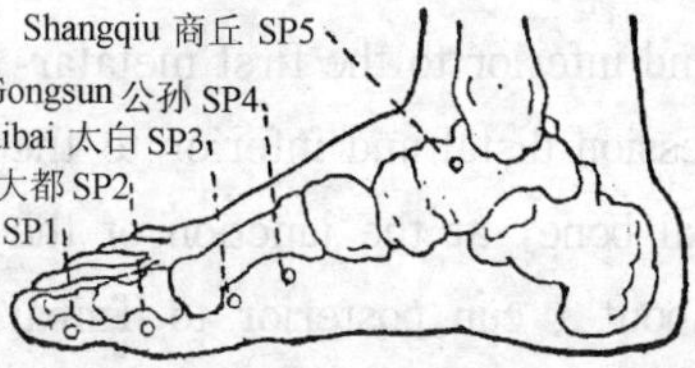

Fig. 38 Foot acupoints on the spleen meridian of foot-taiyin
图38 足太阴脾经足部经穴图

Indications: Unconsciousness, apoplexy, convulsion, abdominal distension, sudden diarrhea, metrorrhagia and metrostaxis, epistaxis and hematochezia.

Note: Jing-Well acupoint of the spleen meridian of foot-taiyin.

【主治】 昏迷,中风,惊风;腹胀,暴泄;崩漏,衄血,便血。

【备注】 足太阴经之"井"穴。

2.1.7.3.2 Dadu (SP 2)

Location: The acupoint is located on the medial side of the great toe, in the depression distal and inferior to the first metatarsodigital joint and the junction of the red and white skin (see Fig. 38).

Indications: Abdominal pain, abdominal distension, diarrhea, vomiting, no sweating in febrile disease and dysphoria.

Note: Ying-Spring acupoint of the spleen meridian of foot-taiyin.

2. 大都 SP2

【位置与取法】 在足内侧缘,当足大趾本节(第一跖趾关节)前下方赤白肉际凹陷处(见图38)。

【主治】 腹痛,腹胀,泄泻,呕吐;热病无汗;烦心。

【备注】 足太阴经之"荥"穴。

2.1.7.3.3 Taibai (SP 3)

Location: The acupoint is located on the medial side of the great toe, in the depression proximal and inferior to the first metatarsodigital joint and the junction of the red and white skin (see Fig. 38).

Indications: Stomachache, abdominal distension,

3. 太白 SP3

【位置与取法】 在足内侧缘,当足大趾本节(第一跖趾关节)后下方赤白肉际凹陷处(见图38)。

【主治】 胃痛,腹胀,呕

vomiting, diarrhea, dysentery, constipation, edema, heaviness of the body, pain of joints and flaccidity syndrome.

吐，泄泻，痢疾，便秘，水肿；体重节痛，痿证。

Note: Shu-Stream and Yuan-Source acupoints of the spleen meridian of foot-taiyin.

【备注】 足太阴经之"输"穴、"原穴"。

2.1.7.3.4 Gongsun (SP 4)

4. 公孙 SP4

Location: The acupoint is located on the medial border of the foot, anterior and inferior to the first metatarsal base, and in the depression distal and inferior to the base of the first metatarsal bone, at the junction of the red and white skin and about 1 cun posterior to Taibai (SP 3). (see Fig. 38)

【位置与取法】 在足内侧缘，当第一跖骨基底的前下方。沿第一跖骨内侧向上方推至有阻挡感，第一跖骨基底部前下方赤白肉际处，约在太白穴后1寸左右。（见图38）

Indications: Abdominal distension, diarrhea, dysentery, edema, acute and chronic stomachache, vomiting, dysphoria and insomnia.

【主治】 腹胀，泄泻，痢疾，水肿；急慢性胃痛，呕吐；烦心，失眠。

Note: Luo-Connecting acupoint of the spleen meridian of foot-taiyin and one of the eight convergent acupoint associating with the thoroughfare vessel.

【备注】 足太阴经之"络"穴；八脉交会穴之一，通于冲脉。

2.1.7.3.5 Shangqiu (SP 5)

5. 商丘 SP5

Location: The acupoint is located in the depression distal and inferior to the medial malleolus, midway between the tuberosity of the navicular bone and the tip of the medial malleolus (see Fig. 38 and 39).

【位置与取法】 在足内踝前下方凹陷中，当舟骨结节与内踝尖连线的中点处。当内踝前缘直线与下缘水平线的交点处（见图38、图39）。

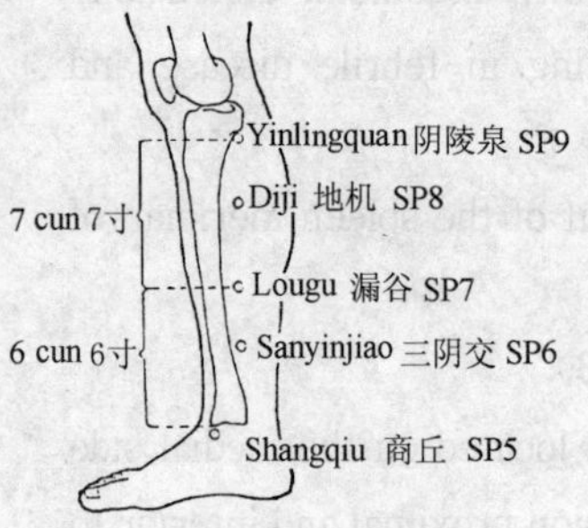

Fig. 39 Lower limb acupoints on the spleen meridian of foot-taiyin
图39 足太阴脾经下肢部经穴图

Indications: Abdominal distension, borborygmus,

【主治】 腹胀，肠鸣，泄

diarrhea, constipation, jaundice, somnolence, stiffness and pain of the tongue as well as tumescent pain of the ankle joint.

泻,便秘;黄疸,嗜卧;舌本强痛;踝关节肿痛。

Note: Jing-River acupoint of the spleen meridian of foot-taiyin.

【备注】 足太阴经之"经"穴。

2.1.7.3.6 Sanyinjiao (SP 6)

6. 三阴交 SP6

Location: The acupoint is located on the medial side of the shank, 3 cun directly above the tip of the medial malleolus, on the posterior border of the medial aspect of the tibia (see Fig. 39).

【位置与取法】 在小腿内侧,当足内踝尖上 3 寸,胫骨内侧缘后方。内踝高点上"一夫",胫骨内侧面后缘(见图 39)。

Indications: Abdominal pain and distension, edema, seminal emission, impotence, retention of urine, irregular menstruation, metrorrhagia and metrostaxis, multicolored leukorrhea, dystocia, amenorrhea, insomnia and hypertension.

【主治】 腹痛,腹胀,水肿;遗精,阳痿;癃闭;月经不调,崩漏,赤白带下,难产,经闭;失眠,高血压病。

Note: ① Crossing acupoint of the foot-taiyin, foot-shaoyin and foot-jueyin meridians. ② To be forbidden to needle for the gravida.

【备注】 ① 足太阴、少阴、厥阴经交会穴。② 孕妇禁针。

2.1.7.3.7 Lougu (SP 7)

7. 漏谷 SP7

Location: The acupoint is located on the medial side of the shank, 6 cun above the tip of medial malleolus and on the line joining the medial malleolus and Yinlingquan (SP 9) (see Fig. 39).

【位置与取法】 在小腿内侧,当内踝尖与阴陵泉的连线上,距内踝尖 6 寸,胫骨内侧缘后方(见图 39)。

Indications: Abdominal pain, abdominal distension, borborygmus and flaccidity and obstruction syndromes of the lower limbs.

【主治】 腹痛,腹胀,肠鸣;下肢痿痹。

2.1.7.3.8 Diji (SP 8)

8. 地机 SP8

Location: The acupoint is located on the medial side of the shank, on the line joining the tip of the medial malleolus and Yinlingquan (SP 9) and 3 cun below Yinlingquan (see Fig. 39).

【位置与取法】 在小腿内侧,当内踝尖与阴陵泉的连线上,阴陵泉下 3 寸(见图 39)。

Indications: Abdominal pain, diarrhea, edema, dysuria, dysmenorrhea, irregular menstruation and flaccidity and obstruction syndromes of the lower limbs.

【主治】 腹痛,泄泻,水肿;小便不利;痛经,月经不调;下肢痿痹。

Note: Xi-Cleft acupoint of the spleen meridian of foot-taiyin.

【备注】 足太阴经之"郄"穴。

2.1.7.3.9　Yinlingquan (SP 9)

9. 阴陵泉　SP9

Location: The acupoint is located on the medial side of the shank, on the lower border of the medial condyle of the tibia and in the depression on the medial border of the tibia (see Fig. 39).

【位置与取法】 在小腿内侧,当胫骨内侧髁后下方凹陷处。当胫骨后缘和腓肠肌之间凹陷中,沿胫骨内侧面后缘向上推时,有明显阻挡感处。(见图 39)

Indications: Abdominal pain, abdominal distension, diarrhea, dysentery, constipation, edema, jaundice, dysuria, and tumescent pain of the knee joint.

【主治】 腹痛,腹胀,泄泻,痢疾,便秘,水肿,黄疸;小便不利;膝关节肿痛。

Note: He Sea acupoint of the spleen meridian of foot-taiyin.

【备注】 足太阴经之"合"穴。

2.1.7.3.10　Xuehai (SP 10)

10. 血海　SP10

Location: When the knee is flexed, the acupoint is located 2 cun above the mediosuperior border of the patella, on the bulge of the medial portion of m. quadriceps femoris. Or when the patient's knee is flexed, the doctor cups the right palm to the left knee of the patient with the thumb on the medial side and with the other four fingers directed proximally. The thumb forms an angle of 45° with the index finger. The acupoint is where the tip of the doctor's thumb rests (see Fig. 40).

【位置与取法】 屈膝,在大腿内侧,髌底内侧端上 2 寸,当股四头肌内侧头的隆起处。正坐垂足,医者以右掌心正对其左膝髌骨顶端,二至五指向上伸直指向膝上,拇指约呈 45°斜置偏向膝内侧,当拇指尖下是穴(见图 40)。

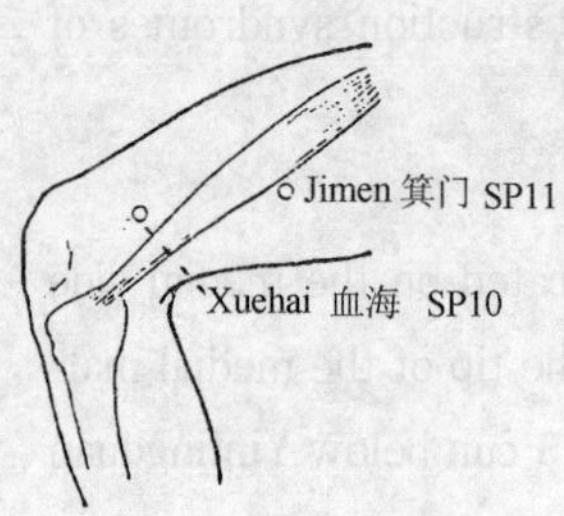

Fig. 40　Lower limb acupoints on the spleen meridian of foot-taiyin

图 40　足太阴脾经下肢部经穴图

Indications: Dysmenorrhea, metrorrhagia and

【主治】 痛经,崩漏,月

metrostaxis, irregular menstruation, urticaria, eczema and tumescent pain of the knee joint.

经不调;瘾疹,皮肤湿疹;膝关节肿痛。

2.1.7.3.11 Chongmen (SP 12)

11. 冲门 SP12

Location: The acupoint is located superior to the lateral end of the inguinal groove, on the lateral side of the femoral artery pulsation and 3.5 cun to the upper border of symphysis pubis (see Fig. 41).

【位置与取法】 在腹股沟外侧,距耻骨联合上缘中点3.5寸,当髂外动脉搏动处的外侧(见图41)。

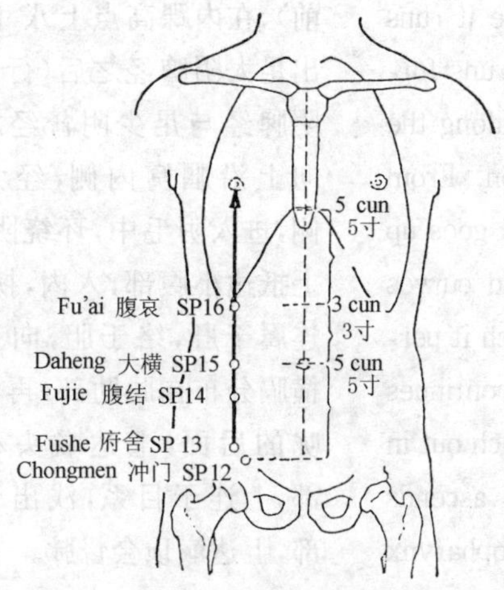

Fig. 41 Abdomen acupoints on the spleen meridian of foot-taiyin

图41 足太阴脾经腹部经穴图

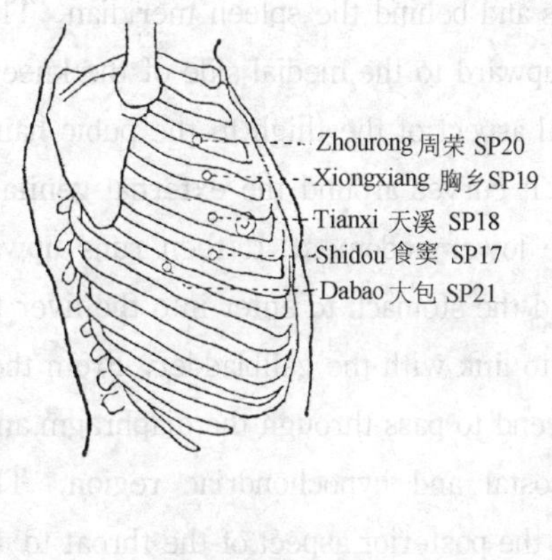

Fig. 42 Chest acupoints on the spleen meridian of foot-taiyin

图42 足太阴脾经胸部经穴图

Indications: Lower abdominal pain, hernia, dysuria, leukorrhagia and irregular menstruaton.

【主治】 少腹痛;疝气,小便不利;带下,月经不调。

2.1.7.3.12 Daheng (SP 15)

12. 大横 SP15

Location: The acupoint is located on the center of the abdomen and 4 cun lateral to the umbilicus (see Fig. 41).

【位置与取法】 在腹中部,距脐中4寸(见图41)。

Indications: Abdominal distension, abdominal pain, diarrhea, dysentery and constipation.

【主治】 腹胀,腹痛,泄泻,痢疾,便秘。

2.1.7.3.13 Dabao (SP 21)

13. 大包 SP21

Location: The acupoint is located on the lateral side of the chest, on the mid-axillary line and at the sixth costal interstice (see Fig. 42).

【位置与取法】 在侧胸部,腋中线上,当第六肋间隙处(见图42)。

Indications: Chest and hypochondriac pain, cough,

【主治】 胸胁痛;咳嗽,

asthma, general pain and flaccidity of the four limbs.

气喘；周身疼痛，四肢无力。

2.1.8 Liver meridian of foot-jueyin

八、足厥阴肝经

2.1.8.1 Cyclical flowing and distribution

（一）循行分布

The liver meridian starts from the dorsal hairy region of the great toe. From there it begins to run upward along the dorsum of the foot. Passing through Zhongfeng (LR 4) and 1 cun in front of the medial malleolus, it ascends to an area 8 cun above the medial malleolus, where it runs across and behind the spleen meridian. Then it runs further upward to the medial side of the knees and along the medial aspect of the thigh to the pubic hair region. From there it curves around the external genitalia and goes up to the lower abdomen. It then runs upward and curves around the stomach to enter into the liver to which it pertains to link with the gallbladder. From there it continues to ascend to pass through the diaphragm and branch out in the costal and hypochondriac region. Then it ascends along the posterior aspect of the throat to the nasopharynx and connects with the eye system. Running further upward, it emerges from the forehead and links with the governor vessel at the vertex.

起于爪甲后的"三毛"中，向上沿足背上缘，过内踝前一寸处，上行小腿内侧（行于足太阴脾经与足少阴肾经之前），在内踝高点上八寸处，交出足太阴脾经之后（行于足太阴脾经与足少阴肾经之间），向上沿腘窝内侧，经大腿内侧，进入阴毛中，环绕阴器，向上抵达小腹部，入内，挟行胃，连属于肝，络于胆，向上通过横膈分布在胁肋部，再沿着喉咙的后面，上达喉头和鼻咽部，上连于目系，浅出于前额部，上达巅顶会督脉。

The branch arising from the eye system runs downward into the cheek and curves around the inner surface of the lips.

分支一：从目系下行面颊的里面（颊粘膜），环绕唇内。

The another branch arising from the liver passes through the diaphragm and runs into the lung to connect with the lung meridian. (see Fig. 43)

分支二：从肝分出向上通过横膈，注入肺中，交手太阴肺经。（见图 43）

Associated viscera: Liver, gallbladder, lung and stomach.

联系脏腑：肝、胆、肺、胃。

Associated organs: Genitalia, throat, pharynx, eyes and mouth.

联系器官：阴器、咽喉、目、口。

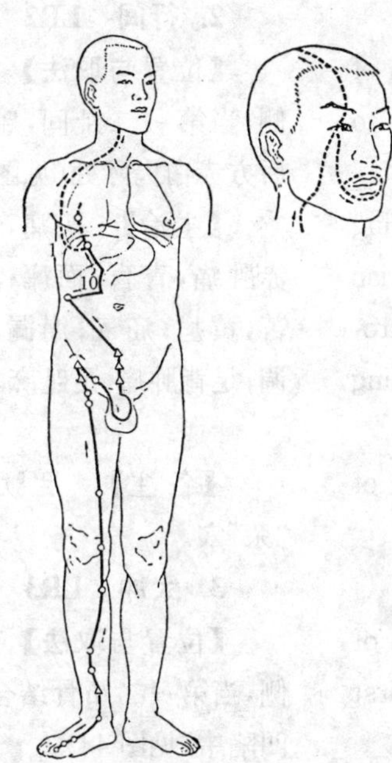

Fig. 43 Flowing route of the liver meridian of foot-jueyin

图 43 足厥阴肝经循行示意图

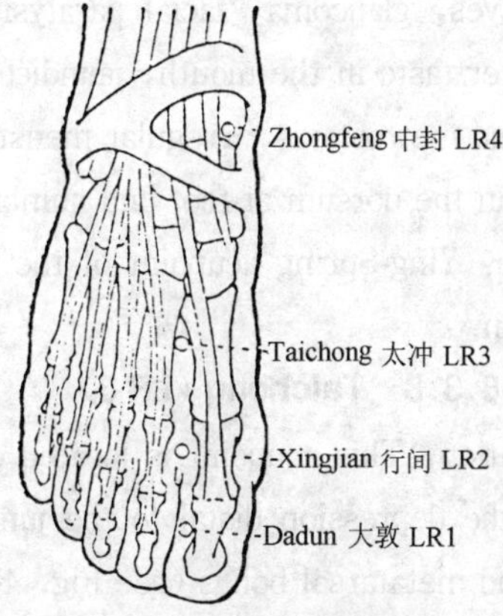

Fig. 44 Foot acupoints on the liver meridian of foot-jueyin

图 44 足厥阴肝经足部经穴图

2.1.8.2 Indications

Liver disease, gynecological disease, genitalia disorder and other diseases involving the areas through which the meridian flows.

(二) 主治要点

本经腧穴主治肝病，妇科、前阴病以及经脉循行部位的其他病证。

2.1.8.3 Commonly used acupoints

(三) 常用腧穴

2.1.8.3.1 Dadun (LR1)

Location: This acupoint is located on the lateral side of the dorsum of the terminal phalanx of the great toe and 0.1 cun to the nail margin (see Fig. 44).

Indications: Apoplexy, coma, epilepsy, hernia, contraction of genitalia, unsmooth urination, irregular menstruation, metrorrhagia and metrostaxis.

Note: Jing-Well acupoint of the liver meridian of foot-jueyin should not be moxibusted before or after labor.

1. 大敦 LR1

【位置与取法】 在足大趾末节外侧，距趾甲角 0.1 寸(见图 44)。

【主治】 中风，昏迷，癫痫；疝气，缩阴证，小便不利；月经不调，崩漏。

【备注】 ① 足厥阴经之“井”穴。② 孕妇产前产后皆不宜灸。

2.1.8.3.2　Xingjian (LR 2)

Location: This acupoint is located on the dorsum of the foot between the first and second toes, proximal to the margin of the web (see Fig. 44).

Indications: Headache, vertigo, redness and swelling pain of eyes, glaucoma, facial paralysis, hypochondriac pain, bitter taste in the mouth, jaundice, hernia, metrorrhagia and metrostaxis, irregular menstruation, swelling and pain in the dorsum of foot and numbness of toes.

Note: Ying-Spring acupoint of the liver meridian of foot-jueyin.

2.1.8.3.3　Taichong (LR 3)

Location: This acupoint is located on the dorsum of foot, in the depression distal to the junction of the first and second metatarsal bones (see Fig. 44).

Indications: Headache, vertigo, redness and swelling pain of eyes, glaucoma, nearsightedness, facial paralysis, apoplexy, epilepsy, infantile convulsion, hernia, metrorrhagia and metrostaxis, irregular menstruation, vomiting, hiccup, stomachache, severe lumbago and flaccidity and obstruction syndromes of lower limbs.

Note: Shu-Stream acupoint and Yuan-Source acupoint of the liver meridian of foot-jueyin.

2.1.8.3.4　Zhongfeng (LR 4)

Location: This acupoint is located on the medial side of the medial malleolus, on the line joining Shangqiu (SP 5) and Jiexi (ST 41) and in the depression on the medial side of the tendon of m. tibialis anterior (see Fig. 44).

Indications: Hernia, seminal emission, dysuria, metrorrhagia and metrostaxis, irregular menstruation, and jaundice.

Note: Jing-River acupoint of the liver meridian of foot-jueyin.

2.1.8.3.5　Ligou (LR 5)

Location: This acupoint is located on the medial side

2. 行间　LR2

【位置与取法】　在足背侧,当第一二趾间,趾蹼缘的后方赤白肉际处(见图 44)。

【主治】　头痛,眩晕;目赤肿痛,青盲;面瘫;胁痛,口苦,黄疸;疝气;崩漏,月经不调;足背肿痛,足趾麻木。

【备注】　足厥阴经之“荥”穴。

3. 太冲　LR3

【位置与取法】　在足背侧,当第一二跖骨结合部之前凹陷中(见图 44)。

【主治】　头痛,眩晕;目赤肿痛,青盲,近视;面瘫;中风,癫痫,小儿惊风;疝气;崩漏,月经不调;呕逆,胃痛;腰痛不可以俯仰,下肢痿痹。

【备注】　足厥阴经之“输”穴、“原”穴。

4. 中封　LR4

【位置与取法】　当足内踝前,商丘与解溪连线上,胫骨前肌腱的内侧凹陷处(见图 44)。

【主治】　疝气,遗精;小便不利;崩漏,月经不调;黄疸。

【备注】　足厥阴经之“经”穴。

5. 蠡沟　LR5

【位置与取法】　在小腿

of the shank, 5 cun above the tip of the medial malleolus and on the medial aspect of the medial border of the tibia (see Fig. 45).

内侧，足内踝尖上 5 寸，胫骨内侧面的中央(见图 45)。

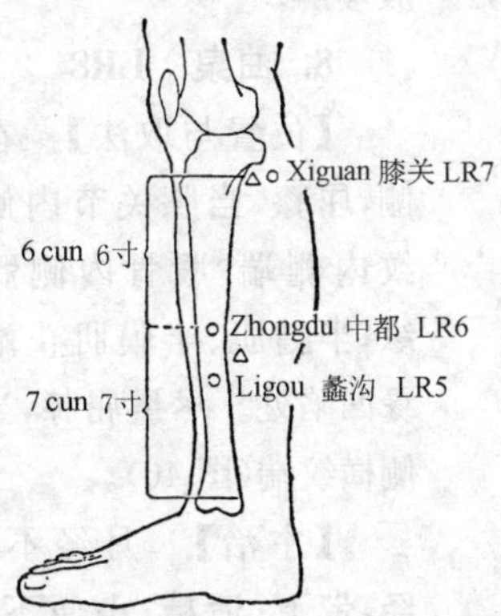

Fig. 45 Lower limb acupoints on the liver meridian of foot-jueyin

图 45 足厥阴肝经下肢部经穴图

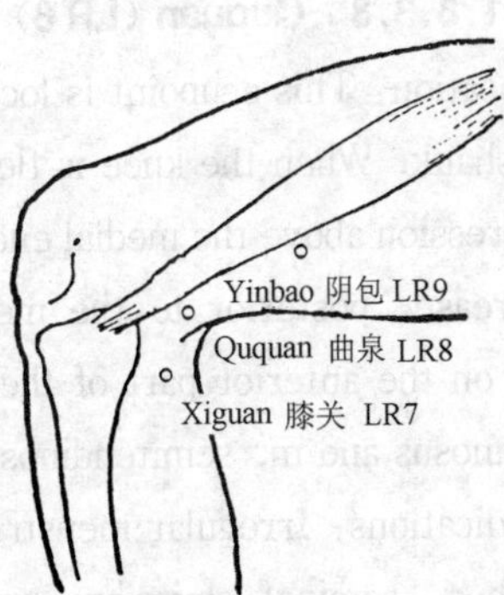

Fig. 46 Medial knee acupoints on the liver meridian of foot-jueyin

图 46 足厥阴肝经膝内侧经穴图

Indications: Irregular menstruation, prolapse of uterus, pudendal pruritus, hernia, unsmooth urination, severe lumbago and lower abdominal pain.

Note: Luo-Connecting acupoint of the liver meridian of foot-jueyin.

【主治】 月经不调，阴挺，阴痒；疝气；小便不利；腰痛不可以俯仰，小腹痛。

【备注】 足厥阴经之"络"穴。

2.1.8.3.6 Zhongdu (LR 6)

Location: This acupoint is located on the medial aspect of the shank, 7 cun above the tip of the medial malleolus and on the centre of the medial border of the tibia (see Fig. 45).

Indications: Hypochondriac pain, abdominal distension and pain, metrorrhagia and metrostaxis, postpartum lochiorrhea and hernia.

Note: Xi-Cleft acupoint of the liver meridian of foot-jueyin.

6. 中都 LR6

【位置与取法】 在小腿内侧，足内踝尖上 7 寸，胫骨内侧面的中央(见图 45)。

【主治】 胁痛，腹痛，腹胀；崩漏，产后恶露不尽；疝气。

【备注】 足厥阴经之"郄穴"。

2.1.8.3.7 Xiguan (LR 7)

Location: This acupoint is located on the medial aspect of the shank, posterior and inferior to the medial condyle of the tibia, 1 cun posterior to Yinlingquan (SP 9)

7. 膝关 LR7

【位置与取法】 在小腿内侧，当胫骨内侧髁的后下方，阴陵泉后 1 寸，腓肠肌内

and in the upper portion of the medial head of m. gastrocnemius (see Fig. 45 and 46).

侧头的上部(见图45、图46)。

Indications: Swelling and pain of knee and flaccidity and obstruction syndromes of lower limbs.

【主治】 膝关节肿痛,下肢痿痹。

2.1.8.3.8 Ququan (LR 8)

8. 曲泉 LR8

Location: This acupoint is located on the medial side of the shank. When the knee is flexed, the acupoint is in the depression above the medial end of the transverse popliteal crease, posterior to the medial epicondyle of the femur, on the anterior part of the insertion of m. semimembranosus and m. semitendinosus (see Fig. 46).

【位置与取法】 在膝内侧,屈膝,当膝关节内侧面横纹内侧端,股骨内侧髁的后缘,半腱肌、半膜肌止端的前缘凹陷处。尽量屈膝,当膝内侧横纹端(图46)。

Indications: Irregular menstruation, dysmenorrhea, leukorrhea, seminal emission, unsmooth urination and swelling and pain of knee.

【主治】 月经不调,痛经,带下;遗精;小便不利;膝髌肿痛。

Note: He-Sea acupoint of the liver meridian of foot-jueyin.

【备注】 足厥阴经之"合"穴。

2.1.8.3.9 Zhangmen (LR 13)

9. 章门 LR13

Location: This acupoint is located on the lateral side of the abdomen, below the free end of the eleventh floating rib. When the shoulder is put down and the elbow is flexed with the tip of the elbow against the hypochondria, the region touched by the elbow tip is the location of this acupoint. (see Fig. 47)

【位置与取法】 在侧腹部,当第十一肋游离端的下方。垂肩屈肘,以肘尖贴于肋部,肘尖处是穴。(见图47)

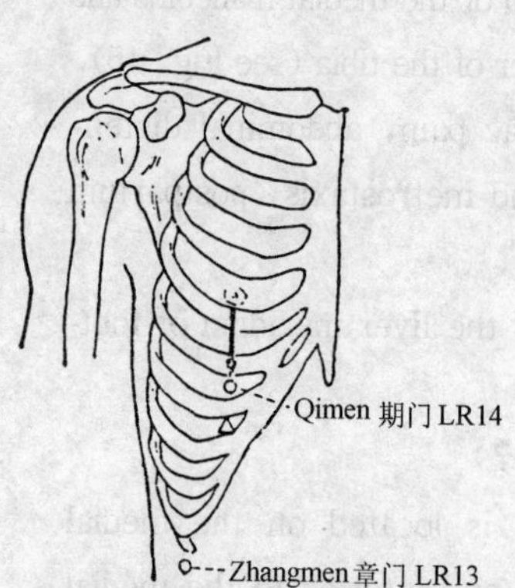

Fig. 47 Hypochondrium and rib-side acupoints on the liver meridian of foot-jueyin

图47 足厥阴肝经胁肋部经穴图

Indications: Abdominal pain, distension and mass, borborygmus, diarrhea, vomiting, hypochondriac pain and pain in the loins and spine.

Note: Front-Mu acupoint of the spleen; one of the eight confluent acupoint associating with the zang organs; crossing acupoint of the liver meridian and gallbladder meridian.

【主治】 腹痛,腹胀,痞块,肠鸣,泄泻,呕吐;胁痛;腰脊痛。

【备注】 脾之"募"穴;八会穴之一,脏会章门;肝经与胆经交会穴。

2.1.8.3.10 Qimen (LR 14)

Location: This acupoint is located on the chest, directly below the nipple, in the sixth intercostal space and 4 cun lateral to the front medium line (see Fig. 47).

Indications: Hypochondriac pain, bitter taste in the mouth, vomiting, hiccup and breast abscess.

Note: Front-Mu acupoint of the liver and crossing acupoint of the liver meridian of foot-jueyin, spleen meridian of foot-taiyin and yin link vessel.

10. 期门 LR14

【位置与取法】 在胸部,当乳头直下,第六肋间隙,前正中线旁开4寸(见图47)。

【主治】 胁痛,口苦;呕吐,呃逆;乳痈。

【备注】 肝之"募"穴;足厥阴、足太阴与阴维脉交会穴。

2.1.9 Kidney meridian of foot-shaoyin

九、足少阴肾经

2.1.9.1 Cyclical flowing and distribution

The kidney meridian starts from the inferior aspect of the small toe and runs obliquely towards the sole. Emerging from the lower aspect of the tuberosity of the navicular bone and running behind the medial malleolus, it enters the heel. From there it ascends along the medial side of the leg to the medial side of the popliteal fossa and goes further upward along the posteromedial aspect of the thigh towards the vertebral column where it enters the kidney to which it pertains, and connects with the bladder. The straight portion of the meridian emerges from the kidney, ascending and passing through the liver and diaphragm. Then it enters the lung, runs along the throat and terminates beside the root of the tongue.

The branch stems from the lung, joins the heart and runs into the chest to link with the pericardium meridian.

(一)循行分布

起于足小趾之下,斜行走向足心,过舟骨粗隆下,沿内踝之后上行,并分出一支进入脚跟中。从内踝之后上行的主干,经小腿内侧后缘,出腘窝内侧,向上沿大腿内侧后缘,穿行脊柱,入内连属于肾,下络于膀胱;其直行的主干从肾向上通过肝、膈,进入肺中,沿着喉咙,挟舌根部。

其分支:从肺分出,络于心,注于胸中,交手厥阴心包

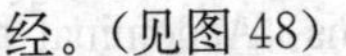

(see Fig. 48)

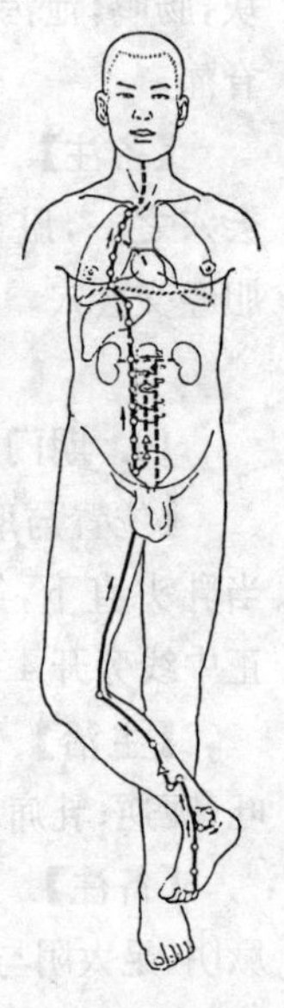

Fig. 48 Flowing route of the kidney meridian of foot-shaoyin

图 48 足少阴肾经循行示意图

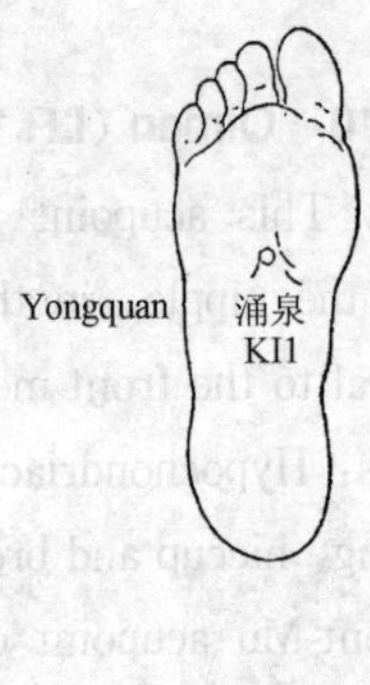

Fig. 49 Sole acupoints on the kidney meridian of foot-shaoyin

图 49 足少阴肾经足底部经穴图

Associated viscera: Kidney, bladder, heart, lung, liver and marrow.

Associated organs: Throat and tongue root.

2.1.9.2 Indications

Gynecological diseases, genital diseases, kidney, lung and throat disorders as well as diseases involving the regions through which the meridian passes.

2.1.9.3 Commonly used acupoints

2.1.9.3.1 Yongquan (KI 1)

Location: This acupoint is located on the sole and in the depression when the foot is in plantar flexion, in the anterior depression when the foot is flexed, approximately at the junction of the anterior one third and posterior two thirds of the sole (see Fig. 49).

Indications: Depressive psychosis, manic psychosis, infantile convulsion, wind stroke, hysteria, headache,

经。(见图 48)

联系脏腑:肾、膀胱、心、肺、肝、髓。

联系器官:喉咙、舌根。

(二) 主治要点

本经腧穴主治妇科、前阴病,肾、肺、咽喉病及经脉循行部位的其他病证。

(三) 常用腧穴

1. 涌泉 KI1

【位置与取法】 在足底部,卷足时足前部凹陷处,约当足底第二三趾缝纹头端与足跟连线的前 1/3 与后 2/3 交点上(见图 49)。

【主治】 癫证,狂证,小儿惊风,中风,癔病;头痛,目

vertigo, sore throat, aphonia, unsmooth urination, constipation and feverish soles.

Note: Jing-Well acupoint of the kidney meridian of foot-shaoyin.

晕;咽喉痛,失音;小便不利,便秘;足心热。

【备注】 足少阴经之"井"穴。

2.1.9.3.2 Rangu (KI 2)

Location: This acupoint is located on the medial side of the foot, on the lower border of the tuberosity of the navicular bone and anterior and inferior to the medial malleolus (see Fig. 50).

2. 然谷 KI2

【位置与取法】 在足内侧,足舟骨粗隆下方,赤白肉际处(见图 50)。

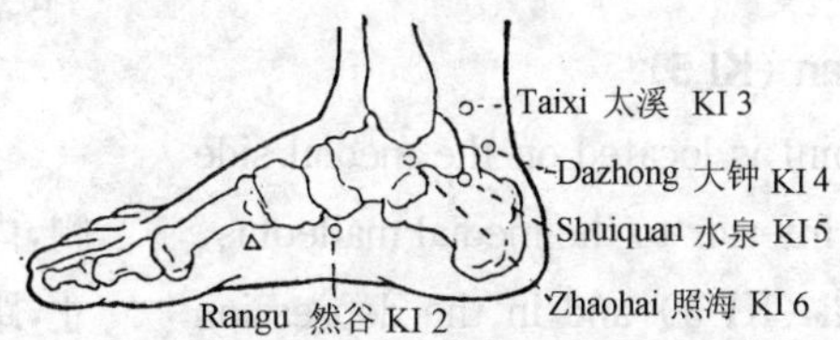

Fig. 50 Foot acupoints on the kidney meridian of foot-shaoyin

图 50 足少阴肾经足部经穴图

Indications: Headache, dizziness, sore throat, diabetes, hemoptysis, irregular menstruation, leukorrhea, prolapse of uterus, seminal emission and unsmooth urination.

Note: Ying-Spring acupoint of the kidney meridian of foot-shaoyin.

【主治】 头痛,头晕;咽喉肿痛;消渴,咳血;月经不调,带下,阴挺;遗精;小便不利。

【备注】 足少阴经之"荥"穴。

2.1.9.3.3 Taixi (KI 3)

Location: This acupoint is located on the medial side of the foot, posterior to the medial malleolus and in the depression between the medial malleolous and tendo calcaneus (see Fig. 50).

Indications: Headache, vertigo, sore throat, toothache due to asthenia-fire, tinnitus, deafness, cough, asthma, hemoptysis, irregular menstruation, seminal emission, impotence, frequent urination and pain in the heel.

Note: Shu-Stream and Yuan-Source acupoints of the kidney meridian of foot-shaoyin.

3. 太溪 KI3

【位置与取法】 在足内侧,内踝后方,当内踝尖与跟腱之间的凹陷处(见图 50)。

【主治】 头痛,眩晕;咽喉疼痛;虚火牙痛;耳鸣,耳聋;咳嗽,气喘,咯血;月经不调;遗精,阳痿,小便频数;足跟痛。

【备注】 足少阴经之"输"、"原"穴。

2.1.9.3.4 Dazhong (KI 4)

Location: This acupoint is located on the medial side of the foot, posterior and inferior to the medial malleolus, and in the depression medial to the attachment of tendo calcaneus (see Fig. 50).

Indications: Cough, asthma, hemoptysis, retention of urine, frequent urination, enuresis, dementia, lumbago and pain in the heel.

Note: Luo-Connecting acupoint of the kidney meridian of foot-shaoyin.

4. 大钟 KI4

【位置与取法】 在足内侧,内踝后下方,当跟腱附着部的内侧前方凹陷处(见图50)。

【主治】 咳嗽,气喘,咳血;癃闭,尿频,遗尿;痴呆;腰痛;足跟痛。

【备注】 足少阴经之“络”穴。

2.1.9.3.5 Shuiquan (KI 5)

Location: This acupoint is located on the medial side of the foot, posterior and inferior to the medial malleolus, 1 cun directly below Taixi (KI 3) and in the depression anterior and superior to the medial side of the tuberosity of the calcaneum (see Fig. 50).

Indications: Irregular menstruation, dysmenorrhea and unsmooth urination.

Note: Xi-Cleft acupoint of the kidney meridian of foot-shaoyin.

5. 水泉 KI5

【位置与取法】 在足内侧,内踝后下方,当太溪直下1寸,跟骨结节的内侧凹陷处。大钟与太溪、水泉适成等腰三角形(见图50)。

【主治】 月经不调,痛经;小便不利。

【备注】 足少阴经之“郄”穴。

2.1.9.3.6 Zhaohai (KI 6)

Location: This acupoint is located on the medial side of the foot and in the depression below the tip of medial malleolus (see Fig. 50).

Indications: Insomnia, somnolence, depressive psychosis and manic psychosis, dry mouth, sore throat, dysmenorrhea, irregular menstruation, multi-colored leukorrhea, unsmooth urination, constipation and swelling and pain in the malleolus joint.

Note: One of the eight convergent acupoints associating with yin heel vessel.

6. 照海 KI6

【位置与取法】 在足内侧,内踝尖下方凹陷处(见图50)。

【主治】 失眠,嗜睡;癫狂;口干,咽喉疼痛;痛经,月经不调,赤白带下;小便不利,便秘;踝关节肿痛。

【备注】 八脉交会穴之一,通于阴蹻脉。

2.1.9.3.7 Fuliu (KI 7)

Location: This acupoint is located on the medial side of the shank, 2 cun directly above Taixi (KI 3) and on the

7. 复溜 KI7

【位置与取法】 在小腿内侧,太溪直上2寸,跟腱

anterior border of tendo calcaneus (see Fig. 51).

前方(见图 51)。

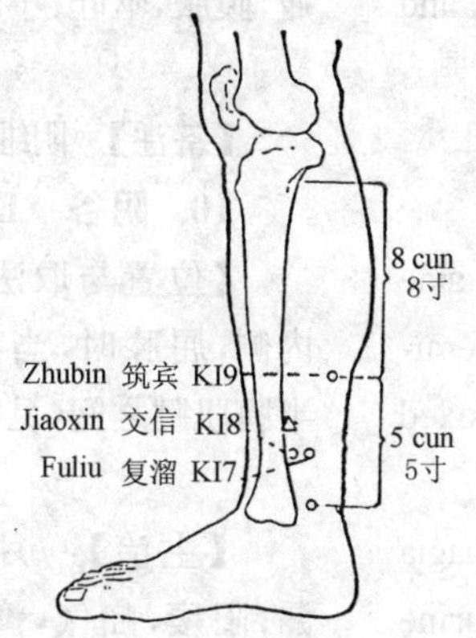

Fig. 51 Lower limb acupoints on the kidney meridian of foot-shaoyin

图 51 足少阴肾经下肢部经穴图

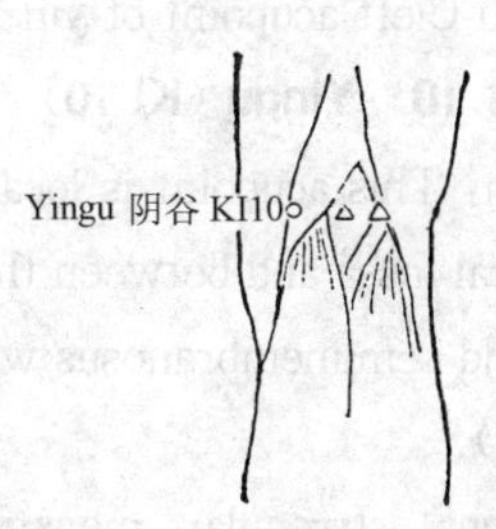

Fig. 52 Popliteal fossa acupoints on the kidney meridian of foot-shaoyin

图 52 足少阴肾经腘窝部经穴图

Indications: Abdominal pain and distension, borborygmus, diarrhea, night sweating, no sweating in febrile disease, stiffness and pain in the loins and spine as well as flaccidity and obstruction syndromes of lower limbs.

【主治】 腹痛,腹胀,肠鸣,泄泻;盗汗,热病汗不出;腰脊强痛,下肢痿痹。

2.1.9.3.8 Jiaoxin (KI 8)

Location: This acupoint is located on the medial side of the shank, 2 cun above Taixi (KI 3), 0.5 cun anterior to Fuliu (KI 7), posterior to the medial border of tibia and between Fuliu (KI 7) and the medial posterior border of the tibia. (see Fig. 51)

Indications: Irregular menstruation, metrorrhagia and metrostaxis, prolapse of uterus, pudendal pruritus, hernia, diarrhea and constipation.

Note: Xi-Cleft acupoint of yin heel vessel.

8. 交信 KI8

【位置与取法】 在小腿内侧,当太溪上 2 寸,复溜前 0.5 寸,胫骨内侧缘的后方。在复溜与胫骨内侧后缘之间取之。(见图 51)

【主治】 月经不调,崩漏,阴挺;阴痒,疝气;泄泻,便秘。

【备注】 阴蹻脉之“郄”穴。

2.1.9.3.9 Zhubin (KI 9)

Location: This acupoint is located on the medial side of the shank, on the line joining Taixi (KI 3) and Yingu (KI 10), 5 cun above Taixi (KI 3) and at the lower end of the belly of m. Gastrocnemius (see Fig. 51).

9. 筑宾 KI9

【位置与取法】 在小腿内侧,当太溪与阴谷的连线上,太溪上 5 寸,腓肠肌肌腹的内下方(见图 51)。

Indications: Depressive psychosis, manic psychosis, epilepsy, abdominal pain and distension, vomiting and pain in the medial side of the shank.

【主治】 癫狂，痫证；腹痛，腹胀，呕吐；小腿内侧痛。

Note: Xi-Cleft acupoint of yin link vessel.

【备注】 阴维脉之"郄"穴。

2.1.9.3.10　Yingu (KI 10)

10. 阴谷　KI10

Location: This acupoint is located on the medial side of the popliteal fossa and between the tendons of m. semitendinosus and semimembranosus when the knee is flexed (see Fig. 52).

【位置与取法】 在腘窝内侧，屈膝时，当半腱肌腱与半膜肌腱之间(见图 52)。

Indications: Irregular menstruation, metrorrhagia and metrostaxis, impotence, hernia, retention of urine and pain in the medial border of knee and popliteal fossa.

【主治】 月经不调，崩漏；阳痿，疝气，癃闭；膝股内廉痛。

Note: He-Sea acupoint of the kidney meridian of foot-shaoyin.

【备注】 足少阴经之"合"穴。

2.1.9.3.11　Henggu (KI 11)

11. 横骨　KI11

Location: This acupoint is located on the lower abdomen, 5 cun below the umbilicus and 0.5 cun lateral to the front medial line (see Fig. 53).

【位置与取法】 在下腹部，当脐中下 5 寸，前正中线旁开 0.5 寸(见图 53)。

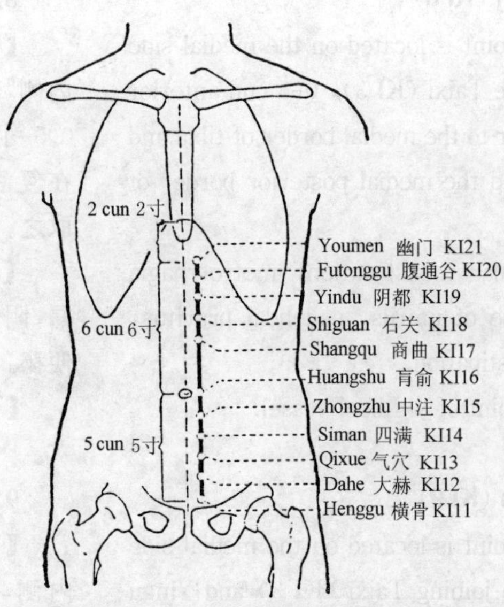

Fig. 53　Abdomen acupoints on the kidney meridian of foot-shaoyin

图 53　足少阴肾经腹部经穴图

Indications: Lower abdominal pain, hernia, impotence, seminal emission, enuresis and unsmooth urination.

【主治】 少腹痛;疝气,阳痿,遗精;遗尿,小便不利。

2.1.9.3.12 Dahe (KI 12)

12. 大赫 KI12

Location: This acupoint is located on the abdomen, 4 cun below umbilicus and and 0.5 cun lateral to the anterior midline (see Fig. 53).

【位置与取法】 在下腹部,当脐中下4寸,前正中线旁开0.5寸(见图53)。

Indications: Lower abdominal pain, irregular menstruation, leukorrhea, prolapse of uterus, seminal emission, impotence and hernia.

【主治】 少腹痛,月经不调,带下,阴挺;遗精,阳痿,疝气。

2.1.9.3.13 Huangshu (KI 16)

13. 肓俞 KI16

Location: This acupoint is located on the center of the abdomen, 0.5 cun lateral to the umbilicus (see Fig. 53).

【位置与取法】 在腹中部,当脐中旁开0.5寸(见图53)。

Indications: Abdominal pain around the umbilicus, abdominal distension, diarrhea, dysentery, constipation, irregular menstruation, hernia and pain in the loins and spine.

【主治】 绕脐腹痛,腹胀,泄泻,痢疾,便秘;月经不调;疝气;腰脊痛。

2.1.9.3.14 Shufu (KI 27)

14. 俞府 KI27

Location: This acupoint is located on the chest, at the lower border of the clavicle and 2 cun lateral to the anterior midline (see Fig. 54).

【位置与取法】 在胸部,当锁骨下缘,前正中线旁开2寸(见图54)。

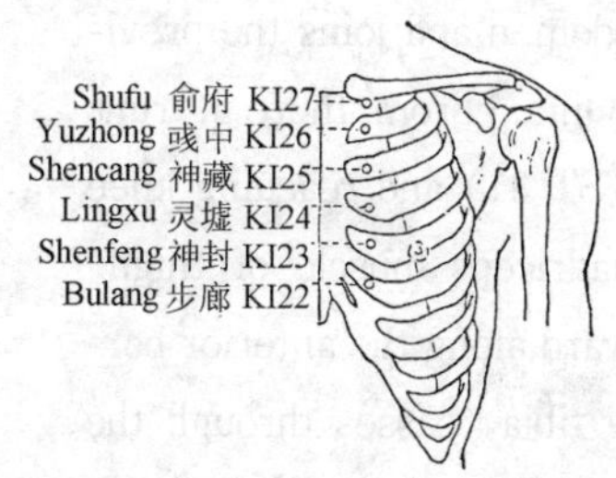

Fig. 54 Chest acupoints on the kidney meridian of foot-shaoyin

图54 足少阴肾经胸部经穴图

Indications: Cough, asthma, chest pain, vomiting and anorexia.

【主治】 咳嗽,气喘;胸痛;呕吐,食欲不振。

2.1.10 Stomach meridian of foot-yangming

十、足阳明胃经

2.1.10.1 Cyclical flowing and distribution

（一）循行分布

The stomach meridian starts from the lateral side of ala nasi. From there it descends to the bridge of the nose and meets with the bladder meridian. Then it turns downward along the lateral side of the nose and enters the upper gum. After reemergence, it curves around the lips and descends to meet with the conception vessel at the mentolabial groove where it runs posterolaterally across the lower portion of the cheek at Daying (ST 5). It then winds along the angle of the mandible and ascends in front of the ear and traverses Shangguan (GB 3). Following the anterior hairline, it reaches the forehead.

起始于鼻，上行至鼻根部，与足太阳经交会于睛明穴，沿鼻外侧下行入上齿中，回出夹口旁，环绕口唇，向下交会于承浆，向后沿着口腮后下方出于下颌大迎（面动脉搏动部），再沿下颌角，上行耳前，经上关穴，沿着发际，至额颅中部。

The externally flowing trunk descends from clavicular fossa and passes by the medial side of the breast, running beside the umbilicus and reaching Qijie.

其外行的主干：从缺盆向下，经过乳房内侧，向下夹脐两旁，进入气街（腹股沟动脉部）。

The first branch emerges in front of Daying (ST 5) and runs downward to Renying (ST 9). From there it goes along the throat and enters the supraclavicular fossa. Then it descends and passes through the diaphragm, entering the stomach to which it pertains and linking with the spleen.

分支一：从大迎前，下走人迎（颈动脉搏动部），沿着喉咙，进入缺盆，向下通过横膈连属于胃，络于脾。

The second branch from the lower orifice of the stomach descends inside the abdomen and joins the previous trunk of the meridian at Qijie. From there it runs downward, traversing Biguan (ST 31) and reaching knee through the prominence of quadriceps muscle of thigh. Then it continues to run downward along the anterior border of the lateral aspect of the tibia, passes through the dorsum of the foot and reaches the lateral side of the tip of the second toe.

分支二：从胃口向下沿着腹里下行至气街部与外行的主干会合，再由此下行经髋关节前，直抵股四头肌隆起处，下向膝髌中，沿着胫骨外侧前缘，下行足背部，进入中趾内侧，出次趾末端。

The third branch stems from the region 3 cun below the knee and enters the lateral side of the middle toe.

分支三：从膝下 3 寸处分出，向下进入足中趾外侧。

The fourth branch emerges from the dorsum of the

分支四：从足背部分出

foot, enters the great toe, comes out from the tip of the great toe and links with the spleen meridian. (see Fig. 55)

进入足大趾，出大趾末端，接足太阴脾经。(见图 55)

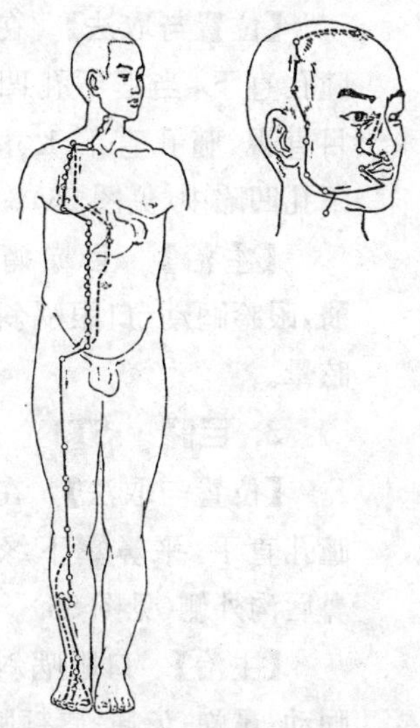

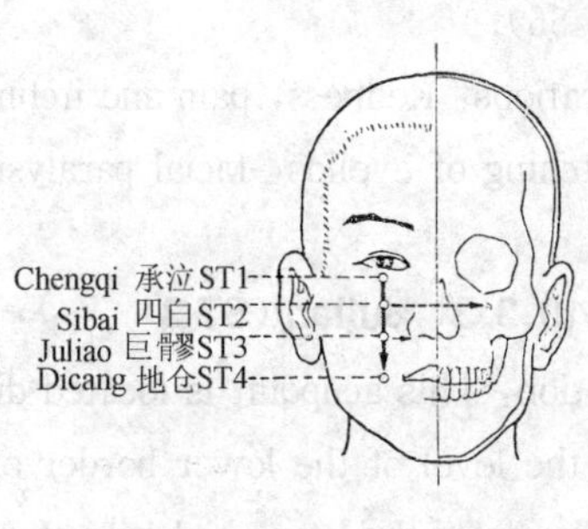

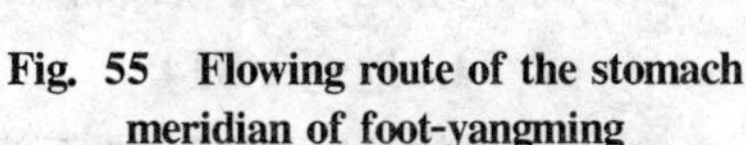

Fig. 55 Flowing route of the stomach meridian of foot-yangming

图 55 足阳明胃经循行示意图

Fig. 56 Head and face acupoints on the stomach meridian of foot-yangming

图 56 足阳明胃经头面部经穴图

Associated viscera: Stomach and spleen.

Associated organs: Eyes, nose, lower teeth, ears, mouth, larynx, and breast.

联系脏腑：胃、脾。

联系器官：目、鼻、下齿、耳、口、喉咙、乳房。

2.1.10.2 Indications

Diseases involving the stomach, intestines, head, face, nose, mouth and tooth as well as mental problems and disorders involving the regions through which the meridian runs.

(二) 主治要点

本经腧穴主治胃肠病，头面、目、鼻、口、齿痛，神志病及经脉循行部位的其他病证。

2.1.10.3 Commonly used acupoints

2.1.10.3.1 Chengqi (ST 1)

Location: This acupoint is located on the face, directly below the pupil, between the eyeball and the infraorbital ridge when the eyes look straight forward (see Fig. 56).

Indications: Redness, swelling and pain of the eyes,

(三) 常用腧穴

1. 承泣 ST1

【位置与取法】 在面部，瞳孔直下，当眼球与眶下缘之间。目直视，瞳孔直下，眼球与眶下缘之间正中(见图 56)。

【主治】 目赤肿痛，流

epiphora, night blindness, twitching of eyelids and facial paralysis.

泪，夜盲，眼睑瞤动，口眼㖞斜。

2.1.10.3.2 Sibai (ST 2)

2. 四白　ST2

Location: This acupoint is located on the face, directly below the pupil and in the depression at the infraorbital foramen when the eyes look straight forward (see Fig. 56).

【位置与取法】 在面部，瞳孔直下，当眶下孔凹陷处。目直视，瞳孔直下1寸，当眶下孔凹陷中(见图56)。

Indications: Redness, pain and itching of eyes, cataract, twitching of eyelids, facial paralysis, headache and vertigo.

【主治】 目赤痛痒，目翳，眼睑瞤动，口眼㖞斜，头痛眩晕。

2.1.10.3.3 Juliao (ST 3)

3. 巨髎　ST3

Location: This acupoint is located directly below the pupil, at the level of the lower border of ala nasi and on the lateral side of the nasolabial groove (see Fig. 56).

【位置与取法】 在面部，瞳孔直下，平鼻翼下缘处，当鼻唇沟外侧(见图56)。

Indications: Facial paralysis, twitching of eyelids, epistaxis, toothache and swelling of lips and cheeks.

【主治】 口眼㖞斜，眼睑瞤动；鼻衄；齿痛；唇颊肿。

2.1.10.3.4 Dicang (ST 4)

4. 地仓　ST4

Location: This acupoint is located lateral to the corner of the mouth and directly below the pupil (see Fig. 56).

【位置与取法】 在面部，口角外侧，上直对瞳孔(见图56)。

Indications: Facial distortion, drooling, toothache and twitching of eyelids.

【主治】 口㖞，流涎；齿痛；眼睑瞤动。

2.1.10.3.5 Jiache (ST 6)

5. 颊车　ST6

Location: This acupoint is one finger-breadth (middle finger) anterior and superior to the lower angle of the mandible where m. masseter attaches at the prominence of the muscle when the teeth are clenched (see Fig. 57).

【位置与取法】 在面颊部，下颌角前上方约一横指(中指)，当咀嚼时咬肌隆起，按之凹陷处(见图57)。

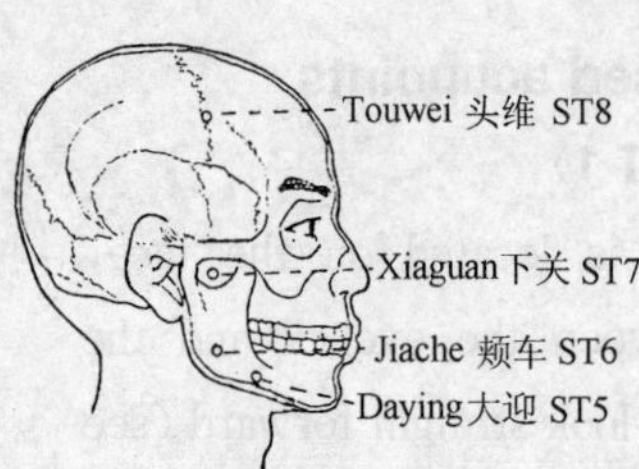

Fig. 57 Head and face acupoints of the stomach meridian of foot-yangming

图57 足阳明胃经头面部经穴图

Indications: Lockjaw, facial distortion, toothache and swelling of cheeks.

【主治】 口噤不语，口㖞；齿痛；颊肿。

2.1.10.3.6 Xiaguan (ST 7)

6. 下关 ST7

Location: This acupoint is located before the ear and in the depression anterior to the condyloid process of the mandible. This acupoint is located with the mouth opened. (see Fig. 57)

【位置与取法】 在面部耳前方，当颧弓与下颌切迹所形成的凹陷中。闭口取穴，合口有孔，张口则闭。(见图 57)

Indications: Deafness, tinnitus, otopyorrhea, toothache, lockjaw, facial distortion and swelling and pain of the cheeks.

【主治】 耳聋，耳鸣，聤耳；齿痛；口噤，口眼㖞斜；面颊肿痛。

2.1.10.3.7 Touwei (ST 8)

7. 头维 ST8

Location: This acupoint is located on the lateral side of the head, 0.5 cun within the anterior hairline at the corner of the forehead, 4.5 cun lateral to the midline of the head (see Fig. 57).

【位置与取法】 在头侧部，当额角发际上 0.5 寸，头正中线旁 4.5 寸(见图 57)。

Indications: Headache, vertigo, epiphora with wind and twitching of eyelids.

【主治】 头痛，目眩；迎风流泪，眼睑瞤动。

2.1.10.3.8 Renying (ST 9)

8. 人迎 ST9

Location: This acupoint is located on the neck, lateral to the Adam's apple, on the anterior border of m. sternocleidomastoideus and at the pulsating point of the common carotid artery (see Fig. 58).

【位置与取法】 在颈部，结喉旁，当胸锁乳突肌的前缘，颈总动脉搏动处(见图 58)。

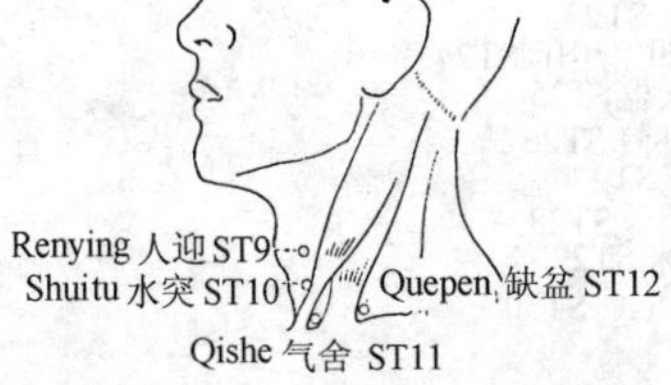

Fig. 58 Neck acupoints on the stomach meridian of foot-yangming

图 58 足阳明胃经颈部经穴图

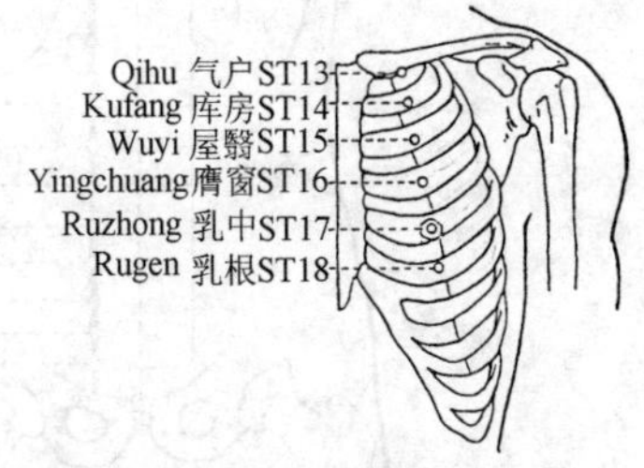

Fig. 59 Chest acupoints on the stomach meridian of foot-yangming

图 59 足阳明胃经胸部经穴图

Indications: Sore throat, asthma, scrofula, goiter and hypertension.

【主治】 咽喉肿痛；气喘；瘰疬，瘿气；高血压病。

2.1.10.3.9 Quepen (ST 12)

Location: This acupoint is located in the midpoint of the supraclavicular fossa and 4 cun lateral to anterior midline (see Fig. 58).

Indications: Cough, dyspnea, sore throat, pain in the supraclavicular fossa and scrofula.

9. 缺盆　ST12

【位置与取法】 在锁骨上窝中央，距前正中线 4 寸(见图 58)。

【主治】 咳嗽，气喘；咽喉肿痛；缺盆中痛；瘰疬。

2.1.10.3.10 Rugen (ST 18)

Location: This acupoint is located directly below the nipple, on the root of breast, in the fifth intercostal space and 4 cun lateral to the anterior midline (see Fig. 59).

Indications: Cough, asthma, hiccup, chest pain, breast abscess and insufficiency of lactation.

10. 乳根　ST18

【位置与取法】 在胸部，当乳头直下，乳房根部，第五肋间隙，距前正中线 4 寸(见图 59)。

【主治】 咳嗽，气喘；呃逆；胸痛；乳痈，乳汁少。

2.1.10.3.11 Liangmen (ST 21)

Location: This acupoint is located 4 cun above the umbilicus and 2 cun lateral to anterior midline (see Fig. 60).

11. 梁门　ST21

【位置与取法】 在上腹部，当脐中上 4 寸，距前正中线 2 寸(见图 60)。

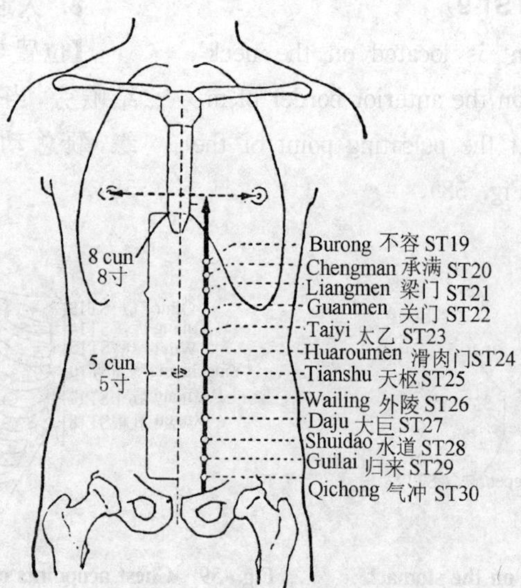

Fig. 60 Abdomen acupoints on the stomach meridian of foot-yangming

图 60　足阳明胃经腹部经穴图

Indications: Stomachache, vomiting, poor appetite, abdominal distension and diarrhea.

【主治】 胃痛，呕吐，食欲不振，腹胀，泄泻。

2.1.10.3.12 Tianshu (ST 25)

Location: This acupoint is located on the center of the abdomen and 2 cun lateral to the center of the umbilicus (see Fig. 60).

Indications: Abdominal distension, borborygmus, pain around the umbilicus, diarrhea, dysentery and irregular menstruation.

Note: Front-Mu acupoint of the large intestine.

12. 天枢 ST25

【位置与取法】 在腹中部,当脐中旁开 2 寸(见图 60)。

【主治】 腹胀肠鸣,绕脐痛,便秘,泄泻,痢疾;月经不调。

【备注】 大肠之"募"穴。

2.1.10.3.13 Shuidao (ST 28)

Location: This acupoint is located 3 cun below the umbilicus and 2 cun lateral to the anterior midline (see Fig. 60).

Indications: Dysmenorrhea, sterility, dysuria, hernia and lower abdominal distension.

13. 水道 ST28

【位置与取法】 在下腹部,当脐中下 3 寸,距前正中线 2 寸(见图 60)。

【主治】 痛经,不孕;小便不利,疝气;小腹胀满。

2.1.10.3.14 Guilai (ST 29)

Location: This acupoint is located 4 cun below the umbilicus and 2 cun lateral to anterior midline (see Fig. 60).

Indications: Irregular menstruation, leukorrhea, hernia, prolapse of uterus and abdominal pain.

14. 归来 ST29

【位置与取法】 在下腹部,当脐中下 4 寸,距前正中线 2 寸(见图 60)。

【主治】 月经不调,白带;疝气,阴挺;腹痛。

2.1.10.3.15 Qichong (ST 30)

Location: This acupoint is located 5 cun below the umbilicus and 2 cun lateral to the anterior midline (see Fig. 60).

Indications: Borborygmus, abdominal pain, irregular menstruation, sterility, hernia, impotence and pudendal swelling.

15. 气冲 ST30

【位置与取法】 在腹股沟稍上方,当脐中下 5 寸,距前正中线 2 寸(见图 60)。

【主治】 肠鸣腹痛;月经不调,不孕;疝气,阳痿,阴肿。

2.1.10.3.16 Futu (ST 32)

Location: This acupoint is located in the front of the thigh, on the line connecting the anterior superior iliac spine and lateral border of the patella, 6 cun above the laterosuperior border of the patella. Or it is located below the tip of the middle finger when the midpoint of the first transverse crease posterior to the palm presses against the

16. 伏兔 ST32

【位置与取法】 在大腿前面,当髂前上棘与髌底外侧端的连线上,髌底上 6 寸。髌骨外上缘上 6 寸(量 2 夫);或以手掌掌后第一横纹正中,按在膝盖上缘正中,手指并拢压

midpoint in the upper border of the knee with the fingers closed together and put on the thigh. (see Fig. 61)

在大腿上，中指尖下是穴。(见图 61)

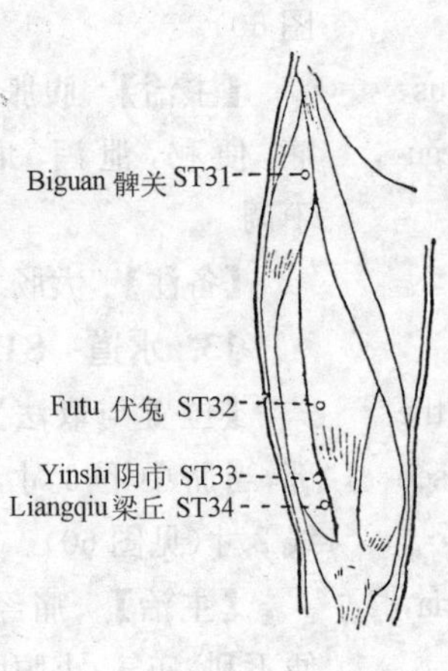

Fig. 61　Lower limb acupoints on the stomach meridian of foot-yangming

图 61　足阳明胃经下肢部经穴图

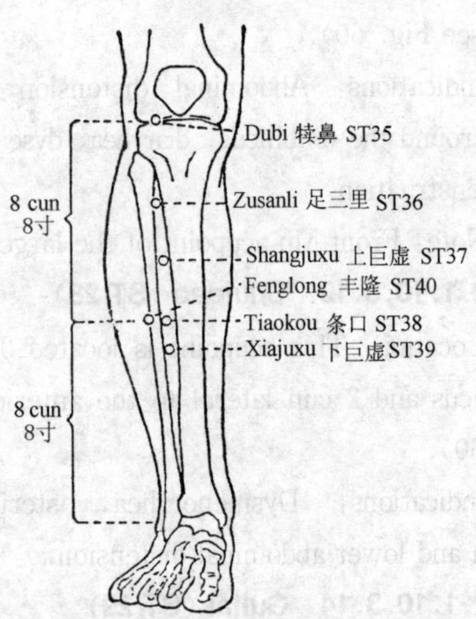

Fig. 62　Lower limb acupoints on the stomach meridian of foot-yangming

图 62　足阳明胃经下肢部经穴图

Indications: Aching loins and cold sensation in the knee, paralysis of the lower limbs, beriberi and hernia.

【主治】　腰痛膝冷，下肢麻痹，脚气；疝气。

2.1.10.3.17　Liangqiu (ST 34)

17. 梁丘　ST34

Location: When the knee is flexed, the acupoint is in the front of the thigh, on the line connecting the anterior superior iliac spine and lateral border of the patella, 2 cun above the laterosuperior border of the patella (see Fig. 61).

【位置与取法】　屈膝，在大腿前面，当髂前上棘与髌底外侧端的连线上，髌底上 2 寸(见图 61)。

Indications: Stomachache, hematuria, breast abscess, swelling and pain of the knee and paralysis of the lower limbs.

【主治】　胃痛；血尿；乳痈；膝肿痛，下肢不遂。

Note: Xi-Cleft acupoint of the stomach meridian of foot-yangming.

【备注】　足阳明经之"郄"穴。

2.1.10.3.18　Dubi (ST 35)

18. 犊鼻　ST35

Location: This acupoint is located in the depression lateral to the patellar ligament when the knee is flexed (See Fig. 62).

【位置与取法】　屈膝，在膝部，髌骨与髌韧带外侧凹陷中(见图 62)。

Indications: Pain of knee, paralysis of the lower limbs, inflexibility and beriberi.

【主治】 膝痛,下肢麻痹,屈伸不利,脚气。

2.1.10.3.19 Zusanli (ST 36)

19. 足三里 ST36

Location: This acupoint is located on the lateral side of the shank, 3 cun below Dubi (ST 35), one finger-breadth (midfinger) from the anterior crest of the tibia, in m. tibialis anterior (see Fig. 62).

【位置与取法】 在小腿前外侧,当犊鼻下 3 寸,距胫骨前缘一横指(中指)(见图 62)。

Indications: Stomachache, vomiting, dysphagia, abdominal distension, diarrhea, dysentery, constipation, intestinal abscess, depressive psychosis and manic psychosis, amnesia, insomnia, breast abscess, swelling and pain of knee, paralysis and pain of lower limbs, beriberi, edema and emaciation due to asthenia consumption.

【主治】 胃痛,呕吐,噎膈;腹胀,泄泻,痢疾,便秘;肠痈;癫狂,健忘,失眠;乳痈;膝关节肿痛,下肢痹痛;脚气;水肿;虚劳羸瘦。

Note: He-Sea acupoint of the stomach meridian of foot-yangming.

【备注】 足阳明经之"合"穴。

2.1.10.3.20 Shangjuxu (ST 37)

20. 上巨虚 ST37

Location: This acupoint is located on the lateral side of the shank, 6 cun below Dubi (ST 35), one finger-breadth (midfinger) from the anterior crest of the tibia, in m. tibialis anterior (see Fig. 62).

【位置与取法】 在小腿前外侧,当犊鼻下 6 寸,距胫骨前缘一横指(中指)(见图 62)。

Indications: Borborygmus, abdominal pain, diarrhea, constipation, intestinal abscess, flaccidity and obstruction syndromes of lower limbs and beriberi.

【主治】 肠鸣,腹痛,泄泻,便秘,肠痈;下肢痿痹,脚气。

Note: Lower He-Sea acupoint of the large intestine meridian of hand-yangming.

【备注】 手阳明经之"下合穴"。

2.1.10.3.21 Tiaokou (ST 38)

21. 条口 ST38

Location: This acupoint is located on the lateral side of the shank, 8 cun below Dubi (ST 35), one finger-breadth from the anterior crest of the tibia, in m. tibialis anterior (see Fig. 62).

【位置与取法】 在小腿前外侧,当犊鼻下 8 寸,距胫骨前缘一横指(中指)(见图 62)。

Indications: Epigastric pain, flaccidity and obstruction syndromes of lower limbs, spasm, swelling of foot and pain in the shoulder and arm.

【主治】 脘腹疼痛;下肢痿痹,转筋,跗肿;肩臂痛。

2.1.10.3.22 Xiajuxu (ST 39)

22. 下巨虚 ST39

Location: This acupoint is located on the lateral side of

【位置与取法】 在小腿

the shank, 9 cun below Dubi (ST 35), one finger-breadth (midfinger) from the anterior crest of the tibia (see Fig. 62).

前外侧，当犊鼻下 9 寸，距胫骨前缘一横指（中指）（见图 62）。

Indications: Lower abdominal pain, diarrhea, dysentery, breast abscess, flaccidity and obstruction syndromes of lower limbs and pain of loins and spine involving scrotum.

【主治】 小腹痛，泄泻，痢疾；乳痛；下肢痿痹；腰脊痛引睾丸。

Note: Lower He-Sea acupoint of the small intestine meridian of hand-taiyang.

【备注】 手太阳经之“下合穴”。

2.1.10.3.23 Fenglong (ST 40)

23. 丰隆 ST40

Location: This acupoint is located on the lateral side of the shank, 8 cun above the tip of external malleolus, lateral to Tiaokou (ST 38) and two finger-breadth (midfinger) from the anterior crest of the tibia (see Fig. 62).

【位置与取法】 在小腿前外侧，当外踝尖上 8 寸，条口外，距胫骨前缘二横指（中指）（见图 62）。

Indications: Vomiting, constipation, edema, headache, vertigo, profuse phlegm and cough, depressive psychosis, manic psychosis, epilepsy, and flaccidity and obstruction syndromes of lower limbs.

【主治】 呕吐，便秘，水肿；头痛，眩晕；痰多咳嗽；癫狂痫；下肢痿痹。

Note: Luo-Connecting acupoint of the stomach meridian of foot-yangming.

【备注】 足阳明经之“络”穴。

2.1.10.3.24 Jiexi (ST 41)

24. 解溪 ST41

Location: This acupoint is located in the depression at the midpoint of the transverse crease of the dorsum of foot and shank, between the tendons of m. extensor digitorum longus and hallucis longus (see Fig. 63).

【位置与取法】 在足背与小腿交界处的横纹中央凹陷中，当踇长伸肌腱与趾长伸肌腱之间（见图 63）。

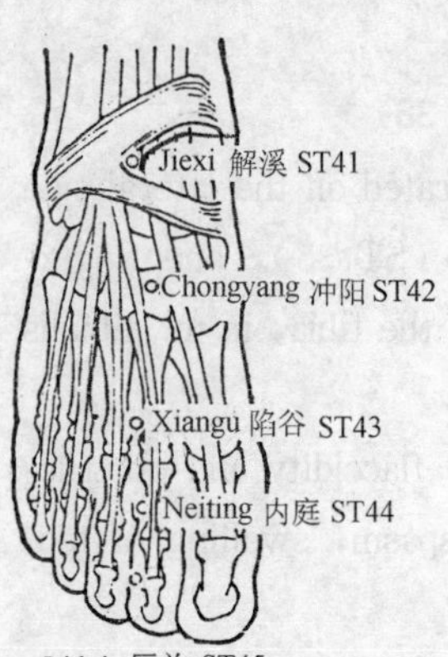

Fig. 63 Foot dorsum acupoints on the stomach meridian of foot-yangming

图 63 足阳明胃经足背部经穴图

Indications: Headache, vertigo, depressive psychosis and manic psychosis, abdominal distension, constipation, flaccidity and obstruction syndromes of lower limbs and swelling and pain of ankle joint.

【主治】 头痛，眩晕；癫狂；腹胀，便秘；下肢痿痹，踝关节肿痛。

Note: Jing-River acupoint of the stomach meridian of foot-yangming.

【备注】 足阳明经之"经"穴。

2.1.10.3.25 Chongyang (ST 42)

25. 冲阳 ST42

Location: This acupoint is located on the prominence of the foot dorsum, in the depression between the second and third metatarsal bones and the cuneiform bone and at the pulsating point of the artery on the dorsum of foot (see Fig. 63).

【位置与取法】 在足背最高处，当踇长伸肌腱与趾长伸肌腱之间，足背动脉搏动处(见图 63)。

Indications: Distortion of face, swelling of cheeks, toothache, depressive psychosis and manic psychosis, epilepsy, and flaccidity of foot.

【主治】 口眼㖞斜；面肿；齿痛；癫狂痫；足痿无力。

Note: Yuan-Source acupoint of the stomach meridian of foot-yangming.

【备注】 足阳明经之"原"穴。

2.1.10.3.26 Xiangu (ST 43)

26. 陷谷 ST43

Location: This acupoint is located on the dorsum of foot and in the depression anterior to the junction of the second and third metatarsal bones (see Fig. 63).

【位置与取法】 在足背，当二三跖骨结合部前方凹陷处(见图 63)。

Indications: Swelling of cheeks, redness, swelling and pain of the eyes, borborygmus, abdominal pain, swelling and pain of the dorsum of foot and febrile disease.

【主治】 面肿，目赤肿痛；肠鸣腹痛；足背肿痛；热病。

Note: Shu-Stream acupoint of the stomach meridian of foot-yangming.

【备注】 足阳明经之"输"穴。

2.1.10.3.27 Neiting (ST 44)

27. 内庭 ST44

Location: This acupoint is located on the dorsum of foot, in the red and white part posterior to the border of toe webs, proximal to the web margin between the second and third toes (see Fig. 63).

【位置与取法】 在足背，当二三趾间，趾蹼缘后方赤白肉际处。足背第二三趾的趾缝端(见图 63)。

Indications: Toothache, sore throat, facial distortion, epistaxis, stomachache, acid regurgitation, abdominal distension, diarrhea, dysentery, constipation, swelling

【主治】 齿痛；咽喉肿痛；口㖞；鼻衄；胃痛吐酸，腹胀，泄泻，痢疾，便秘；足背肿

and pain of dorsum of foot and febrile disease.

Note: Ying-Spring acupoint of the stomach meridian of foot-yangming.

痛;热病。

【备注】 足阳明经之"荥"穴。

2.1.10.3.28 Lidui (ST 45)

28. 厉兑 ST45

Location: This acupoint is located on the lateral side of the second toe, 0.1 cun latero-posterior to the corner of the nail (see Fig. 63).

Indications: Epistaxis, toothache, sore throat, dreaminess, mania and febrile disease.

Note: Jing-Well acupoint of the stomach meridian of foot-yangming.

【位置与取法】 在足第二趾末节外侧,当趾甲角0.1寸(见图63)。

【主治】 鼽衄;齿痛;咽喉肿痛;多梦,癫狂;热病。

【备注】 足阳明经之"井"穴。

2.1.11 Gallbladder meridian of foot-shaoyang

十一、足少阳胆经

2.1.11.1 Cyclical flowing and distribution

(一)循行分布

The gallbladder meridian starts from the outer canthus, ascends to the corner of the forehead, curves downward to the retroauricular region and runs along the side of the neck in front of the triple energizer meridian. Then it turns back, traverses and passes behind the triple energizer meridian down to the supraclavicular fossa. From there it runs downward from the supraclavicular fossa, passes in front of the axilla along the lateral aspect of the chest and through the free ends of the floating ribs to the hip region where it meets the previous branch and descends along the lateral aspect of the thigh to the lateral side of the knee. Then it goes further downward along the anterior aspect of the fibula all the way to its lower end, reaching the anterior aspect of the external malleolus. Finally it runs along the dorsum of the foot to the lateral side of the tip of the fourth toe.

起于目外眦,上行到额角,下行于耳后完骨,沿着颈部行于手少阳经之前,至肩上,再交出手少阳经之后,进入缺盆,从缺盆部下走腋前,沿着侧胸部,经过季胁,向下与行于躯干内的分支会合于髋关节部;沿着大腿外侧,出于膝部外侧,下行于腓骨小头之前,直下至腓骨下端,经外踝的前面,沿着足背部进入第四趾外侧端。

The first branch stems from the retroauricular region and enters the ear. Emerging before the ear, it runs to the posterior aspect of the outer canthus.

分支一:从耳后进入耳中,出走耳前,至目外眦的后方。

The second branch stems from the outer canthus and

分支二:从目外眦处分

runs downward to Daying (ST 5) and meets with the triple energizer meridian in the infraorbital region. Then it runs over Jiache (ST 6) and descends to the neck and enters the supraclavicular fossa to meet with the main trunk of the meridian. Then it further descends into the chest, passes through the diaphragm to link with the liver and enters the gallbladder to which it pertains. Running inside the hypochondriac region, it emerges from the lateral side of the lower abdomen near the femoral artery at the inguinal region. Finally it runs superficially along the margin of the pubes and goes transversely into the hip region.

出，下走至大迎部，会手少阳经抵目眶下，向后下覆盖于颊车部至颈，与主干会合于缺盆部；然后向下进入胸中，通过横膈，络于肝，连属于胆，沿着胁里，出于少腹两侧的腹股沟动脉部，绕行阴部毛际，横向后进入髋关节部。

The third branch stems from the dorsum of the foot and runs between the first and second metatarsal bones to the distal portion of the great toe and ends at its hairy region and links with the liver meridian. (see Fig. 64)

分支三：从足背部分出，进入第一二趾之间，出大趾端，回过来穿过趾甲出于趾背毫毛部，接足厥阴肝经。(见图 64)

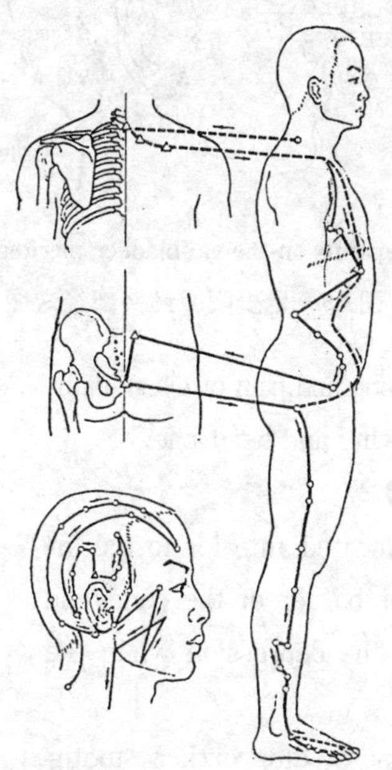

Fig. 64 Flowing route of the gallbladder meridian of foot-shaoyang

图 64 足少阳胆经循行示意图

Associated viscera: Gallbladder and liver.

联系脏腑：胆、肝。

Associated organs: Eyes and ears.

联系器官：目、耳。

2.1.11.2 Indications

（二）主治要点

Disorders of the lateral side of the head, eyes, ears and throat as well as mental problems, febrile disease and other diseases involving the areas through which the meridian passes.

本经腧穴主治侧头、目、耳、咽喉病，神志病，热病以及经脉循行部位的其他病证。

2.1.11.3 Commonly used acupoints

（三）常用腧穴

1.1.11.3.1 Tongziliao (GB 1)

1. 瞳子髎　GB1

Location: This acupoint is located lateral to the outer canthus and at the lateral side of the orbit (see Fig. 65).

【位置与取法】　在面部，目外眦旁，当眶外侧缘处（见图 65）。

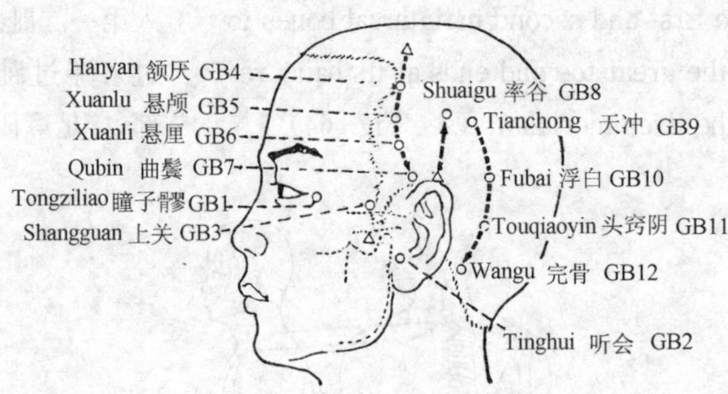

Fig. 65　Head acupoints on the gallbladder meridian of foot-shaoyang

图 65　足少阳胆经头部经穴图

Indications: Redness, swelling and pain of eyes, cataract, glaucoma, epiphora with wind and headache.

【主治】　目赤肿痛，目翳，青盲，迎风流泪；头痛。

2.1.11.3.2 Tinghui (GB 2)

2. 听会　GB2

Location: This acupoint is located anterior to the intertragic notch, at the posterior border of the condyloid process of the mandible and in the depression when the mouth is open (see Fig. 65).

【位置与取法】　在面部，当耳屏间切迹的前方，下颌骨髁状突的后缘，张口有凹陷处（见图 65）。

Indications: Tinnitus, deafness, otopyorrhea, toothache, facial distortion, headache and swelling and pain of the cheeks.

【主治】　耳鸣，耳聋，聤耳；齿痛，口眼㖞斜；头痛，面颊肿痛。

2.1.11.3.3 Shangguan (GB 3)

3. 上关　GB3

Location: This acupoint is located in front of the ear,

【位置与取法】　在耳前

directly above Xiaguan (ST 7) and in the depression at the upper border of the zygomatic arch (see Fig. 65).

下关直上，当颧弓的上缘凹陷处(见图 65)。

Indications: Tinnitus, deafness, facial distortion, lockjaw, toothache and migraine.

【主治】 耳鸣，耳聋；口眼㖞斜，口噤不开；齿痛；偏头痛。

2.1.11.3.4 Xuanlu (GB 5)

4. 悬颅 GB5

Location: This acupoint is located on the hairline of the temporal region and at the midpoint of the line joining Touwei (ST 8) and Qubin (GB 7) (see Fig. 65).

【位置与取法】 在头部鬓发上，当头维与曲鬓弧形连线的中点处(见图 65)。

Indications: Migraine, redness, swelling and pain of eyes and toothache.

【主治】 偏头痛；目赤肿痛，齿痛。

2.1.11.3.5 Qubin (GB 7)

5. 曲鬓 GB7

Location: This acupoint is located on the midpoint on the junction of the vertical line at the posterior border of the pre-auricular hairline with the level line of the tip of the ear, above one finger-breadth anterior to Jiaosun (TE 20) (see Fig. 65).

【位置与取法】 在头部，当耳前鬓角发际后缘的垂线与耳尖水平线交点处。约当角孙(三焦经)前一横指处之鬓发内(见图 65)。

Indications: Migraine, toothache, lockjaw and sudden loss of voice.

【主治】 偏头痛；齿痛，牙关紧闭；暴喑。

2.1.11.3.6 Shuaigu (GB 8)

6. 率谷 GB8

Location: This acupoint is located 1.5 cun from the tip of ear straightly into the hairline, directly above Jiaosun (TE 20) and two finger-breadth (the index and middle fingers closed together) directly above the ear tip when the ear is folded or the midpoint between Jiaosun (TE 20) and the parietale tubercle (see Fig. 65).

【位置与取法】 在头部，当耳尖直上入发际 1.5 寸，角孙直上方。将耳折叠，于耳尖直上约两指(食、中指并拢之宽度)处。或在角孙与顶骨结节的中点处(见图 65)。

Indications: Migraine, vertigo, acute and chronic infantile convulsion.

【主治】 偏头痛，眩晕；小儿急、慢惊风。

2.1.11.3.7 Wangu (GB 12)

7. 完骨 GB12

Location: This acupoint is located in the depression posterior and inferior to the mastoid process (see Fig. 65).

【位置与取法】 在头部，当耳后乳突的后下方凹陷处(见图 65)。

Indications: Headache, stiffness and pain of neck, toothache, facial distortion, epilepsy and malaria.

【主治】 头痛，颈项强痛；齿痛，口歪；癫痫；疟疾。

2.1.11.3.8 Yangbai (GB 14)

Location: This acupoint is located on the forehead, 1 cun directly above the midpoint of the eyebrow (see Fig. 66).

8. 阳白　GB14

【位置与取法】 在前额部,当瞳孔直上,眉上1寸(见图66)。

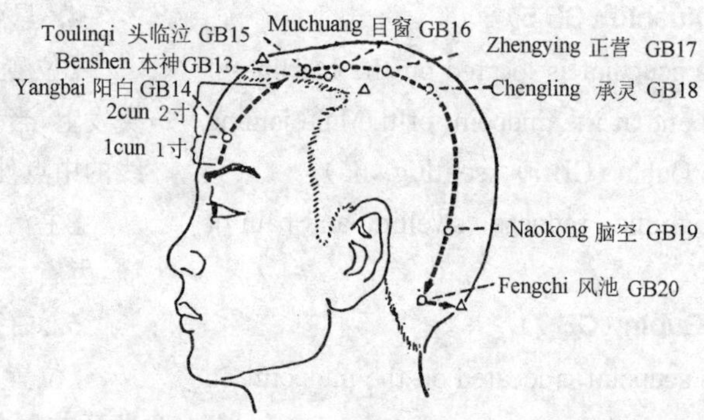

Fig. 66 Head acupoints on the gallbladder meridian of foot-shaoyang
图66 足少阳胆经头部经穴图

Indications: Pain of eyes, blurred vision, twitching of eyelids, facial distortion, headache and facial pain.

【主治】 目痛,视物模糊,眼睑瞤动,口眼㖞斜;头痛,面痛。

2.1.11.3.9 Toulinqi (GB 15)

Location: This acupoint is directly above the pupil and 0.5 cun from the anterior hairline and on the midpoint between Shenting (GV 24) and Touwei (ST 8) (see Fig. 66).

Indications: Headache, vertigo, redness, swelling and pain of eyes, epiphora, cataract, nasal obstruction, rhinorrhea, tinnitus, deafness and infantile convulsion.

9. 头临泣　GB15

【位置与取法】 在头部当瞳孔直上入前发际0.5寸神庭与头维连线的中点处(见图66)。

【主治】 头痛,目眩;目赤肿痛,流泪,目翳;鼻塞,鼻渊;耳鸣,耳聋;小儿惊风。

2.1.11.3.10 Fengchi (GB 20)

Location: This acupoint is located below the occipital bone, parallel to Fengfu (GV 16) and in the depression between the upper portion of m. sternocleidomastoideus and m. trapezius or at the midpoint between Yifeng (TE 17) and Fengfu (GV 16) or at the upper part of the trapezius on both sides with the thumb and index finger parallel

10. 风池　GB20

【位置与取法】 在项部当枕骨之下,与风府(督脉)相平,胸锁乳突肌与斜方肌上端之间的凹陷处。翳风(三焦经)与风府连线的中点。或以拇指与食指沿患者两侧斜方

to the external occipital protuberance. (see Fig. 66)

肌的上端，平枕外粗隆处(风府)。(见图 66)

Indications: Headache, vertigo, redness, swelling and pain of eyes, nearsightedness, epiphora with wind, night blindness, nasal obstruction, rhinorrhea, epistaxis, tinnitus, deafness, epilepsy, apoplexy, stiffness and pain of neck, common cold, febrile disease, malaria and goiter.

【主治】 头痛，眩晕；目赤肿痛，近视，迎风流泪，雀目；鼻塞，鼻渊，鼽衄；耳鸣，耳聋；癫痫，中风；颈项强痛；感冒，热病，疟疾，瘿气。

2.1.11.3.11 Jianjing (GB 21)

11. 肩井 GB21

Location: This acupoint is located on the shoulder and at the midway between Dazhui (GV 14) and the acromion (see Fig. 67).

【位置与取法】 在肩上，当大椎(督脉)与肩峰端连线的中点上(见图 67)。

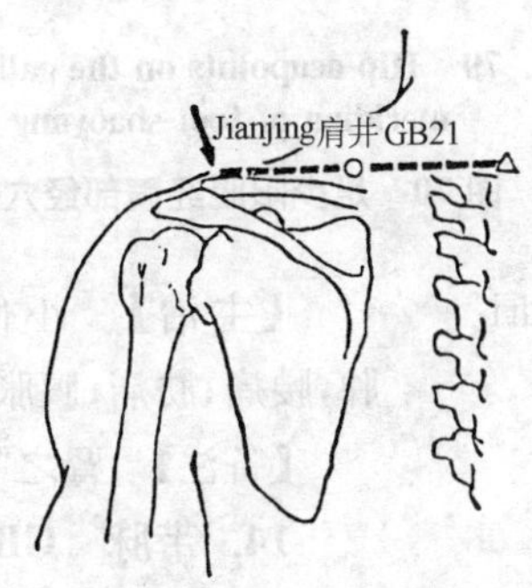

Fig. 67 Shoulder acupoints on the gallbladder meridian of foot-shaoyang

图 67 足少阳胆经肩部经穴图

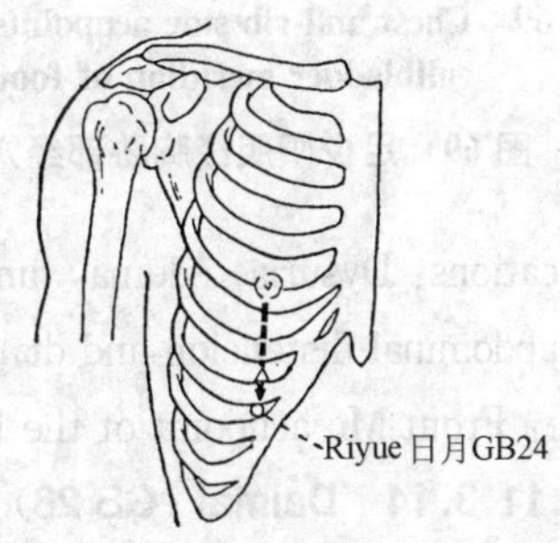

Fig. 68 Chest acupoints on the gallbladder meridian of foot-shaoyang

图 68 足少阳胆经胸部经穴

Indications: Stiffness and pain of neck, shoulder and back, paralysis of upper limbs, breast abscess, agalactia, dystocia and scrofula.

【主治】 头项强痛，肩背疼痛，上肢不遂；乳痈，乳汁不下；难产；瘰疬。

2.1.11.3.12 Riyue (GB 24)

12. 日月 GB24

Location: This acupoint is located on the upper abdomen, directly below the nipple, in the seventh intercostal space and 4 cun lateral to the anterior midline (see Fig. 68).

【位置与取法】 在上腹部，当乳头直下，第七肋间隙，前正中线旁开 4 寸(见图 68)。

Indications: Jaundice, hypochondriac pain, vomiting and acid regurgitation.

【主治】 黄疸，胁肋疼痛，呕逆，吞酸。

Note: Front-Mu acupoint of the gallbladder.

【备注】 胆之"募"穴。

2.1.11.3.13 Jingmen (GB 25)

Location: This acupoint is located lateral to the waist, 1.8 cun posterior to Zhangmen (LR 13) and on the lower border of the free end of the twelfth rib (see Fig. 69).

13. 京门 GB25

【位置与取法】 在侧腰部,章门后1.8寸,当第十二肋骨游离端的下方(见图 69)。

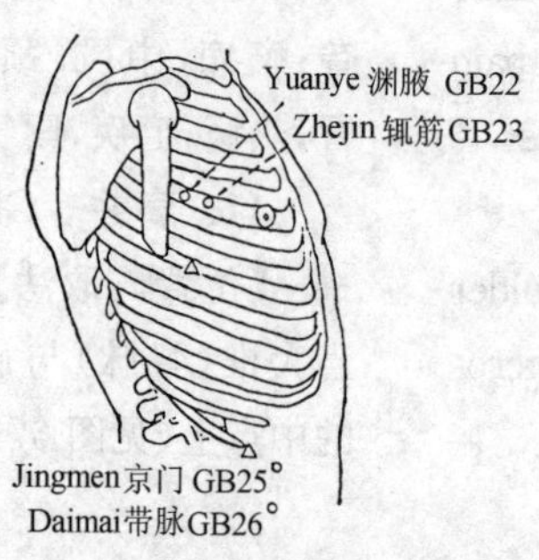

Fig. 69 Chest and rib-side acupoints on the gallbladder meridian of foot-shaoyang

图 69 足少阳胆经胸胁部经穴图

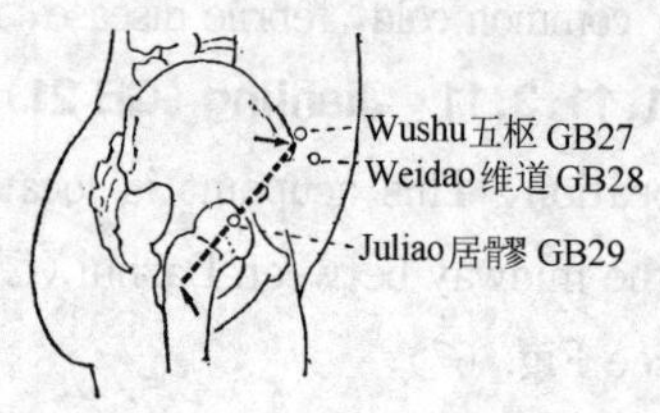

Fig. 70 Hip acupoints on the gallbladder meridian of foot-shaoyang

图 70 足少阳胆经髋部经穴图

Indications: Dysuria, edema, lumbago, hypochondriac pain, abdominal distension and diarrhea.

Note: Front-Mu acupoint of the kidney.

【主治】 小便不利,水肿,腰痛;胁痛;腹胀,泄泻。

【备注】 肾之"募"穴。

2.1.11.3.14 Daimai (GB 26)

Location: This acupoint is located lateral to the abdomen, 1.8 cun below Zhangmen (LR 13), directly below the free end of the eleventh rib and at the level with the umbilicus (see Fig. 69).

Indications: Amenorrhea, irregular menstruation, leukorrhea, hernia, abdominal pain and pain in the loins and hypochondria.

14. 带脉 GB26

【位置与取法】 在侧腹部,章门下1.8寸,当第十一肋骨游离端下方垂线与脐水平线的交点上(见图 69)。

【主治】 经闭,月经不调,带下病;疝气;腹痛,腰胁痛。

2.1.11.3.15 Juliao (GB 29)

Location: This acupoint is located on the midpoint between the anterosuperior iliac spine and the great trochanter (see Fig. 70).

Indications: Lumbago, flaccidity and obstruction syndromes of lower limbs and hernia.

15. 居髎 GB29

【位置与取法】 在髋部,当髂前上棘与股骨大转子最凸点连线的中点处(见图 70)。

【主治】 腰痛,下肢痿痹;疝气。

2.1.11.3.16 Huantiao (GB 30)

Location: This acupoint is located lateral to the

16. 环跳 GB30

【位置与取法】 在股外

thigh. When the thigh is flexed, the acupoint is at the junction of the lateral 1/3 and medial 2/3 of the distance between the most protruding point of the great trochanter and the hiatus of the sacrum (see Fig. 71).

侧部,侧卧屈股,当股骨大转子最凸点与骶管裂孔连线的外 1/3 与中 1/3 交点处。取本穴应侧卧,伸下腿屈上腿,以使股骨大转子暴露更明显(见图 71)。

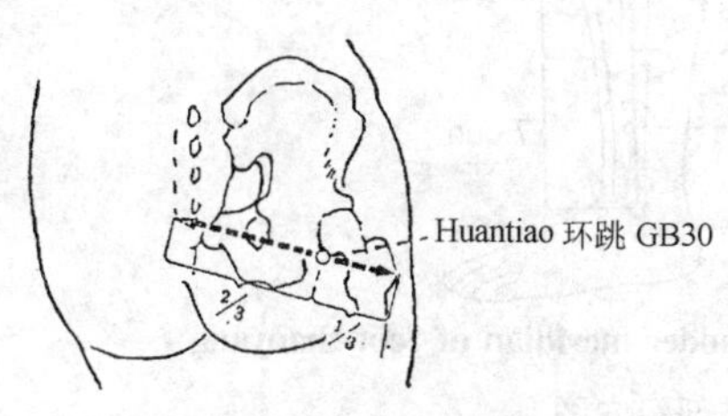

Fig. 71 Hip acupoints on the gallbladder meridian of foot-shaoyang

图 71 足少阳胆经髋部经穴图

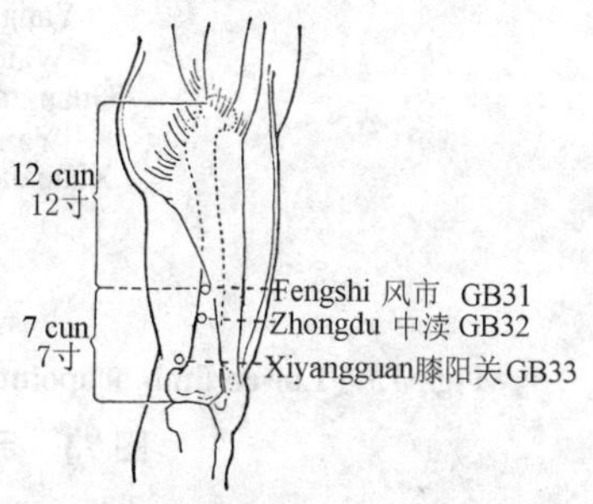

Fig. 72 Lower limb acupoints on the gallbladder meridian of foot-shaoyang

图 72 足少阳胆经下肢部经穴图

Indications: Pain in the loins and legs, flaccidity and obstruction syndromes of lower limbs, sprain of waist and urticaria.

【主治】 腰腿痛,下肢痿痹,腰扭伤;风疹。

2.1.11.3.17 Fengshi (GB 31)

17. 风市 GB31

Location: This acupoint is located on the midline lateral to the thigh, 7 cun above the transverse popliteal crease. Or when the patient stands erect with the hands close to the sides, the point is where the tip of the middle finger touches (see Fig. 72).

【位置与取法】 在大腿外侧部的中线上,当腘横纹上 7 寸,或直立垂手时,中指尖处(见图 72)。

Indications: Flaccidity and obstruction syndromes of lower limbs, general pruritus and beriberi.

【主治】 下肢痿痹;遍身瘙痒;脚气。

2.1.11.3.18 Xiyangguan (GB 33)

18. 膝阳关 GB33

Location: This acupoint is located lateral to the knee, 3 cun above Yanglingquan (GB 34) and in the depression above external epicondyle of the femur (see Fig. 72).

【位置与取法】 在膝外侧,当阳陵泉上 3 寸,股骨外上髁上方的凹陷处(见图 72)。

Indications: Swelling, pain and spasm of knees and numbness of shank.

【主治】 膝髌肿痛挛急,小腿麻木。

2.1.11.3.19 Yanglingquan (GB 34)

Location: This acupoint is located lateral to the shank and in the depression anterior and inferior to the head of the fibula (see Fig. 73).

19. 阳陵泉 GB34

【位置与取法】 在小腿外侧,当腓骨头前下方凹陷处(见图 73)。

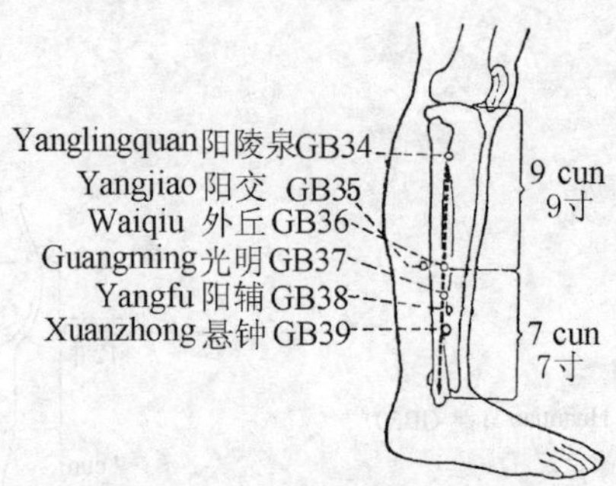

Fig. 73 Lower limb acupoints on the gallbladder meridian of foot-shaoyang

图 73 足少阳胆经下肢部经穴图

Indications: Hypochondriac pain, bitter taste in the mouth, jaundice, vomiting, pain in the loins and legs, flaccidity and obstruction syndromes of lower limbs, acute and chronic sprain of waist and stiffness of neck.

Note: He-Sea acupoint of the gallbladder meridian of foot-shaoyang and one of the eight confluent acupoints associating with tendons.

【主治】 胁痛,口苦,黄疸,呕吐;腰腿痛,下肢痿痹;急、慢性腰扭伤,落枕。

【备注】 足少阳经之"合"穴;八会穴之"筋会"。

2.1.11.3.20 Yangjiao (GB 35)

Location: This acupoint is located lateral to the shank, 7 cun above the tip of the external malleolus and on the posterior border of the fibula (see Fig. 73).

Indications: Distension and fullness in the chest and hypochondria, flaccidity and obstruction syndromes of lower limbs and depressive psychosis and manic psychosis.

Note: Xi-Cleft acupoint of yang link vessel.

20. 阳交 GB35

【位置与取法】 在小腿外侧,当外踝尖上 7 寸,腓骨后缘(见图 73)。

【主治】 胸胁胀满,下肢痿痹;癫狂。

【备注】 阳维脉之"郄"穴。

2.1.11.3.21 Waiqiu (GB 36)

Location: This acupoint is located lateral to the shank, 7 cun above the tip of the external malleolus, on the anterior border of the fibula and parallel to Yangjiao (GB 35) (see Fig. 73).

21. 外丘 GB36

【位置与取法】 在小腿外侧,当外踝尖上 7 寸,腓骨前缘,平阳交(见图 73)。

Indications: Distension and fullness in the chest and hypochondria, flaccidity and obstruction syndromes of lower limbs and depressive psychosis and manic psychosis.

Note: Xi-Cleft acupoint of the gallbladder meridian of foot-shaoyang.

【主治】 胸胁胀满,下肢痿痹;癫狂。

【备注】 足少阳经之"郄"穴。

2.1.11.3.22 Guangming (GB 37)

Location: This acupoint is located lateral to the shank, 5 cun above the tip of the external malleolus, on the anterior border of the fibula (see Fig. 73).

Indications: Pain of eyes, night blindness, nearsightedness, epiphora with wind, distending pain in the breast and flaccidity and obstruction syndromes of lower limbs.

Note: Luo-Connecting acupoint of the gallbladder meridian of foot-shaoyang.

22. 光明 GB37

【位置与取法】 在小腿外侧,当外踝尖上 5 寸,腓骨前缘(见图 73)。

【主治】 目痛,夜盲,近视,迎风流泪;乳房胀痛;下肢痿痹。

【备注】 足少阳经之"络"穴。

2.1.11.3.23 Yangfu (GB 38)

Location: This acupoint is located lateral to the shank, 4 cun above the tip of the external malleolus, slightly anterior to the anterior border of the fibula (see Fig. 73).

Indications: Migraine, pain of the outer canthus, swelling and pain in the axillary region, distending pain in the chest and hypochondria, flaccidity and obstruction syndromes of lower limbs, sore throat, scrofula and beriberi.

Note: Jing-River acupoint of the gallbladder meridian of foot-shaoyang.

23. 阳辅 GB38

【位置与取法】 在小腿外侧,当外踝尖上 4 寸,腓骨前缘稍前方(见图 73)。

【主治】 偏头痛,目外眦痛,腋下肿痛,胸胁胀痛,下肢痿痹;咽喉肿痛;瘰疬;脚气。

【备注】 足少阳经之"经"穴。

2.1.11.3.24 Xuanzhong (GB 39)

Location: This acupoint is located lateral to the shank, 3 cun above the tip of the external malleolus, on the anterior border of the fibula (see Fig. 73).

Indications: Stiffness of neck, distending pain in the chest and hypochondria, flaccidity and obstruction syndromes of lower limbs, sore throat, beriberi and hemorrhoids.

Note: One of the eight confluent acupoints associating with marrow.

24. 悬钟 GB39

【位置与取法】 在小腿外侧,当外踝尖上 3 寸,腓骨前缘(见图 73)。

【主治】 项强,胸胁胀痛,下肢痿痹;咽喉肿痛;脚气;痔疾。

【备注】 八会穴之"髓会"。

2.1.11.3.25　Qiuxu（GB 40）

Location：This acupoint is located anterior and inferior to the external malleolus，in the depression on the lateral side of the tendon of m. extensor digitorum longus.（see Fig. 74）

25. 丘墟　GB40

【位置与取法】 在足外踝的前下方，当趾长伸肌腱的外侧凹陷处。踝关节背屈呈直角，当外踝前缘垂直线与外踝下缘水平线的相交处的凹陷中。（见图 74）

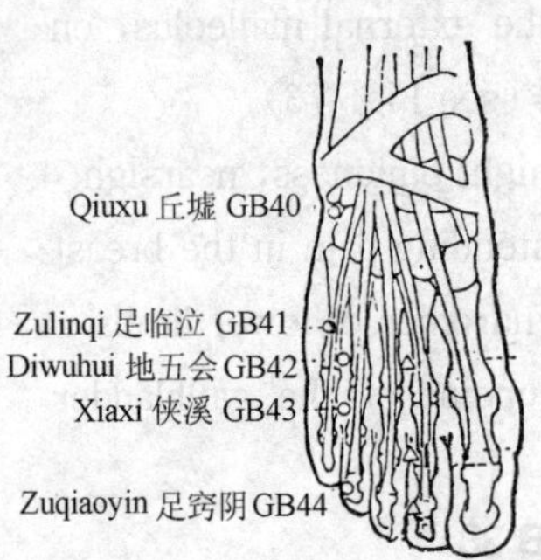

Fig. 74　Foot acupoints on the gallbladder meridian of foot-shaoyang

图 74　足少阳胆经足部经穴图

Indications：Distending pain in the chest and hypochondria，swelling in the axillary region，flaccidity and obstruction syndromes of the lower limbs，swelling and pain of the external malleolus，redness，swelling and pain of eyes，cataract and malaria.

Note：Yuan-Source acupoint of the gallbladder meridian of foot-shaoyang.

【主治】 胸胁胀痛，腋下肿，下肢痿痹，外踝肿痛；目赤肿痛，目翳；疟疾。

【备注】 足少阳经之“原”穴。

2.1.11.3.26　Zulinqi（GB 41）

Location：This acupoint is located lateral to the dorsum of foot，posterior to the fourth metatarsophalangeal joint and in the depression lateral to the extensor muscle tendon of the small toe（see Fig. 74）.

Indications：Hypochondriac pain；flaccidity of foot；pain of foot dorsum；numbness of toes；irregular menstruation；multi-coloured leukorrhagia；redness，pain and swelling of eyes；breast abscess；scrofula and malaria.

26. 足临泣　GB41

【位置与取法】 在足背外侧，当第四趾本节（第四跖趾关节）的后方，小趾伸肌腱的外侧凹陷处(见图 74)。

【主治】 胁肋疼痛，足痿不用，足跗疼痛，足趾麻木；月经不调，赤白带下；目赤肿痛；乳痈；瘰疬；疟疾。

Note: Shu-Stream acupoint of the gallbladder meridian of foot-shaoyang and one of the convergent acupoints associating with the belt vessel.

【备注】 足少阳经之"输"穴;八脉交会穴之一,通于带脉。

2.1.11.3.27 Xiaxi (GB 43)

27. 侠溪 GB43

Location: This acupoint is located laterally on the foot dorsum, between the 4th and 5th toes and posterior to the red and white margin behind the toe web (see Fig. 74).

【位置与取法】 在足背外侧,当第四五趾间,趾蹼缘后方赤白肉际(见图 74)。

Indications: Headache, vertigo, redness, swelling and pain of the eyes, tinnitus, deafness, pain in the hypochondria, breast abscess and febrile disease.

【主治】 头痛,目眩;目赤肿痛;耳鸣,耳聋;胁肋疼痛;乳痈;热病。

Note: Ying-Spring acupoint of the gallbladder meridian of foot-shaoyang.

【备注】 足少阳经之"荥"穴。

2.1.11.3.28 Zuqiaoyin (GB 44)

28. 足窍阴 GB44

Location: This acupoint is located on the lateral side of the fourth toe, about 0.1 cun latero-posterior to the corner of the nail (see Fig. 74).

【位置与取法】 在足第四趾末节外侧,距趾甲角0.1寸(见图 74)。

Indications: Headache, redness, swelling and pain of eyes, deafness, sore throat, hypochondriac pain, apoplexy, syncope, insomnia, febrile disease and cough.

【主治】 头痛;目赤肿痛;耳聋;咽喉肿痛;胁痛;中风,昏厥,失眠;热病;咳逆。

Note: Jing-Well acupoint of the gallbladder meridian of foot-shaoyang.

【备注】 足少阳经之"井"穴。

2.1.12 Bladder meridian of foot-taiyang

十二、足太阳膀胱经

2.1.12.1 Cyclical flowing and distribution

(一) 循行分布

The bladder meridian starts from the inner canthus, ascends to the forehead and joins the governor vessel at the vertex. From there it enters the brain, reemerges and runs superficially from the vertex to the medial side of the scapular region. Then it runs to the loins along the spinal column and enters the abdominal cavity from the deep layer of muscles to link with the kidney and joins the bladder to which it pertains.

起于目内眦,上行额部,交会于巅顶,从巅顶入络脑,复出浅表,经过项部,沿着肩胛部的内侧,挟脊柱两侧抵达腰中,进入脊柱两侧的肌肉并深入腹内,络于肾,连属膀胱。

The first branch stems from the vertex and runs to areas above the ears.

分支一:从巅顶分出到耳上角。

The second branch stems from the waist, descends through the gluteal region and ends in the popliteal fossa.

The third branch stems from the posterior aspect of the neck, runs straight downward along the medial border of the scapula. Then it passes through the gluteal region downward along the lateral aspect of the thigh and meets with the preceding branch descending from the lumbar region in the popliteal fossa. From there it descends to the leg and further to the posterior aspect of the external malleolus. Finally it runs along the tuberosity of the fifth metatarsal bone and reaches the lateral side of the tip of the little toe to link with the kidney meridian. (see Fig. 75)

分支二:从腰中分出,向下挟脊两旁,穿过臀部,至腘窝中。

分支三:自项部分出,从肩胛内缘直下通过肩胛,挟行于脊柱两侧,通过臀部,沿大腿外侧后缘,与腰中下来的支脉会合于腘窝中;两脉相合由此向下,穿过腓肠肌,出外踝后面,沿第五跖骨粗隆,至足小趾外侧端,接足少阴肾经。(见图 75)

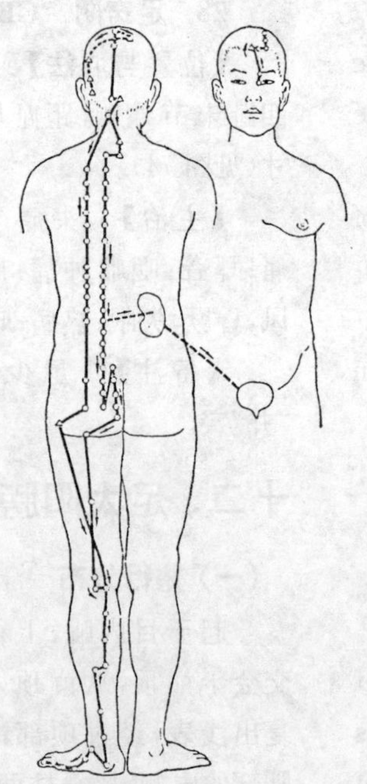

Fig. 75 Flowing route of the bladder meridian of foot-taiyang

图 75 足太阳膀胱经循行示意图

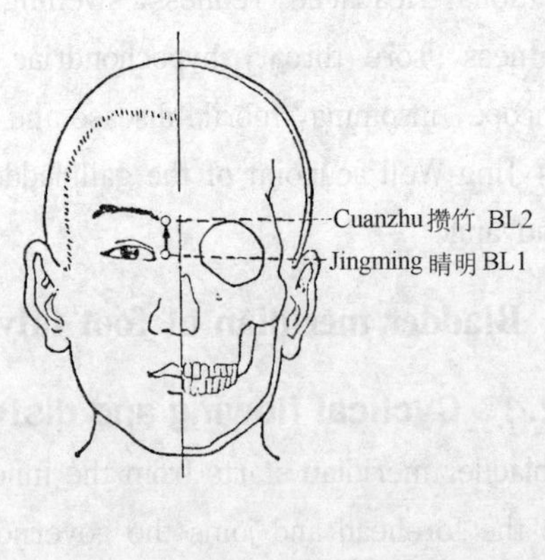

Fig. 76 Head and face acupoints on the bladder meridian of foot-taiyang

图 76 足太阳膀胱经头面部经穴图

Associated viscera: Bladder, kidney, and brain.

Associated organs: Eyes, nose, and ears.

联系脏腑:膀胱、肾、脑。

联系器官:目、鼻、耳。

2.1.12.2 Indications

(二)主治要点

Diseases of the head, neck, eyes, back, waist and

本经腧穴主治头、项、目

lower limbs as well as mental problems. The indications of the Back-Shu acupoints on the first lateral line of the back and the acupoints on the second line parallel to the first lateral line include the disorders of the related viscera, tissues and organs.

背、腰、下肢部病证以及神志病，背部第一侧线的背俞穴及第二侧线相平的腧穴，主治与其相关的脏腑病证和有关的组织器官病证。

2.1.12.3 Commonly used acupoints

（三）常用腧穴

2.1.12.3.1 Jingming (BL 1)

Location: This acupoint is located in the depression slightly superior to the inner canthus (see Fig. 76).

Indications: Redness, swelling and pain of eyes, epiphora, blurred vision, dizziness, nearsightedness, night blindness and color blindness.

1. 睛明 BL1

【位置与取法】 在面部，目内眦角稍上方的凹陷处(见图 76)。

【主治】 目赤肿痛，流泪，视物不明，目眩，近视，夜盲，色盲。

2.1.12.3.2 Cuanzhu (BL 2)

Location: This acupoint is located in the depression of the eyebrow or on the supraorbial notch (see Fig. 76).

Indications: Facial distortion, blurred vision, epiphora, redness, swelling and pain of the eyes, twitching of eyelids, prolapse of eyelids, pain in the supraorbital region and headache.

2. 攒竹 BL2

【位置与取法】 在面部，当眉头陷中，眶上切迹处。睛明直上眉头凹陷中。(见图 76)

【主治】 口眼㖞斜，目视不明，流泪，目赤肿痛，眼睑瞤动，眼睑下垂；眉棱骨痛，头痛。

2.1.12.3.3 Tianzhu (BL 10)

Location: This acupoint is located in the depression on the lateral aspect of m. trapezius and 1.3 cun lateral to the midpoint of the posterior hairline, about two finger-breadth to Yamen (GV 15). (see Fig. 77)

3. 天柱 BL10

【位置与取法】 在后头部，大筋(斜方肌)外缘之后发际凹陷中，约当后发际正中旁开1.3寸。在哑门穴旁约两横指，斜方肌外缘处。(见图 77)

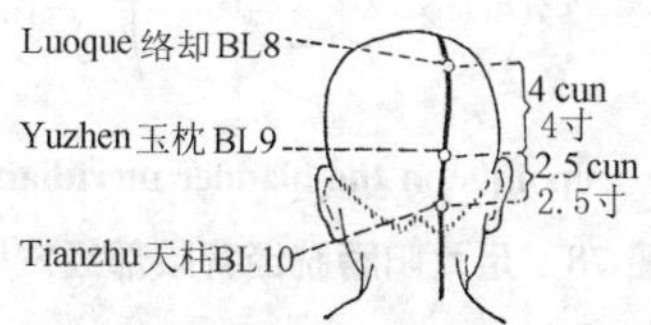

Fig. 77 Head and face acupoints on the bladder meridian of foot-taiyang

图 77 足太阳膀胱经头部经穴图

Indications: Headache, stiff neck, pain in the shoulder and back, nasal obstruction, depressive psychosis and manic psychosis, epilepsy and febrile disease.

【主治】　头痛，项强，肩背痛；鼻塞；癫狂痫证；热病。

2.1.12.3.4　Dazhu (BL 11)

4. 大杼　BL11

Location: This acupoint is located below and 1.5 cun lateral to the spinous process of the first thoracic vertebra (see Fig. 77).

【位置与取法】　在背部，当第一胸椎棘突下，旁开 1.5 寸（见图 77）。

Indications: Stiff neck, pain in the shoulder and back, headache, nasal obstruction, sore throat, cough and fever.

【主治】　项强，肩背痛；头痛，鼻塞，咽喉肿痛；咳嗽；发热。

Note: One of the eight confluent acupoints associating with bones.

【备注】　八会穴之"骨会"。

2.1.12.3.5　Fengmen (BL 12)

5. 风门　BL12

Location: This acupoint is located below and 1.5 cun lateral to the spinous process of the second thoracic vertebra (see Fig. 78).

【位置与取法】　在背部，当第二胸椎棘突下，旁开 1.5 寸（见图 78）。

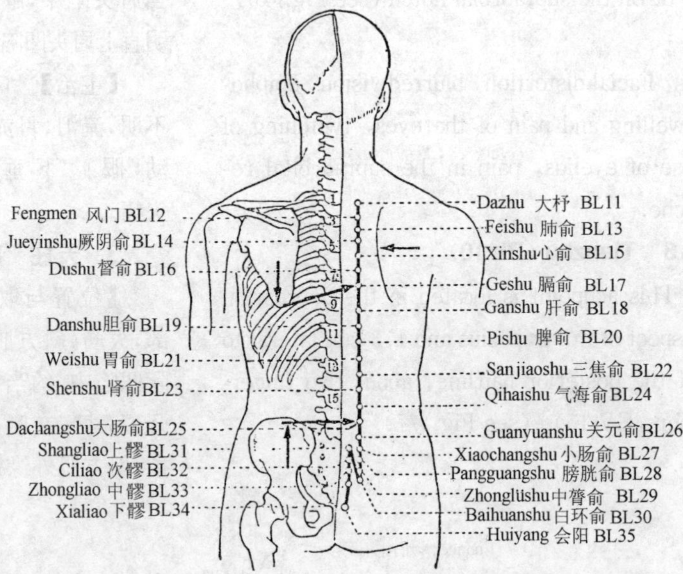

Fig. 78　Back acupoints on the bladder meridian of foot-taiyang

图 78　足太阳膀胱经背腰部经穴图

Indications: Common cold, cough, nasal obstruction, running nose, fever, headache, stiff neck and pain in the

【主治】　伤风，咳嗽，鼻塞，流涕，发热头痛；项强，胸

chest and back.

背痛。

2.1.12.3.6 Feishu (BL 13)

Location: This acupoint is located below and 1.5 cun lateral to the spinous process of the third thoracic vertebra (see Fig. 78).

Indications: Cough, asthma, hematemesis, hemoptysis, bone-steaming fever, tidal fever, night sweating and nasal obstruction.

6. 肺俞 BL13

【位置与取法】 在背部，当第三胸椎棘突下，旁开 1.5 寸(见图 78)。

【主治】 咳嗽，气喘；咯血，咳血；骨蒸，潮热，盗汗；鼻塞。

2.1.12.3.7 Jueyinshu (BL 14)

Location: This acupoint is located below and 1.5 cun lateral to the spinous process of the fourth thoracic vertebra (see Fig. 78).

Indications: Angina pectoris, palpitation, vomiting, cough and chest oppression.

7. 厥阴俞 BL14

【位置与取法】 在背部，当第四胸椎棘突下，旁开 1.5 寸(见图 78)。

【主治】 心痛，心悸；呕吐；咳嗽，胸闷。

2.1.12.3.8 Xinshu (BL 15)

Location: This acupoint is located below and 1.5 cun lateral to the spinous process of the fifth thoracic vertebra (see Fig. 78).

Indications: Angina pectoris, palpitation, hematemesis, insomnia, amnesia, dreaminess, epilepsy, cough and night sweating.

8. 心俞 BL15

【位置与取法】 在背部，当第五胸椎棘突下，旁开 1.5 寸(见图 78)。

【主治】 心痛，惊悸，吐血；失眠，健忘，多梦，癫痫；咳嗽，盗汗。

2.1.12.3.9 Dushu (BL 16)

Location: This acupoint is located below and 1.5 cun lateral to the spinous process of the sixth thoracic vertebra (see Fig. 78).

Indications: Angina pectoris, chest oppression, asthma, abdominal pain and alternate chills and fever.

9. 督俞 BL16

【位置与取法】 在背部，当第六胸椎棘突下，旁开 1.5 寸(见图 78)。

【主治】 心痛；胸闷，气喘；腹痛；寒热。

2.1.12.3.10 Geshu (BL 17)

Location: This acupoint is located below and 1.5 cun lateral to the spinous process of the seventh thoracic vertebra. It is on the level with both interior angles of scapulas. (see Fig. 78)

Indications: Vomiting, hiccup, hematemesis, asthma, cough, tidal fever and night sweating.

10. 膈俞 BL17

【位置与取法】 在背部，当第七胸椎棘突下，旁开 1.5 寸。平两肩胛下角(见图 78)。

【主治】 呕吐，呃逆，吐血；气喘，咳嗽，潮热，盗汗。

Note: One of the eight confluent acupoints associating with blood.

【备注】 八会穴之“血会”。

2.1.12.3.11 Ganshu (BL 18)

11. 肝俞　BL18

Location: This acupoint is located below and 1.5 cun lateral to the spinous process of the ninth thoracic vertebra (see Fig. 78).

【位置与取法】 在背部，当第九胸椎棘突下，旁开1.5寸(见图78)。

Indications: Jaundice, hypochondriac pain, hematemesis, redness of eyes, dizziness, night blindness, depressive psychosis, manic psychosis, epilepsy and pain in the back and spine.

【主治】 黄疸，胁痛，吐血；目赤，目眩，雀目；癫狂痫证；脊背痛。

2.1.12.3.12 Danshu (BL 19)

12. 胆俞　BL19

Location: This acupoint is located below and 1.5 cun lateral to the spinous process of the tenth thoracic vertebra (see Fig. 78).

【位置与取法】 在背部，当第十胸椎棘突下，旁开1.5寸(见图78)。

Indications: Jaundice, bitter taste in the mouth, hypochondriac pain, lung tuberculosis and tidal fever.

【主治】 黄疸，口苦，胁痛；肺痨，潮热。

2.1.12.3.13 Pishu (BL 20)

13. 脾俞　BL20

Location: This acupoint is located below and 1.5 cun lateral to the spinous process of the eleventh thoracic vertebra (see Fig. 78).

【位置与取法】 在背部，当第十一胸椎棘突下，旁开1.5寸(见图78)。

Indications: Abdominal distension, jaundice, vomiting, diarrhea, dysentery, hematochezia, edema and backache.

【主治】 腹胀，黄疸，呕吐，泄泻，痢疾，便血，水肿；背痛。

2.1.12.3.14 Weishu (BL 21)

14. 胃俞　BL21

Location: This acupoint is located below and 1.5 cun lateral to the spinous process of the twelfth thoracic vertebra (see Fig. 78).

【位置与取法】 在背部，当第十二胸椎棘突下，旁开1.5寸(见图78)。

Indications: Stomachache, vomiting, hiccup, abdominal distension, borborygmus and pain in the chest and back.

【主治】 胃脘痛，呕吐，呃逆，腹胀，肠鸣；胸背痛。

2.1.12.3.15 Sanjiaoshu (BL 22)

15. 三焦俞　BL22

Location: This acupoint is located below and 1.5 cun lateral to the spinous process of the first lumbar vertebra (see Fig. 78).

【位置与取法】 在腰部，当第一腰椎棘突下，旁开1.5寸(见图78)。

Indications: Borborygmus, abdominal distension,

【主治】 肠鸣，腹胀，呕

vomiting, diarrhea, dysentery, edema and stiffness and pain in the loins and back.

吐,泄泻,痢疾,水肿;腰背强痛。

2.1.12.3.16 Shenshu (BL 23)

Location: This acupoint is located below and 1.5 cun lateral to the spinous process of the second lumbar vertebra (see Fig. 78).

Indications: Enuresis, seminal emission, impotence, irregular menstruation, leukorrhea, edema, tinnitus, deafness and lumbago.

16. 肾俞 BL23

【位置与取法】 在腰部,当第二腰椎棘突下,旁开 1.5 寸。平两肋弓下缘(见图 78)。

【主治】 遗尿;遗精,阳痿;月经不调,带下;水肿;耳鸣,耳聋;腰痛。

2.1.12.3.17 Qihaishu (BL 24)

Location: This acupoint is located below and 1.5 cun lateral to the spinous process of the third lumbar vertebra (see Fig. 78).

Indications: Borborygmus, abdominal distension, hemorrhoids, dysmenorrhea and lumbago.

17. 气海俞 BL24

【位置与取法】 在腰部,当第三腰椎棘突下,旁开 1.5 寸(见图 78)。

【主治】 肠鸣腹胀,痔漏;痛经;腰痛。

2.1.12.3.18 Dachangshu (BL 25)

Location: This acupoint is located below and 1.5 cun lateral to the spinous process of the fourth lumbar vertebra. It is on the level with both iliac crest. (see Fig. 78)

Indications: Abdominal distension, borborygmus, diarrhea, constipation, dysentery and lumbago.

18. 大肠俞 BL25

【位置与取法】 在腰部,当第四腰椎棘突下,旁开 1.5 寸。平两髂嵴(见图 78)。

【主治】 腹胀,肠鸣,泄泻,便秘,痢疾;腰痛。

2.1.12.3.19 Guanyuanshu (BL 26)

Location: This acupoint is located below and 1.5 cun lateral to the spinous process of the fifth lumbar vertebra (see Fig. 78).

Indications: Abdominal distension, diarrhea, frequent or unsmooth urination, enuresis and lumbago.

19. 关元俞 BL26

【位置与取法】 在腰部,当第五腰椎棘突下,旁开 1.5 寸(见图 78)。

【主治】 腹胀,泄泻;小便频数或不利,遗尿;腰痛。

2.1.12.3.20 Xiaochangshu (BL 27)

Location: This acupoint is located 1.5 cun lateral to median sacral crest and at the level of the first posterior sacral foramen (see Fig. 78).

Indications: Abdominal distension, diarrhea, dysentery, enuresis, hematuria, seminal emission, irregular menstruation, leukorrhea and lumbago.

20. 小肠俞 BL27

【位置与取法】 在骶部,当骶正中嵴旁开 1.5 寸,平第一骶后孔(见图 78)。

【主治】 腹胀,泄泻,痢疾;遗尿,尿血;遗精;月经不调,带下;腰痛。

2.1.12.3.21 Pangguangshu (BL 28)

Location: This acupoint is located 1.5 cun lateral to median sacral crest and on the level with the second posterior sacral foramen (see Fig. 78).

Indications: Dysuria, enuresis, retention of urine, diarrhea, constipation and stiffness and pain in the loins and spine.

21. 膀胱俞　BL28

【位置与取法】 在骶部，当骶正中嵴旁开1.5寸，平第二骶后孔(见图78)。

【主治】 小便不利，遗尿，癃闭；泄泻，便秘；腰脊强痛。

2.1.12.3.22 Zhonglüshu (BL 29)

Location: This acupoint is located 1.5 cun lateral to median sacral crest and on the level with the third posterior sacral foramen (see Fig. 78).

Indications: Diarrhea, hernia and stiffness and pain in the loins and spine.

22. 中膂俞　BL29

【位置与取法】 在骶部，当骶正中嵴旁开1.5寸，平第三骶后孔(见图78)。

【主治】 泄泻，疝气；腰脊强痛。

2.1.12.3.23 Baihuanshu (BL 30)

Location: This acupoint is located 1.5 lateral to median sacral crest and on the level with the fourth posterior sacral foramen (see Fig. 78).

Indications: Enuresis, hernia, seminal emission, irregular menstruation, leukorrhea and pain in lumbosacral region.

23. 白环俞　BL30

【位置与取法】 在骶部，当骶正中嵴旁开1.5寸，平第四骶后孔(见图78)。

【主治】 遗尿，疝气，遗精；月经不调，带下；腰骶疼痛。

2.1.12.3.24 Shangliao (BL 31)

Location: This acupoint is located between posterior superior iliac and the posterior midline and in the first posterior sacral foramen (see Fig. 78).

Indications: Dysuria, seminal emission, impotence, irregular menstruation, leukorrhea, prolapse of uterus and lumbago.

24. 上髎　BL31

【位置与取法】 在骶部，当髂后上棘与后正中线之间，适对第一骶后孔处(见图78)。

【主治】 小便不利，遗精，阳痿；月经不调，带下，阴挺；腰痛。

2.1.12.3.25 Ciliao (BL 32)

Location: This acupoint is located medial and inferior to the posterior superior iliac and the posterior midline, in the second posterior sacral foramen and approximately the midpoint of Pangguangshu (BL 28) and the midline on the back (see Fig. 78).

Indications: Irregular menstruation, dysmenorrhea,

25. 次髎　BL32

【位置与取法】 在骶部，当髂后上棘内下方，适对第二骶后孔处。约当膀胱俞与背正中线的中点(见图78)。

【主治】 月经不调，痛

leukorrhea, hernia, dysuria, seminal emission, impotence, lumbago and flaccidity and obstruction syndromes of lower limbs.

经;带下;疝气;小便不利;遗精;腰痛,下肢痿痹。

2.1.12.3.26 Zhongliao (BL 33)

Location: This acupoint is located medial and inferior to Ciliao (BL 32) and in the third posterior sacral foramen (see Fig. 78).

Indications: Constipation, diarrhea, unsmooth urination, irregular menstruation, leukorrhea and lumbago.

26. 中髎 BL33

【位置与取法】 在骶部,当次髎下内方,适对第三骶后孔处(见图 78)。

【主治】 便秘,泄泻;小便不利;月经不调;带下;腰痛。

2.1.12.3.27 Xialiao (BL 34)

Location: This acupoint is located inferior to Zhongliao (BL 33) and in the fourth posterior sacral foramen (see Fig. 78).

Indications: Abdominal pain, constipation, unsmooth urination, leukorrhea, irregular menstruation and lumbago.

27. 下髎 BL34

【位置与取法】 在骶部,当中、下髎内方,适对第四骶后孔处(见图 78)。

【主治】 腹痛,便秘;小便不利;带下;月经不调;腰痛。

2.1.12.3.28 Huiyang (BL 35)

Location: This acupoint is located 0.5 cun lateral to the coccyx (see Fig. 78).

Indications: Diarrhea, hematochezia, hemorrhoids, impotence and leukorrhea.

28. 会阳 BL35

【位置与取法】 在骶部,尾骨端旁开 0.5 寸(见图 78)。

【主治】 泄泻,便血,痔疾;阳痿;带下。

2.1.12.3.29 Chengfu (BL 36)

Location: This acupoint is located posterior to the thigh and in the midpoint of the transverse gluteal crease (see Fig. 79).

29. 承扶 BL36

【位置与取法】 在大腿后面,臀下横纹的中点(见图79)。

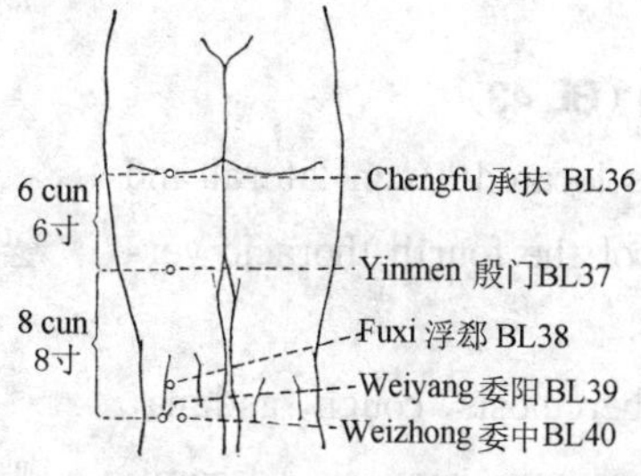

Fig. 79 Lower limb acupoints on the bladder meridian of foot-taiyang

图 79 足太阳膀胱经下肢部经穴图

Indications: Hemorrhoids, pain in the waist, sacrum, buttocks and thigh.

【主治】 痔疾;腰、骶、臀、股部疼痛。

2.1.12.3.30 Yinmen (BL 37)

30. 殷门 BL37

Location: This acupoint is located posterior to the thigh, on the line joining Chengfu (BL 36) and Weizhong (BL 40) and 6 cun below Chengfu (BL 36).

【位置与取法】 在大腿后面,当承扶与委中的连线上,承扶下6寸(见图79)。

Indications: Lumbago and flaccidity and obstruction syndromes of lower limbs.

【主治】 腰痛,下肢痿痹。

2.1.12.3.31 Weiyang (BL 39)

31. 委阳 BL39

Location: This acupoint is located on the lateral side of the popliteal transverse crease and on the medial border of the tendon of m. biceps femoris (see Fig. 79).

【位置与取法】 在腘横纹外侧端,当股二头肌腱的内侧(见图79)。

Indications: Abdominal fullness, dysuria, stiffness and pain in the waist and spine as well as spasmodic pain in the legs and foot.

【主治】 腹满,小便不利;腰脊强痛,腿足挛痛。

Note: Lower He-Sea acupoint of the triple energizer meridian of hand-shaoyang.

【备注】 手少阳经之"下合穴"。

2.1.12.3.32 Weizhong (BL 40)

32. 委中 BL40

Location: This acupoint is located on the midpoint of the popliteal transverse crease and between the tendons of m. biceps femoris and m. semitendinosus (see Fig. 79 and 81).

【位置与取法】 在腘横纹中点,当股二头肌腱与半腱肌肌腱的中间(见图79、图81)。

Indications: Lumbago, flaccidity and obstruction syndromes of lower limbs, dysuria, enuresis, abdominal pain, vomiting, diarrhea and erysipelas.

【主治】 腰痛,下肢痿痹;小便不利,遗尿;腹痛,吐泻;丹毒。

Note: He-Sea acupoint of the bladder meridian of foot-taiyang.

【备注】 足太阳经之"合"穴。

2.1.12.3.33 Gaohuang (BL 43)

33. 膏肓 BL43

Location: This acupoint is located 3 cun lateral and inferior to the spinous process of the fourth thoracic vertebra (see Fig. 80).

【位置与取法】 在背部,当第四胸椎棘突下,旁开3寸(见图80)。

Indications: Pulmonary tuberculosis, cough, asthma, hemoptysis, night sweating, insomnia, amnesia, dreaminess, seminal emission and dyspepsia.

【主治】 肺痨,咳嗽,气喘,咳血,盗汗;失眠,健忘,多梦;遗精;完谷不化。

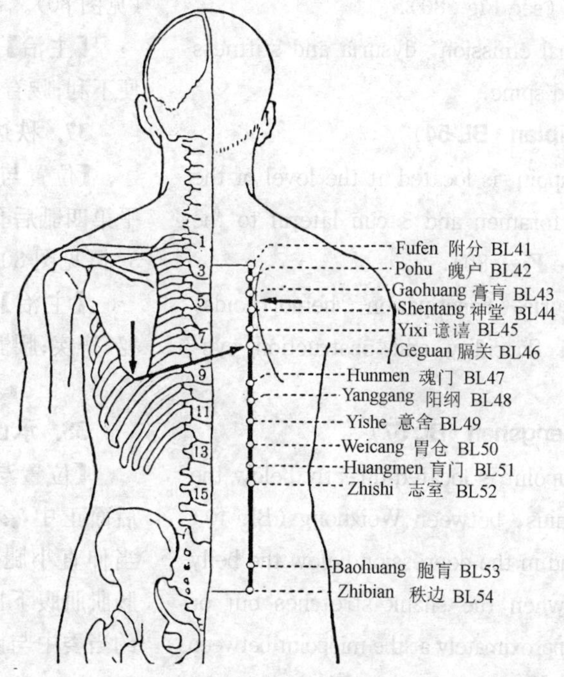

Fig. 80 Back acupoints on the bladder meridian of foot-taiyang

图 80 足太阳膀胱经背腰部经穴图

2.1.12.3.34 Geguan (BL 46)

Location: This acupoint is located 3 cun lateral and nferior to the spinous process of the seventh thoracic verebra (see Fig. 80).

Indications: Vomiting, belching, hiccup, chest opression and stiffness and pain in the spine and back.

2.1.12.3.35 Yanggang (BL 48)

Location: This acupoint is located 3 cun lateral and nferior to the spinous process of the tenth thoracic vertera (see Fig. 80).

Indications: Borborygmus, abdominal pain, diarrhea, undice, hypochondriac pain and diabetes.

2.1.12.3.36 Zhishi (BL 52)

Location: This acupoint is located on the waist and 3 n lateral and inferior to the spinous process of the

34. 膈关 BL46

【位置与取法】 在背部，当第七胸椎棘突下，旁开 3 寸(见图 80)。

【主治】 呕吐，嗳气，呃逆；胸闷；脊背强痛。

35. 阳纲 BL48

【位置与取法】 在背部，当第十胸椎棘突下，旁开 3 寸(见图 80)。

【主治】 肠鸣，腹痛，泄泻；黄疸；胁痛；消渴。

36. 志室 BL52

【位置与取法】 在腰部，当第二腰椎棘突下，旁开 3 寸

second lumbar vertebra (see Fig. 80).

（见图 80）。

Indications: Seminal emission, dysuria and stiffness and pain in the loins and spine.

【主治】 遗精，阳痿，小便不利；腰脊强痛。

2.1.12.3.37 Zhibian (BL 54)

37. 秩边 BL54

Location: This acupoint is located at the level of the fourth posterior sacral foramen and 3 cun lateral to the median sacral crest (see Fig. 80).

【位置与取法】 在臀部，平第四骶后孔，骶正中嵴旁开 3 寸(见图 80)。

Indications: Dysuria, constipation, hemorrhoids, lumbosacral pain, and flaccidity and obstruction syndromes of lower limbs.

【主治】 小便不利，便秘，痔疾；腰骶痛，下肢痿痹。

2.1.12.3.38 Chengshan (BL 57)

38. 承山 BL57

Location: This acupoint is located directly below the belly of m. gastrocnemius, between Weizhong (BL 40) and Kunlun (BL 60) and in the depression below the belly of m. gastrocnemius when the shank stretches out or when the heel lifts up, approximately at the midpoint between Weizhong (BL 40) and tendo calcaneus (see Fig. 81).

【位置与取法】 在小腿后面正中，委中与昆仑之间，当伸直小腿或足跟上提时腓肠肌肌腹下出现尖角凹陷处。约当委中与跟腱之中点(见图 81)。

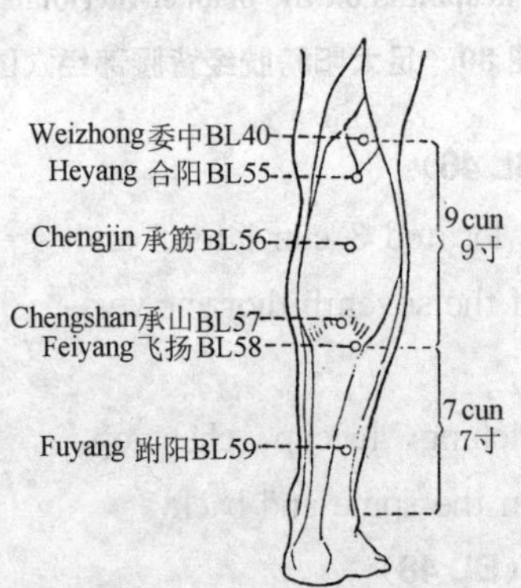

Fig. 81 Lower limb acupoints on the bladder meridian of foot-taiyang

图 81 足太阳膀胱经下肢部经穴图

Indications: Spasmodic pain in the loins and legs, spasm of gastrocnemius, hemorrhoids, constipation, hematochezia and prolapse of rectum.

【主治】 腰腿拘急疼痛转筋；痔疾，便秘，便血，脱肛。

2.1.12.3.39 Feiyang (BL 58)

39. 飞扬 BL58

Location: This acupoint is located on the posterior side of the shank, posterior to the external malleolus, 7

【位置与取法】 在小腿后面，当外踝后，昆仑穴直上

cun directly above Kunlun (BL 60) and 1 cun lateral and inferior to Chengshan (BL 57) (see Fig. 81).

寸，承山外下方 1 寸处(见图 81)。

Indications: Headache, dizziness, epistaxis, pain in the waist and leg and hemorrhoids.

【主治】 头痛，目眩，鼽衄；腰腿疼痛；痔疾。

Note: Luo-Connecting acupoint of the bladder meridian of foot-taiyang.

【备注】 足太阳经之“络”穴。

2.1.12.3.40 Fuyang (BL 59)

40. 跗阳 BL59

Location: This acupoint is located on the back of the shank posterior to the external malleolus and 3 cun directly above Kunlun (BL 60).

【位置与取法】 在小腿后面，外踝后，昆仑直上 3 寸(见图 82)。

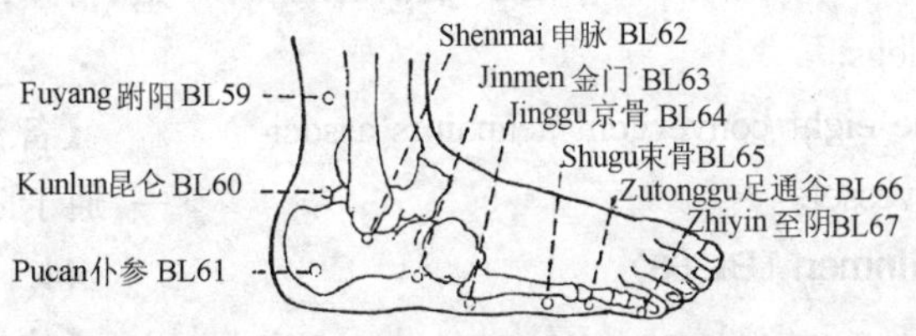

Fig. 82 Foot acupoints on the bladder meridian of foot-taiyang

图 82 足太阳膀胱经足部经穴图

Indications: Headache, lumbosacral pain, flaccidity and obstruction syndromes of lower limbs and swelling and pain of external malleolus.

【主治】 头痛；腰骶疼痛，下肢痿痹，外踝肿痛。

Note: Xi-Cleft acupoint of the yang heel vessel.

【备注】 阳蹻脉之“郄”穴。

2.1.12.3.41 Kunlun (BL 60)

41. 昆仑 BL60

Location: This acupoint is located posterior to the external malleolus and in the depression between the external malleolus and tendo calcaneus (see Fig. 82).

【位置与取法】 在足部外踝后方，当外踝尖与跟腱之间的凹陷处(见图 82)。

Indications: Headache, stiffness of neck, dizziness, epistaxis, epilepsy, dystocia, lumbosacral pain and swelling and pain in heel.

【主治】 头痛，项强；目眩；鼻衄；癫痫；难产；腰骶疼痛，脚跟肿痛。

Note: Jing-River acupoint of the bladder meridian of foot-taiyang.

【备注】 足太阳经之“经”穴。

2.1.12.3.42 Pucan (BL 61)

42. 仆参 BL61

Location: This acupoint is located on the lateral side of the foot, posterior to the external malleolus, directly

【位置与取法】 在足外侧部，外踝后下方，昆仑直下，

below Kunlun (BL 60), lateral to calcaneus and at the junction of the red and white skin (see Fig. 82).

Indications: Flaccidity and obstruction syndromes of lower limbs, pain in the heel and epilepsy.

跟骨外侧，赤白肉际处(见图82)。

【主治】 下肢痿痹，足跟痛；癫痫。

2.1.12.3.43 Shenmai (BL 62)

Location: This acupoint is located lateral to the foot and in the depression directly below the external malleolus (see Fig. 82).

Indications: Headache, dizziness, redness and pain of eyes, twitching of eyelids, depressive psychosis, manic psychosis, epilepsy, insomnia, somnolence and aching pain in the loins and legs.

Note: One of the eight convergent acupoints associating with yang heel vessel.

43. 申脉 BL62

【位置与取法】 在足外侧部，外踝直下方凹陷中(见图82)。

【主治】 头痛，眩晕，目赤痛，眼睑瞤动；癫狂痫，失眠，嗜睡；腰腿酸痛。

【备注】 八脉交会穴之一，通于阳蹻脉。

2.1.12.3.44 Jinmen (BL 63)

Location: This acupoint is located lateral to the foot, directly below the anterior border of the external malleolus and below the border of femur (see Fig. 82).

Indications: Headache, epilepsy, infantile convulsion, lumbago, flaccidity and obstruction syndromes of lower limbs and pain in the external malleolus.

Note: Xi-Cleft acupoint of the bladder meridian of foot-taiyang.

44. 金门 BL63

【位置与取法】 在足外侧，当外踝前缘直下，骰骨下缘处(见图82)。

【主治】 头痛；癫痫，小儿惊风；腰痛，下肢痿痹，外踝痛。

【备注】 足太阳经之"郄"穴。

2.1.12.3.45 Jinggu (BL 64)

Location: This acupoint is located lateral to the foot, below the tuberosit of the fifth metatarsal bone and at the junction of the red and white skin (see Fig. 82).

Indications: Headache, stiffness of neck, cataract, epilepsy and lumbago.

Note: Yuan-Source acupoint of the bladder meridian of foot-taiyang.

45. 京骨 BL64

【位置与取法】 在足外侧，第五跖骨粗隆下方，赤白肉际处(见图82)。

【主治】 头痛，项强；目翳；癫痫；腰痛。

【备注】 足太阳经之"原"穴。

2.1.12.3.46 Shugu (BL 65)

Location: This acupoint is located lateral to the foot, posterior to the head of the fifth metatarsal bone and at

46. 束骨 BL65

【位置与取法】 在足外侧，足小趾本节(第五跖趾关节)的

the junction of the red and white skin (see Fig. 82).

后方，赤白肉际处(见图82)。

Indications: Headache, stiffness of neck, dizziness, depressive psychosis, manic psychosis, and pain in the loins and legs.

【主治】 头痛，项强；目眩；癫狂；腰腿痛。

Note: Shu-Stream acupoint of the bladder meridian of foot-taiyang.

【备注】 足太阳经之“输”穴。

2.1.12.3.47 Zutonggu (BL 66)

47. 足通谷 BL66

Location: This acupoint is located lateral to the foot, anterior to the head of the fifth metatarsal bone and at the junction of the red and white skin (see Fig. 82).

【位置与取法】 在足外侧，足小趾本节(第五跖趾关节)的前方，赤白肉际处(见图82)。

Indications: Headache, stiffness of neck, dizziness, epistaxis, depressive psychosis, and manic psychosis.

【主治】 头痛，项强；目眩；鼻衄；癫狂。

Note: Ying-Spring acupoint of the bladder meridian of foot-taiyang.

【备注】 足太阳经之“荥”穴。

2.1.12.3.48 Zhiyin (BL 67)

48. 至阴 BL67

Location: This acupoint is located on the lateral side of the small toe, about 0.1 cun posterior to the corner of the nail (see Fig. 82).

【位置与取法】 在足小趾末节外侧，距趾甲角 0.1 寸(见图82)。

Indications: Headache, pain of eyes, nasal obstruction, epistaxis, malposition of fetus and dystocia.

【主治】 头痛；目痛；鼻塞，鼻衄；胎位不正，难产。

Note: Jing-Well acupoint of the bladder meridian of foot-taiyang.

【备注】 足太阳经之“井”穴。

2.2 Eight extraordinary vessels

第二节 奇经八脉

2.2.1 Governor vessel

一、督脉

2.2.1.1 Cyclical flowing and distribution

(一) 经脉循行

The governor vessel starts from the uterus, runs downward to the central region of the pelvis around the genitals and into the external orifice of the urethra in women and around penis in men. It joins the conception and thoroughfare vessels over perineum, passes by the anus, moves upward from inside the coccyx and sacrum,

督脉起于胞宫，下向骨盆的中央，络循阴器——在女子入系溺孔、男子循阴茎，与任、冲脉会合于会阴，绕过肛门之后，从尾骶沿脊内上行，到项后风府穴进入脑内，连属于

and enters the brain from Fengfu (GV 16). The external portion runs to the lower end of the nose bridge from the vertex through the forehead and ends at the gum. The first branch runs side by side with the kidney meridian, enters the spine from the coccyx and sacrum region and links with the kidney. The second branch runs side by side with the trunk of the bladder meridian, ascends from the inner canthus, reaches the vertex and links with the brain. Then it runs downward the neck beside the spine, reaches the waist, enters the muscles beside the spine, connects with the kidney and joins the branches of the bladder and kidney meridians in the kidney. The third branch arises directly from the uterus and through the umbilicus. Then it passes through the heart, enters the throat, comes to the mandible, runs around the lips and ends below the eyes (see Fig. 83).

脑,其外从头顶正中经前额到鼻柱下端,至龈交而止。督脉循行的旁支:一支在下部与足少阴肾经同行,在肛门之后尾骶部贯脊,连属于肾;一支在上部与足太阳膀胱经的主干同行,从目内眦上行,交巅顶,络脑,下项,挟脊两旁,抵达腰中,入循脊柱两旁肌肉,连络于肾,足太阳、足少阴同行支在肾中会合;一支前行,自少腹中之胞宫直上,穿过脐中央,经过心,入于喉咙,上至下颌部,环绕唇口,上系于两目之下(见图 83)。

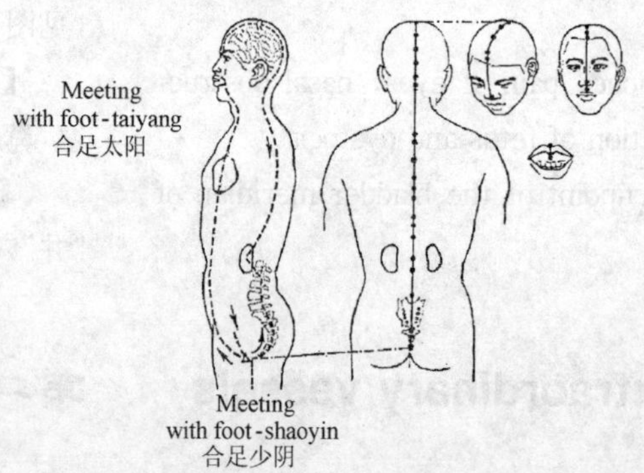

Fig. 83 Flowing route of the governor vessel

图 83 督脉循行示意图

Associated viscera: Heart, kidney, brain and marrow.

Associated organs: Nose, eyes, lips, throat, genitalia and anus.

联系脏腑:心、肾、脑、髓。

联系器官:鼻、目、唇口、喉咙、阴器、肛门。

2.2.1.2 Indications

(二)主治要点

Mental problems, febrile disease, disorders of the lumbosacral region, back and head as well as diseases of

本经腧穴主治神志病,热病,腰骶、背、头项局部病证及

the related viscera.

2.2.1.3 Commonly used acupoints

2.2.1.3.1 Changqiang (GV 1)

Location: This acupoint is at the midpoint between the tip of the coccyx and the anus in prone position when patient kneels or touches the knees with the chest (see Fig. 84).

相应的内脏疾病。

（三）常用腧穴

1. 长强 GV1

【位置与取法】 跪伏，或胸膝位，在尾骨端下，当尾骨端与肛门连线的中点处（见图 84）。

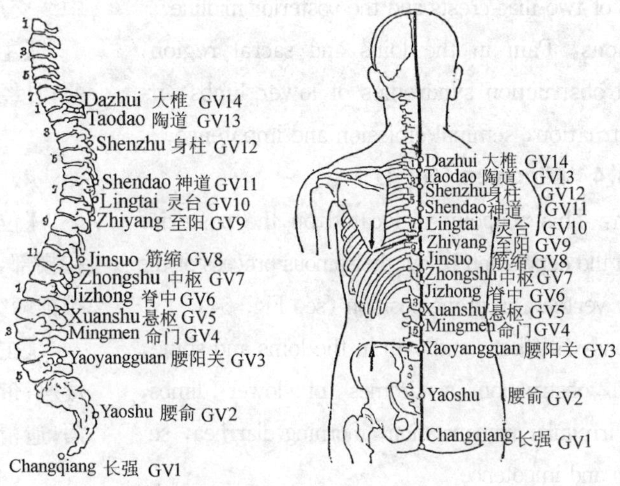

Fig. 84 Back acupoints on the governor vessel

图 84 督脉背腰部经穴图

Indications: Constipation, hematochezia, hemorrhoids, prolapse of rectum, depressive psychosis, manic psychosis, epilepsy, rigid and arched back, and pain in the coccyx and sacrum region.

Note: Luo-Connecting acupoint of the governor vessel.

2.2.1.3.2 Yaoshu (GV 2)

Location: This acupoint is located on the posterior midline and in the hiatus of the sacrum in prone or side-prone position. Or it is located on the midline posterior to the level of the lower borders of two sacral corners when they are pressed (see Fig. 84).

【主治】 便秘，便血，痔疾，脱肛；癫狂痫证；脊强反折，尾骶部疼痛。

【备注】 督脉之“络”穴。

2. 腰俞 GV2

【位置与取法】 俯卧或侧卧位，在骶部，当后正中线上，适对骶管裂孔处（见图 84）。或先按取尾骨上方左右的骶角，在两骶角下缘平齐的后正中线上取穴。

Indications: Stiffness and pain in the loins and spine, flaccidity and obstruction syndromes of lower limbs, irregular menstruation, hemorrhoids and epilepsy.

【主治】 腰脊强痛，下肢痿痹；月经不调；痔疾；癫痫。

2.2.1.3.3 Yaoyangguan (GV 3)

3. 腰阳关 GV3

Location: This acupoint is located on the posterior midline and in the depression below the spinous process of the fourth lumbar vertebra in prone position (see Fig. 84) or in the depression on the midpoint of the line joining the highest points of two iliac crests and the posterior midline.

【位置与取法】 俯卧位，在腰部，当后正中线上，第四腰椎棘突下凹陷中(见图 84)。或两髂嵴高点的连线与后正中线交点处的凹陷中取穴。

Indications: Pain in the loins and sacral region, flaccidity and obstruction syndromes of lower limbs, irregular menstruation, seminal emission and impotence.

【主治】 腰骶痛，下肢痿痹；月经不调；遗精，阳痿。

2.2.1.3.4 Mingmen (GV 4)

4. 命门 GV4

Location: This acupoint is located on the posterior midline and in the depression below the spinous process of the second lumbar vertebra in prone position (see Fig. 84).

【位置与取法】 俯卧位，在腰部，当后正中线上，第二腰椎棘突下凹陷中(见图 84)。

Indications: Stiffness and pain in the loins and spine, flaccidity and obstruction syndromes of lower limbs, leukorrhagia, irregular menstruation, morning diarrhea, seminal emission and impotence.

【主治】 腰脊强痛，下肢痿痹；带下；月经不调；五更肾泻；遗精，阳痿。

2.2.1.3.5 Jizhong (GV 6)

5. 脊中 GV6

Location: This acupoint is located on the posterior midline and in the depression below the spinous process of the eleventh thoracic vertebra in prone position (see Fig. 84).

【位置与取法】 俯卧位，在背部，当后正中线上，第十一胸椎棘突下凹陷中(见图 84)。

Indications: Hemorrhoids, prolapse of rectum, stiffness and pain in the loins and spine, epilepsy, diarrhea, jaundice and infantile malnutrition.

【主治】 痔疾，脱肛；腰脊强痛；癫痫；泄泻；黄疸；小儿疳积。

2.2.1.3.6 Jinsuo (GV 8)

6. 筋缩 GV8

Location: This acupoint is located on the posterior midline and in the depression below the spinous process of the ninth thoracic vertebra in prone position (see Fig. 84).

【位置与取法】 俯卧位，在背部，当后正中线上，第九胸椎棘突下凹陷中(见图 84)。

Indications: Stiffness of spine, flaccidity of limbs, spasm, depressive psychosis, manic psychosis, epilepsy, stomachache and jaundice.

【主治】 脊强，四肢不收，筋挛拘急；癫狂痫证；胃痛，黄疸。

2.2.1.3.7 Zhiyang (GV 9)

Location: This acupoint is located on the posterior midline and in the depression below the spinous process of the seventh thoracic vertebra in prone position (see Fig. 84). Or in the depression on the midpoint on the line joining the line between two infra-scapular angles and the posterior midline.

Indications: Distending pain in the chest and hypochondria, jaundice, cough, stiffness of spine and pain in the back.

7. 至阳 GV9

【位置与取法】 俯卧位，在背部，当后正中线上，第七胸椎棘突下凹陷中(见图 84)。在两肩胛骨下角连线与后正中线的交点处凹陷中取穴。

【主治】 胸胁胀痛，黄疸；咳嗽；脊强，背痛。

2.2.1.3.8 Lingtai (GV 10)

Location: This acupoint is located on the posterior midline and in the depression below the spinous process of the sixth thoracic vertebra in prone position (see Fig. 84).

Indications: Cough, asthma, stiffness and pain in the spine and back as well as carbuncle.

8. 灵台 GV10

【位置与取法】 俯卧位，在背部，当后正中线上，第六胸椎棘突下凹陷中(见图 84)。

【主治】 咳嗽，气喘；脊背强痛；疔疮。

2.2.1.3.9 Shendao (GV 11)

Location: This acupoint is located on the posterior midline and in the depression below the spinous process of the fifth thoracic vertebra in prone position (see Fig. 84).

Indications: Angina pectoris, palpitation, amnesia, insomnia, cough, asthma and stiffness and pain in the spine and back.

9. 神道 GV11

【位置与取法】 俯卧位，在背部，当后正中线上，第五胸椎棘突下凹陷中(见图 84)。

【主治】 心痛，心悸，健忘，失眠；咳嗽，气喘；脊背强痛。

2.2.1.3.10 Shenzhu (GV 12)

Location: This acupoint is located on the posterior midline and in the depression below the spinous process of the third thoracic vertebra in prone position (see Fig. 84). It is located in the depression on the point between the line connecting the two superior points of the scapulae and the posterior midline.

Indications: Cough, asthma, epilepsy and stiffness and pain in the spine and back.

10. 身柱 GV12

【位置与取法】 俯卧位，在背部，当后正中线上，第三胸椎棘突下凹陷中(见图 84)。在两肩胛冈高点连线与后正中线交点处凹陷中取穴。

【主治】 咳嗽，气喘；癫痫；脊背强痛。

2.2.1.3.11 Taodao (GV 13)

Location: This acupoint is located on the posterior midline and in the depression below the spinous process of the first thoracic vertebra in prone position (see Fig. 84).

Indications: Headache, stiff neck, stiffness of spine, aversion to cold, fever, cough, asthma, bone-steaming fever, tidal fever, mania and epilepsy, malaria and back carbuncle.

11. 陶道　GV13

【位置与取法】 俯卧位，在背部，当后正中线上，第一胸椎棘突下凹陷中(见图 84)。

【主治】 头痛，项强，脊强；恶寒发热，咳嗽，气喘，骨蒸潮热；狂痫证；疟疾；疔疮发背。

2.2.1.3.12 Dazhui (GV 14)

Location: This acupoint is located on the posterior midline and in the depression below the spinous process of the seventh cervical vertebra in prone position (see Fig. 84).

Indications: Headache, stiffness of neck, cough, asthma, bone-steaming fever, night sweating, epilepsy, febrile disease, malaria, urticaria and emaciation due to consumptive disease.

12. 大椎　GV14

【位置与取法】 俯卧位，当后正中线上，第七颈椎棘突下凹陷中(见图 84)。

【主治】 头痛项强；咳嗽，气喘，骨蒸盗汗；癫痫；热病；疟疾；风疹；虚劳羸瘦。

2.2.1.3.13 Yamen (GV 15)

Location: This acupoint is located 0.5 cun directly above the midpoint of the posterior hairline and below the first cervical vertebra when the patient sits upright (see Fig. 85).

13. 哑门　GV15

【位置与取法】 正坐位，在项部，当后发际正中直上 0.5 寸，第一颈椎下(见图 85)。

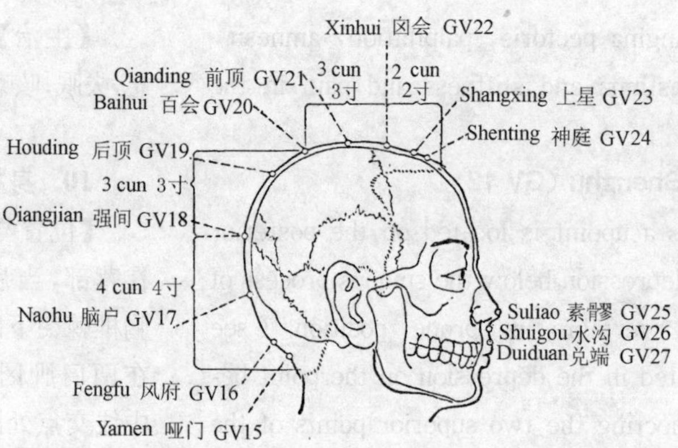

Fig. 85　Head and neck acupoints on the governor vessel

图 85　督脉头颈部经穴图

Indications: Sudden loss of voice, stiff tongue due to apoplexy, headache, stiff neck, depressive psychosis, manic psychosis, and epilepsy.

【主治】 暴喑,中风舌强不语;头痛项强;癫狂痫。

2.2.1.3.14 Fengfu (GV 16)

Location: This acupoint is located 1 cun directly above the midpoint of the posterior hairline, directly below the external occipital protuberance, in the depression between m. trapezius of both sides when the patient sits upright (see Fig. 85).

Indications: Epilepsy, inability to speak after apoplectic seizure, stiff neck, headache, dizziness, sore throat, loss of voice and epistaxis.

14. 风府 GV16

【位置与取法】 正坐位,在项部,当后发际正中直上1寸,枕外粗隆直下,两侧斜方肌之间凹陷中(见图85)。

【主治】 癫痫,中风不语;项强;头痛,眩晕;咽喉肿痛,失音;鼻衄。

2.2.1.3.15 Naohu (GV 17)

Location: This acupoint is located 2.5 cun directly above the posterior hairline, 1.5 cun above Fengfu (GV 16) and in the depression at the upper border of the external occipital protuberance when the patient sits upright (see Fig. 85).

Indications: Headache, dizziness, loss of voice, stiff neck and depressive psychosis and manic psychosis.

15. 脑户 GV17

【位置与取法】 正坐位,在头部,当后发际正中直上2.5寸,风府上1.5寸,枕外粗隆上缘凹陷处(见图85)。

【主治】 头痛,头晕;失音;项强;癫狂。

2.2.1.3.16 Qiangjian (GV 18)

Location: This acupoint is located 4 cun directly above the posterior hairline, 1.5 cun above Naohu (GV 17) (see Fig. 85) and on the midpoint of the line joining Fengfu (GV 16) and Baihui (GV 20) when the patient sits upright.

Indications: Headache, vertigo, facial distortion, stiff neck, epilepsy and insomnia.

16. 强间 GV18

【位置与取法】 正坐位,在头部,当后发际正中直上4寸(脑户上1.5寸)(见图85)。当风府与百会连线的中点取穴。

【主治】 头痛,目眩,口㖞;项强;癫痫,失眠。

2.2.1.3.17 Houding (GV 19)

Location: This acupoint is located 5.5 cun directly above the posterior hairline, 3 cun above Naohu (GV 17) (see Fig. 85) and 0.5 cun posterior to the line joining the anterior and posterior hairlines when the patient sits upright.

17. 后顶 GV19

【位置与取法】 正坐位,在头部,当后发际正中直上5.5寸(脑户上3寸)(见图85)。当前、后发际连线中点向后0.5寸是穴。

Indications: Headache, vertigo, stiffness and pain in the neck, depressive psychosis, manic psychosis, and epilepsy as well as insomnia.

【主治】 头痛，眩晕；颈项强痛；癫狂痫证；失眠。

2.2.1.3.18 Baihui (GV 20)

18. 百会 GV20

Location: This acupoint is located 7 cun directly above the posterior hairline when the patient sits upright (see Fig. 85) or 1 cun anterior to the midpoint on the line joining the anterior and posterior hairlines.

【位置与取法】 正坐位，在头部，当后发际正中直上7寸(见图85)。或于两耳尖连线与头部中线的交点处取穴；或于前、后发际连线中点向前1寸处取穴。

Indications: Headache, vertigo, wind stroke, depressive psychosis, manic psychosis, insomnia, prolapse of rectum, prolapse of uterus, gastroptosis, prolapse of kidney and prolonged diarrhea.

【主治】 头痛，眩晕；中风，癫狂，不寐；脱肛；阴挺；胃下垂；肾下垂；久泄。

2.2.1.3.19 Qianding (GV 21)

19. 前顶 GV21

Location: This acupoint is located 3.5 cun directly above the anterior hairline, 1.5 cun anterior to Baihui (GV 20) when the patient sits upright (see Fig. 85).

【位置与取法】 正坐位，在头部，当前发际正中直上3.5寸(百会前1.5寸)(见图85)。

Indications: Headache, vertigo, nasosinusitis, redness, swelling and pain of eyes as well as epilepsy.

【主治】 头痛，眩晕；鼻渊；目赤肿痛；癫痫。

2.2.1.3.20 Xinhui (GV 22)

20. 囟会 GV22

Location: This acupoint is located 2 cun directly above the anterior hairline, 3 cun anterior to Baihui (GV 20) when the patient sits upright (see Fig. 85).

【位置与取法】 正坐位，在头部，当前发际正中直上2寸(百会前3寸)(见图85)。

Indications: Headache, vertigo, nasosinusitis, epistaxis, nasal polyp, redness, swelling and pain of eyes as well as epilepsy.

【主治】 头痛，眩晕；鼻渊，鼻衄，鼻痔；目赤肿痛；癫痫。

2.2.1.3.21 Shangxing (GV 23)

21. 上星 GV23

Location: This acupoint is located 1 cun directly above the anterior hairline when the patient sits with the back leaning against the chair (see Fig. 85).

【位置与取法】 仰靠坐位，在头部，当前发际正中直上1寸(见图85)。

Indications: Nasal obstruction, nasosinusitis, epistaxis, headache, vertigo, pain of eyes, epiphora with wind, epilepsy, malaria and febrile disease.

【主治】 鼻塞，鼻渊，鼻衄；头痛，眩晕；目痛，迎风流泪；癫痫；疟疾，热病。

2.2.1.3.22 Shenting (GV 24)

Location: This acupoint is located 0.5 cun directly above the anterior hairline when the patient sits with the back leaning against the chair (see Fig. 85).

Indications: Headache, vertigo, nasosinusitis, epistaxis, cataract, epiphora with wind, insomnia and depressive psychosis and manic psychosis.

22. 神庭 GV24

【位置与取法】 仰靠坐位,在头部,当前发际正中直上0.5寸(见图85)。

【主治】 头痛,眩晕;鼻渊,鼻衄;目翳,迎风流泪;失眠,癫狂。

2.2.1.3.23 Suliao (GV 25)

Location: This acupoint is located on the center of the nose tip when the patient sits with the back leaning against the chair (see Fig. 85).

Indications: Nasosinusitis, epistaxis, nasal polyp, running nose, unconsciousness, convulsion and suffocation of the newborn.

23. 素髎 GV25

【位置与取法】 仰靠坐位,在面部,当鼻尖的正中央处(见图85)。

【主治】 鼻渊,鼻衄,鼻痔,鼻流清涕;昏迷,惊厥,新生儿窒息。

2.2.1.3.24 Shuigou (GV 26)

Location: This acupoint is located a little above the midpoint of the philtrum where the superior 1/3 of the philtrum meets with the middle 1/3 when the patient sits with the back leaning against the chair (see Fig. 85).

Indications: Apoplexy, unconsciousness, depressive psychosis and manic psychosis, epilepsy, infantile convulsion, facial distortion, toothache, lockjaw, nasal obstruction, epistaxis, acute sprain of waist, stiff neck and infantile enuresis.

24. 水沟 GV26

【位置与取法】 仰靠坐位,在面部,当人中沟的上1/3与中1/3交点处(见图85)。

【主治】 中风,昏迷,癫狂痫,小儿惊风;口眼㖞斜,齿痛,口噤;鼻塞,鼻衄;急性腰扭伤,落枕;小儿遗尿。

2.2.1.3.25 Yinjiao (GV 28)

Location: This acupoint is located at the junction of the gum and the frenulum of the upper lip when the patient sits with the back leaning against the chair (see Fig. 86).

25. 龈交 GV28

【位置与取法】 仰靠坐位,在上唇内,唇系带与上齿龈的相接处(见图86)。

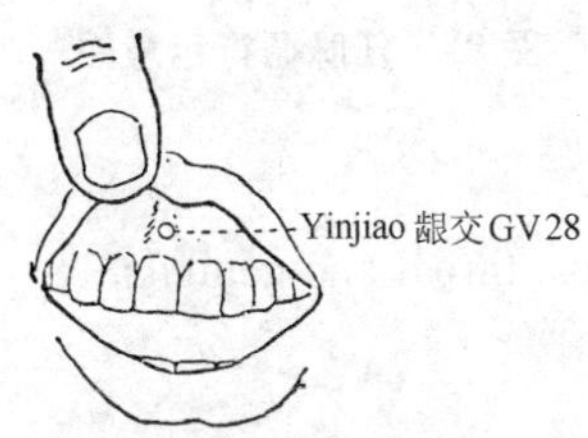

Fig. 86 Acupoint behind the upper lip on the governor vessel

图86 督脉上唇内经穴图

Indications: Swelling and pain of the gum, oral sore, halitosis and depressive psychosis and manic psychosis.

【主治】 齿龈肿痛，口疮，口臭；癫狂。

2.2.2 Conception vessel

二、任脉

2.2.2.1 Cyclical flowing and distribution

（一）循行分布

The conception vessel starts from the uterus and emerges from the perineum. It goes anteriorly to the pubic region and ascends along the interior of the abdomen, passing through Guanyuan (CV 4) and the other points along the front midline to the throat. Ascending further, it curves around the lips, passes through the cheek and enters the infraorbital region. One of its branch runs along with the thoroughfare vessel upward in the spine (see Fig. 87).

任脉起始于胞宫，下出会阴部，经阴器向上到阴毛处，沿腹里，上出关元，沿胸腹正中线上至咽喉部，再经下颌络唇口，沿面部入眼内；一支与冲脉同沿着背脊的里面上行（见图 87）。

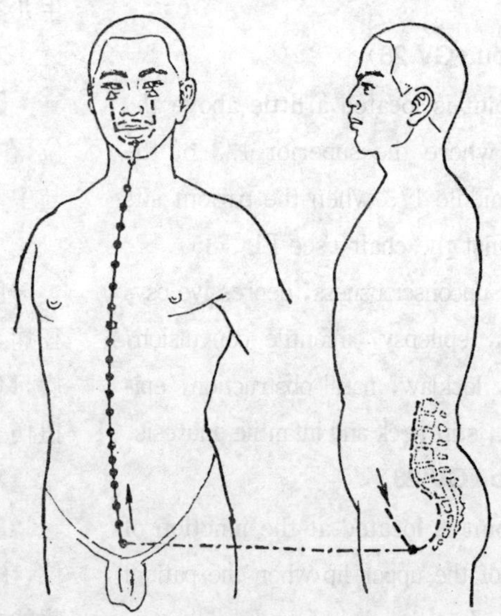

Fig. 87　Flowing route of the conception vessel

图 87　任脉循行示意图

Associated viscus: Uterus.

Associated organs: Lips, eyes, throat and genitals.

联系脏腑：胞宫。

联系器官：唇口、目、咽喉、阴器。

2.2.2.2 Indications

（二）主治要点

Local disorders of the abdomen, chest, neck and

本经腧穴主治腹、胸、颈、

head and diseases of the related viscera. A few of the acupoints on the conception vessel are effective in strengthening the body.

头面的局部病证及相应的内脏器官病证，少数腧穴有强壮作用。

2.2.2.3 Commonly used acupoints

（三）常用腧穴

2.2.2.3.1 Qugu（CV 2）

Location：This acupoint is located on the anterior midline and the midpoint of the upper border of the symphysis pubis in supine position（see Fig. 88）.

Indications：Irregular menstruation，leukorrhea，unsmooth urination，enuresis，seminal emission and impotence.

1. 曲骨 CV2

【位置与取法】 仰卧位，在前正中线上，耻骨联合上缘的中点处(见图 88)。

【主治】 月经不调，带下；小便不利，遗尿；遗精，阳痿。

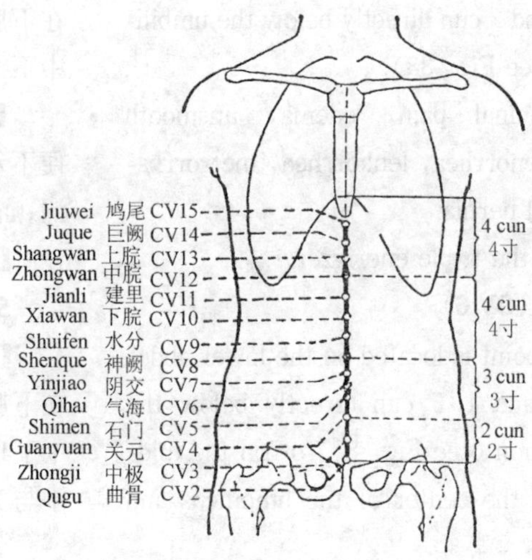

Fig. 88 Abdomen acupoints on the conception vessel

图 88 任脉腹部经穴图

2.2.2.3.2 Zhongji（CV 3）

Location：This acupoint is located on the lower abdomen，anterior midline and 4 cun directly below the umbilicus in supine position（see Fig. 88）.

Indications：Irregular menstruation，metrorrhagia and metrostaxis，leukorrhea，prolapse of uterus，sterility，enuresis，unsmooth urination，hernia，seminal emission and impotence.

Note：Front-Mu acupoint of the bladder.

2. 中极 CV3

【位置与取法】 仰卧位，在下腹部，前正中线上，当脐中下 4 寸(见图 88)。

【主治】 月经不调，崩漏；带下；阴挺；不孕；遗尿，小便不利；疝气；遗精，阳痿。

【备注】 膀胱之“募”穴。

2.2.2.3.3 Guanyuan (CV 4)

Location: This acupoint is located on the lower abdomen, anterior midline and 3 cun directly below the umbilicus in supine position (see Fig. 88).

Indications: Diarrhea, irregular menstruation, leukorrhea, sterility, enuresis, frequent urination, anuria, seminal emission, impotence, hernia and emaciation due to consumptive disease.

Note: Front-Mu acupoint of the small intestine.

2.2.2.3.4 Shimen (CV 5)

Location: This acupoint is located on the lower abdomen, anterior midline and 2 cun directly below the umbilicus in supine position (see Fig. 88).

Indications: Abdominal pain, edema, unsmooth urination, diarrhea, amenorrhea, leukorrhea, metrorrhagia and metrostaxis, and hernia.

Note: Front-Mu of the triple energizer.

2.2.2.3.5 Qihai (CV 6)

Location: This acupoint is located on the lower abdomen, anterior midline and 1.5 cun directly below the umbilicus in supine position (see Fig. 88) or on the midpoint of the line joining the center of the umbilicus and Guanyuan (CV 4).

Indications: Dysmenorrhea, amenorrhea, irregular menstruation, enuresis, seminal emission, hernia, abdominal pain, diarrhea, constipation and prostration.

Note: Yuan-Source acupoint of Huang (middle medialsternum).

2.2.2.3.6 Shenque (CV 8)

Location: This acupoint is located on the center of the abdomen and the umbilicus in supine position (see Fig. 88).

Indications: Abdominal pain, diarrhea, prolapse of rectum, edema and prostration.

3. 关元　CV4

【位置与取法】 仰卧位，在下腹部，前正中线上，当脐中下3寸(见图88)。

【主治】 泄泻；月经不调，带下，不孕；遗尿，小便频数，尿闭；遗精，阳痿，疝气；虚劳羸瘦。

【备注】 小肠之“募”穴。

4. 石门　CV5

【位置与取法】 仰卧位，在下腹部，前正中线上，当脐中下2寸(见图88)。

【主治】 腹痛，水肿，小便不利，泄泻；经闭，带下，崩漏；疝气。

【备注】 三焦之“募”穴。

5. 气海　CV6

【位置与取法】 仰卧位，在下腹部，前正中线上，当脐中下1.5寸(见图88)。或当脐中与关元连线之中点处取穴。

【主治】 痛经，经闭，月经不调；遗尿；遗精；疝气；腹痛，泄泻，便秘；虚脱。

【备注】 肓之“原”穴。

6. 神阙　CV8

【位置与取法】 仰卧位，在腹中部，脐中央(见图88)。

【主治】 腹痛，泄泻，脱肛；水肿；虚脱。

2.2.2.3.7 Shuifen (CV 9)

Location: This acupoint is located on the upper abdomen, anterior midline and 1 cun directly above the umbilicus in supine position (see Fig. 88).

Indications: Abdominal pain, regurgitation, vomiting, diarrhea, anuria and edema.

2.2.2.3.8 Xiawan (CV 10)

Location: This acupoint is located on the upper abdomen, anterior midline and 2 cun directly above the umbilicus in supine position (see Fig. 88).

Indications: Abdominal pain and distension, dyspepsia, vomiting, diarrhea and abdominal mass.

2.2.2.3.9 Jianli (CV 11)

Location: This acupoint is located on the upper abdomen, anterior midline and 3 cun directly above the umbilicus in supine position (see Fig. 88).

Indications: Stomachache, abdominal distension, vomiting, poor appetite and edema.

2.2.2.3.10 Zhongwan (CV 12)

Location: This acupoint is located on the upper abdomen and anterior midline, 4 cun directly above the umbilicus in supine position and at the midpoint between the xiphoid process and the umbilicus (see Fig. 88).

Indications: Stomachache, abdominal distension, vomiting, hiccup, hematemesis, acid regurgitation, jaundice, borborygmus, diarrhea, edema, anorexia, dyspepsia, depressive psychosis, manic psychosis, postpartum syncope due to blood loss, syncope, insomnia, consumptive disease and asthma.

Note: Front-Mu acupoint of the stomach and one of the eight confluent acupoints associating with the fu organs.

2.2.2.3.11 Shangwan (CV 13)

Location: This acupoint is located on the upper abdomen, anterior midline and 5 cun directly above the umbilicus

7. 水分 CV9

【位置与取法】 仰卧位，在上腹部，前正中线上，当脐中上1寸(见图88)。

【主治】 腹痛，翻胃吐食，泄泻；小便不通；水肿。

8. 下脘 CV10

【位置与取法】 仰卧位，在上腹部，前正中线上，当脐中上2寸(见图88)。

【主治】 腹痛，腹胀，食谷不化，呕吐，泄泻；痞块。

9. 建里 CV11

【位置与取法】 仰卧位，在上腹部，前正中线上，当脐中上3寸(见图88)。

【主治】 胃痛，腹胀，呕吐，食欲不振，水肿。

10. 中脘 CV12

【位置与取法】 仰卧位，在上腹部，前正中线上，当脐中上4寸(见图88)。当胸剑联合与脐中连线的中点处是穴。

【主治】 胃痛，腹胀，呕吐，呃逆，吐血，吞酸；黄疸，肠鸣，泄泻，水肿，纳呆，食谷不化；癫狂，产后血晕，晕厥；失眠；虚劳；哮喘。

【备注】 胃之"募"穴，八会穴之"腑会"。

11. 上脘 CV13

【位置与取法】 仰卧位，在上腹部，前正中线上，当脐

in supine position (see Fig. 88).

中上 5 寸(见图 88)。

Indications: Stomachache, vomiting, abdominal distension and epilepsy.

【主治】 胃痛,呕吐,腹胀;癫痫。

2.2.2.3.12 Juque (CV 14)

12. 巨阙　CV14

Location: This acupoint is located on the upper abdomen, anterior midline and 6 cun directly above the umbilicus in supine position (see Fig. 88).

【位置与取法】 仰卧位,在上腹部,前正中线上,当脐中上 6 寸(见图 88)。

Indications: Angina pectoris, dysphoria, palpitation, amnesia, vomiting, acid regurgitation, hiccup, dysphagia, jaundice, depressive psychosis, manic psychosis, and epilepsy.

【主治】 心痛,心烦,心悸,健忘;呕吐,吞酸,呃逆,噎膈,黄疸;癫狂痫证。

Note: Front-Mu acupoint of the heart.

【备注】 心之"募"穴。

2.2.2.3.13 Jiuwei (CV 15)

13. 鸠尾　CV15

Location: This acupoint is located on the upper abdomen, anterior midline and 1 cun directly below the xiphoid process in supine position (see Fig. 88).

【位置与取法】 仰卧位,在上腹部,前正中线上,当胸剑结合部下 1 寸(见图 88)。

Indications: Angina pectoris, dysphoria, palpitation, depressive psychosis, manic psychosis, epilepsy, cough, asthma, chest pain, abdominal distension, vomiting, hiccup, jaundice and diarrhea.

【主治】 心痛,心烦,心悸;癫狂痫证;咳嗽,气喘,胸痛;腹胀,呕吐,呃逆,黄疸,泄利。

Note: Luo-Connecting acupoint of the conception vessel and Yuan-Source acupoint of gao (middle medialsternum).

【备注】 任脉之"络"穴,膏之"原"穴。

2.2.2.3.14 Tanzhong (CV 17)

14. 膻中　CV17

Location: This acupoint is located on the anterior midline in women, at the level with the fourth intercostal space and midway between the nipples in men (see Fig. 89).

【位置与取法】 仰卧位在胸部,女性在前正中线上平第四肋间隙;男性在两乳头连线的中点(见图 89)。

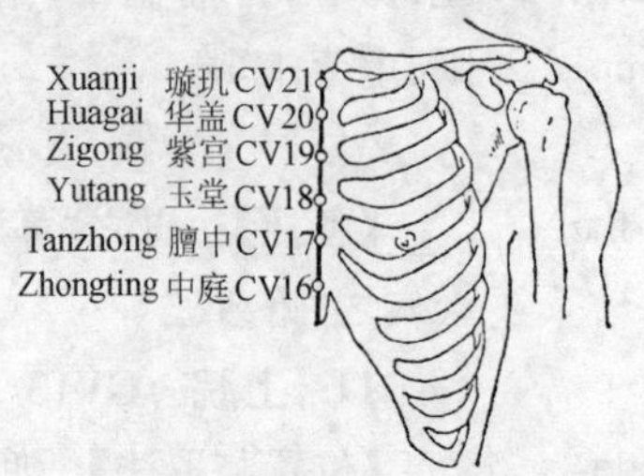

Fig. 89　Chest acupoints on the conception vessel
图 89　任脉胸部经穴图

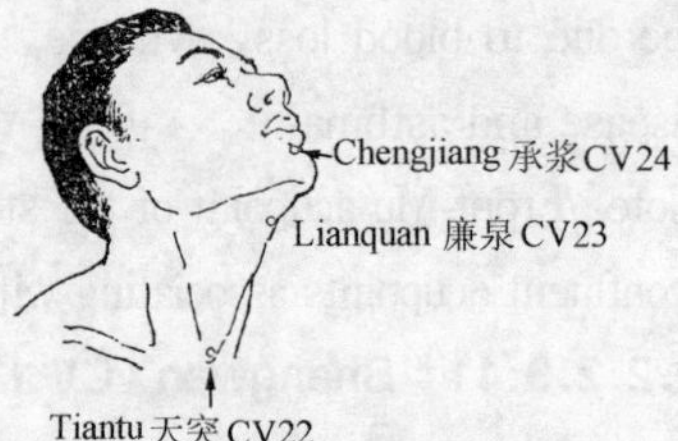

Fig. 90　Neck acupoints on the conception vess
图 90　任脉颈颏部经穴图

Indications: Cough, asthma, chest pain, angina pectoris, palpitation, dysphoria, insomnia, insufficiency of lactation, breast abscess, vomiting and dysphagia.

【主治】 咳嗽,气喘,胸痛;心痛,心悸,心烦,失眠;乳少,乳痛;呕吐,噎膈。

Note: Front-Mu acupoint of the pericardium and one of the eight confluent acupoints associating with qi.

【备注】 心包之"募"穴,八会穴之"气会"。

2.2.2.3.15 Yutang (CV 18)

15. 玉堂 CV18

Location: This acupoint is located on the anterior midline and on the level with the third intercostal space (see Fig. 89).

【位置与取法】 仰卧位,在胸部,当前正中线上,平第三肋间隙(见图 89)。

Indications: Cough, asthma, chest pain and vomiting.

【主治】 咳嗽,气喘,胸痛;呕吐。

2.2.2.3.16 Xuanji (CV 21)

16. 璇玑 CV21

Location: This acupoint is located on the anterior midline and 1 cun below the suprasternal fossa (see Fig. 89).

【位置与取法】 仰卧位,在胸部,当前正中线上,胸骨上窝中央下 1 寸(见图 89)。

Indications: Cough, asthma, chest pain and sore throat.

【主治】 咳嗽,气喘,胸痛;咽喉肿痛。

2.2.2.3.17 Tiantu (CV 22)

17. 天突 CV22

Location: This acupoint is located on the anterior midline and in the suprasternal fossa (see Fig. 90).

【位置与取法】 仰靠坐位,在颈部,当前正中线上,胸骨上窝中央(见图 90)。

Indications: Cough, asthma, chest pain, sore throat, sudden loss of voice, goiter, dysphagia and plum-pit obstructive sensation in the throat.

【主治】 咳嗽,气喘,胸痛;咽喉肿痛,暴喑;瘿气;噎膈;梅核气。

2.2.2.3.18 Lianquan (CV 23)

18. 廉泉 CV23

Location: This acupoint is located on the anterior midline, above the Adam's apple and in the depression of the upper border of the hyoid bone (see Fig. 90).

【位置与取法】 仰靠坐位,在颈部,当前正中线上,喉结上方,舌骨上缘凹陷处(见图 90)。

Indications: Sublingual swelling and pain, sluggish movement of the tongue, drooling, aphasia due to stiff tongue, sudden loss of voice and difficulty in swallowing.

【主治】 舌下肿痛,舌缓流涎,舌强不语,暴喑,吞咽困难。

2.2.2.3.19 Chengjiang (CV 24)

19. 承浆 CV24

Location: This acupoint is located in the depression

【位置与取法】 仰靠坐

in the center of the mentolabial groove (see Fig. 90).

位，在面部，当颏唇沟的正中凹陷处(见图 90)。

Indications: Facial distortion, swelling and pain of gum, drooling and epilepsy.

【主治】 口㖞；齿龈肿痛；流涎；癫痫。

2.2.3 Thoroughfare vessel

三、冲脉

2.2.3.1 Cyclical flowing and distribution

(一) 循行分布

The thoroughfare vessel starts from the uterus. One branch runs along with the conception vessel upwards in the spine. Another branch stems from the uterus, passes through perineum and genitals and comes out from Qijie (pathway of qi). The branch running upward runs with the kidney and stomach meridians upward to the abdomen from Qijie, distributes over the chest, reaches the throat and emerges from the upper part of the throat and posterior part of the nose canal. From there it forks sub-branches to link the lips and mouth and other yang meridians over the head and face. The branch running downward moves downward from Qijie along the medial side of the thigh and enters the popliteal fossa. From there it runs into the deep layer of the muscles over the medial side of the tibia and forks into two sub-branches posterior to the internal malleolus. One sub-branch combines with the kidney meridian and flows into the three yin meridians of the foot, ending at the bottom of the foot. The other sub-branch obliquely enters the internal malleolus, runs deep into the ankle joint, emerges from the dorsum of foot and enters the great toe. (see Fig. 91)

冲脉起始于胞宫，一支与任脉同循背脊的里面上行；一支自胞宫，经会阴，过阴器，出气街。其上行者，从气街与足少阴、足阳明经并行，循腹上行，散布于胸中，上行至咽喉，出于咽喉上部和后鼻道，分出分支联络唇口，渗灌头面诸阳经与目。其下行者，从气街沿大腿内侧下行，进入腘中，下行于胫骨内侧的深部，至足内踝之后而分成两支：下行者并少阴之经，渗灌足三阴经，入于足下；前行者，斜行进入内踝，深行于踝关节，出足背，进入足大趾间。(见图 91)

Associated viscus: Uterus.

联系脏腑：胞宫。

Associated organs: Lips, mouth, throat, eyes and genitals.

联系器官：唇口、咽喉(颃颡)、眼、阴器。

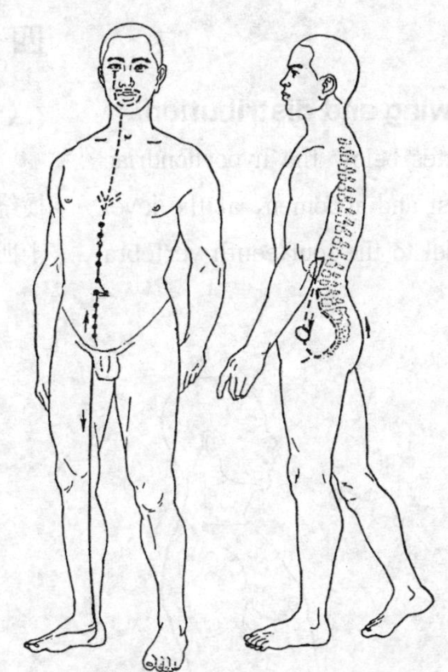

Fig. 91 Flowing route of the thoroughfare vessel

图 91 冲脉循行示意图

2.2.3.2 Indications

Gynecological diseases, syndromes of the chest, abdomen, stomach, intestines and kidney as well as disorders involving the areas through which the meridian passes.

2.2.3.3 Crossing acupoints

Conception vessel: Huiyin (CV 1) and Yinjiao (CV 7).

Stomach meridian: Qichong (ST 30).

Kidney meridian: Henggu (KI 11), Dahe (KI 12), Qixue (KI 13), Siman (KI 14), Zhongzhu (KI 15), Huangshu (KI 16), Shangqu (KI 17), Shiguan (KI 18), Futonggu (KI 20) and Youmen (KI 21).

Besides, Gongsun (SP 4) of the spleen meridian is also connected with the thoroughfare vessel.

(二) 主治要点

本经在临床上主要治疗妇科疾病,胸腹部的胃肠、肾等脏器的综合病症以及经脉所过部位的其他病证。

(三) 交会穴

任脉:会阴,阴交。

足阳明经:气冲。

足少阴经:横骨,大赫,气穴,四满,中注,肓俞,商曲,石关,腹通谷,幽门。

此外,足太阴脾经的公孙穴通于冲脉。

2.2.4 Belt vessel

2.2.4.1 Cyclical flowing and distribution

The belt vessel originates below the hypochondriac region, runs around the waist and abdomen, at the level with the umbilicus and parallel to the fourteenth vertebra (see Fig. 92).

四、带脉

(一) 循行分布

带脉起于季肋部的下面，横绕腰腹一周，前平脐，后平十四椎(见图 92)。

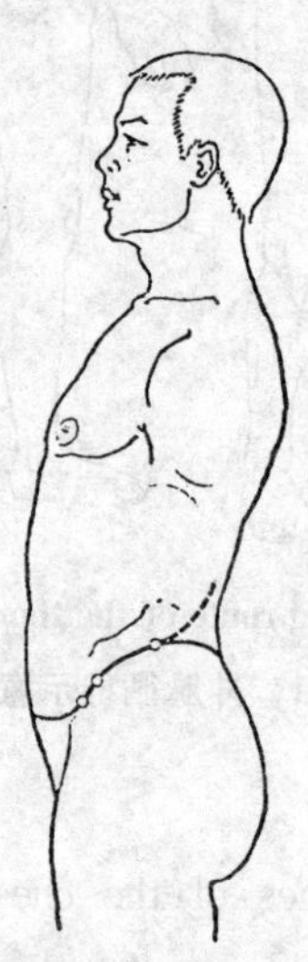

Fig. 92　Flowing route of the belt vessel

图 92　带脉循行示意图

2.2.4.2 Indications

Gynecological diseases, disorders of the loins and abdomen as well as flaccidity syndrome.

2.2.4.3 Crossing acupoints

Gallbladder meridian: Daimai (GB 26), Wushu (GB 27) and Weidao (GB 28).

Besides, Zulinqi (GB 41) of the gallbladder meridian is also connected with the belt vessel.

(二) 主治要点

本经在临床上主要治疗妇科疾病，腰腹部病证以及痿证等。

(三) 交会穴

足少阳经：带脉，五枢，维道。

此外，足少阳胆经的足临泣通于带脉。

2.2.5 Yin heel and yang heel vessels

2.2.5.1 Cyclical flowing and distribution

2.2.5.1.1 Yin heel vessel

Yin heel vessel starts from below the medial malleolus and ascends to the upper portion of the medial malleolus. Then it runs straight upward along the posterior border of the medial aspect of the thigh to the external genitalia. From there it goes upward along the chest to the supraclavicular fossa and runs further upward lateral to throat. There it converges with the thoroughfare vessel, passes by the nose and combines with yang heel vessel at the inner canthus. Then it runs upward with yang heel vessel and enters the brain between the two tendons in the nape (see Fig. 93).

五、阴蹻脉与阳蹻脉

(一)循行分布

1. 阴蹻脉

起于足内踝之下,上行于内踝上方,向上沿大腿内侧,进入阴器,上行腹,沿着胸里、缺盆,抵达咽喉,左右交会贯穿冲脉,上行鼻外,与阳蹻脉会于目内眦,会合阳蹻而上行,在项中两筋间入脑(见图93)。

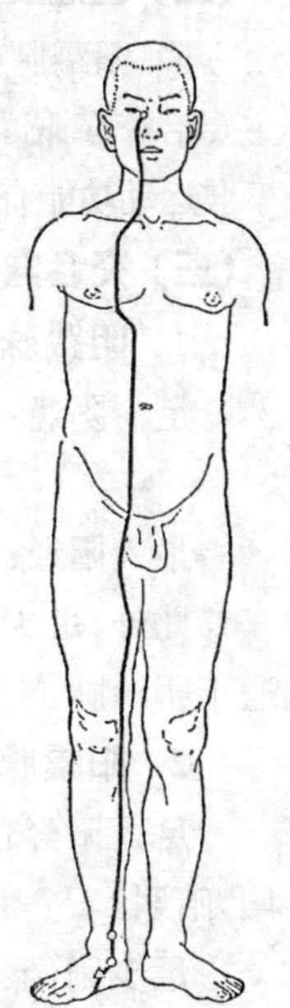

Fig. 93 Flowing route of the yin heel vessel

图 93 阴蹻脉循行示意图

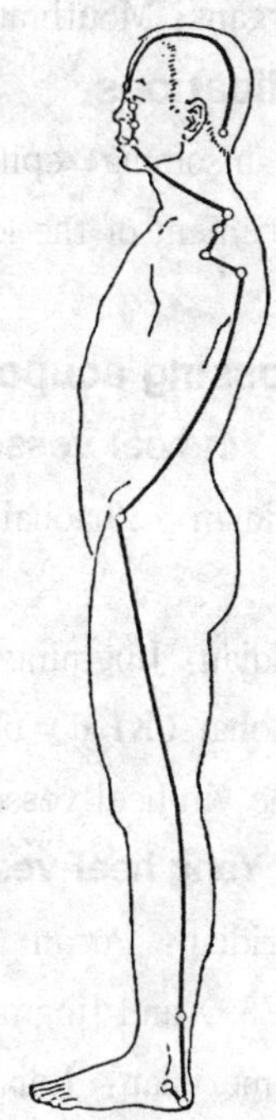

Fig. 94 Flowing route of the yang heel vessel

图 94 阳蹻脉循行示意图

Associated viscus: Brain.

Associated organs: Genitalia, throat and eyes.

2.2.5.1.2 Yang heel vessel

Yang heel vessel starts from the lateral and inferior side of the heel. It runs upward from behind the external malleolus, passes the lateral side of the shank and the thigh, moves upward along the posterior side of the hypochondria and reaches the shoulder from the posterior region of the axillary fold. From there, it ascends along the neck to the corner of the mouth. Then it enters the inner canthus along the lateral side of the nose to combine with the yin heel vessel. Running further upward along the bladder meridian to Fengchi (GB 20), it enters the brain between the two tendons in the nape (see Fig. 94).

Associated viscus: Brain.

Associated organs: Mouth and eyes.

2.2.5.2 Indications

Somnolence, insomnia, epilepsy and other disorders related to the movement of the lower limbs.

2.2.5.3 Crossing acupoints

2.2.5.3.1 Yin heel vessel

Kidney meridian: Zhaohai (KI 6) and Jiaoxin (KI 8).

Bladder meridian: Jingming (BL 1).

Besides, Zhaohai (KI 6) of the kidney meridian is connected with the yin heel vessel.

2.2.5.3.2 Yang heel vessel

Bladder meridian: Pucan (BL 61), Shenmai (BL 62), Fuyang (BL 59) and Jingming (BL 1).

Gallbladder meridian: Juliao (GB 29) and Fengchi (GB 20) [according to *Nanjing* (*Canon of Difficulties*)].

Stomach meridian: Dicang (ST 4), Juliao (ST 3) and Chengqi (ST 1).

联系脏腑:脑。

联系器官:阴器、咽喉、目。

2. 阳蹻脉

起于跟中之外下方,经外踝下,过小腿外侧,直上循大腿外侧,上行胁肋后侧,从腋后上肩,循颈,挟口,上循鼻外,至目内眦,与阴蹻脉会合,沿足太阳经上行入风池,在项中两筋间入脑(见图94)。

联系脏腑:脑。

联系器官:口、目。

(二)主治要点

阴、阳蹻脉相对,在临床上主要治疗多眠、不寐,癫痫和与下肢运动功能有关的疾病。

(三)交会穴

1. 阴蹻脉

足少阴经:照海,交信。

足太阳经:睛明。

此外,足少阴肾经的照海通于阴蹻脉。

2. 阳蹻脉

足太阳经:仆参,申脉,跗阳,睛明。

足少阳经:居髎,风池(依《难经》)。

足阳明经:地仓,巨髎,承泣。

Large intestine meridian: Jianyu (LI 15) and Jugu (LI 16).

手阳明经:肩髃,巨骨。

Small intestine meridian: Naoshu (SI 10).

手太阳经:臑俞。

Governor vessel: Fengfu (GV 16) [according to *Lingshu* (*Spiritual Pivot*)].

督脉:风府(据《灵枢》)。

Besides, Shenmai (BL 62) of the bladder meridian is connected with the yang heel vessel.

此外,足太阳膀胱经的申脉通于阳蹻脉。

2.2.6 Yin link and yang link vessels

六、阴维脉与阳维脉

2.2.6.1 Cyclical flowing and distribution

(一)循行分布

2.2.6.1.1 Yin link vessel

1. 阴维脉

The yin link vessel starts from the medial aspect of the leg and ascends along the medial aspect of the thigh to the abdomen to combine with the spleen meridian. Then it runs along the chest and combines with the conception vessel (see Fig. 95).

起于小腿内侧,沿大腿内侧上行到腹部,与足太阴经相合,循胸在颈部合于任脉(见图 95)。

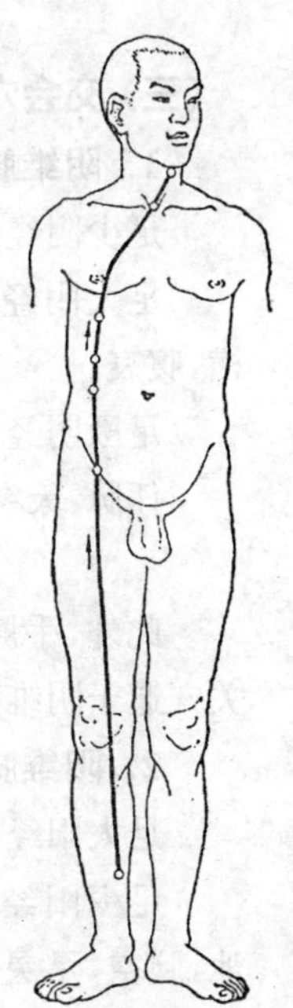

Fig. 95 Flowing route of the yin link vessel

图 95 阴维脉循行示意图

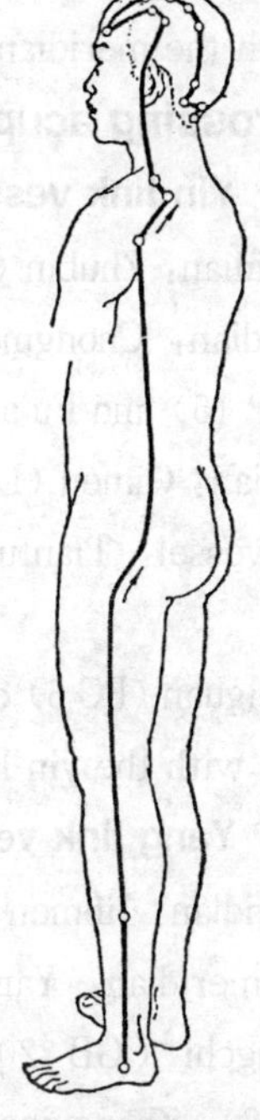

Fig. 96 Flowing route of the yang link vessel

图 96 阳维脉循行示意图

2.2.6.1.2 Yang link vessel

The yang link vessel starts from the heel and emerges from the external malleolus. From there, it ascends along the lateral side of the lower limbs to the posterior side of the hypochondriac and costal regions. From the posterior aspect of the axilla, it moves up to the shoulder. Then it runs to the forehead and turns backward to the back of the neck to combine with the governor vessel (see Fig. 96).

2. 阳维脉

起于足外踝下，上向下肢外侧，上行胁肋后侧，从腋后上肩，循颈额角再到后项，合于督脉(见图 96)。

2.2.6.2 Indications

Yin link and yang link vessels govern the superficies of the whole body. Clinically the indication of yin link vessel mainly includes interior sthenia syndromes, such as the disorders of the heart, chest and stomach; while the indication of yang link vessel mainly includes exterior asthenia syndromes, such as aversion to cold and fever, exogenous febrile disease and the disorders involving the areas through which the meridian passes.

(二) 主治要点

阴、阳维脉互相维系，主一身之表里。在临床上阴维脉主要治疗里实证，如心、胸、胃的病证；阳维脉主要治疗营卫不和的表证，如恶寒发热、外感热病，以及经脉循行所过部位的病证。

2.2.6.3 Crossing acupoints

2.2.6.3.1 Yin link vessel

Kidney meridian: Zhubin (KI 9).

Spleen meridian: Chongmen (SP 12), Fushe (SP 13), Daheng (SP 15) and Fu'ai (SP 16).

Liver meridian: Qimen (LR 14).

Conception vessel: Tiantu (CV 22) and Lianquan (CV 23).

Besides, Neiguan (PC 6) of the pericardium meridian is also connected with the yin link vessel.

(三) 交会穴

1. 阴维脉

足少阴经：筑宾。

足太阴经：冲门，府舍，大横，腹哀。

足厥阴经：期门。

任脉：天突，廉泉。

此外，手厥阴心包经的内关穴通于阴维脉。

2.2.6.3.2 Yang link vessel

Bladder meridian: Jinmen (BL 63).

Gallbaldder meridian: Yangjiao (GB 35), Jianjing (GB 21), Fengchi (GB 20), Naokong (GB 19), Chengling (GB 18), Zhengying (GB 17), Muchuang (GB 16), Toulinqi (GB 15), Benshen (GB 13) and Yangbai

2. 阳维脉

足太阳经：金门。

足少阳经：阳交，肩井，风池，脑空，承灵，正营，目窗，头临泣，本神，阳白。

(GB 14).

Small intestine meridian: Naoshu (SI 10).

Triple energizer meridian: Tianliao (TE 15).

Governor vessel: Fengfu (GV 16) and Yamen (GV 15).

手太阳经:臑俞。

手少阳经:天髎。

督脉:风府,哑门。

Besides, Waiguan (TE 15) of the triple energizer meridian is also connected with the yang link vessel.

此外,手少阳三焦经的外关穴通于阳维脉。

2.3 Extraordinary acupoints

第三节 经外奇穴

2.3.1 Acupoints on the head and neck

一、头颈部穴

2.3.1.1 Sishencong (EX-HN 1)

Location: A group of four acupoints, at the vertex, 1 cun respectively posterior, anterior, and lateral to Baihui (GV 20) (see Fig. 97).

1. 四神聪 EX-HN1

【位置与取法】 在头顶部,当百会前后左右各1寸,共四穴(见图97)。

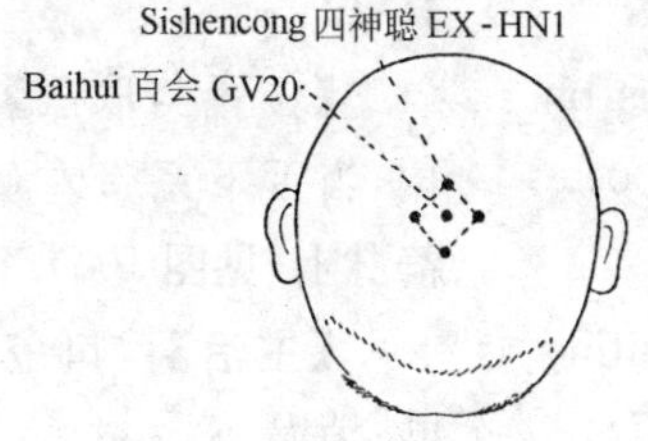

Fig. 97 Extraordiary acupoints on the head and neck

图97 头项部奇穴图

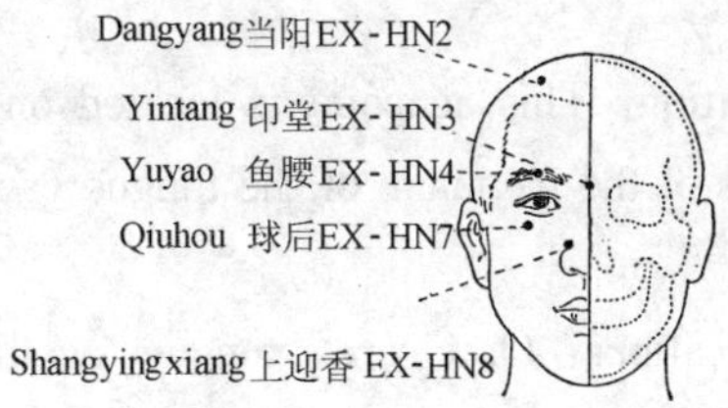

Dangyang 当阳 EX-HN2

Yintang 印堂 EX-HN3

Yuyao 鱼腰 EX-HN4

Qiuhou 球后 EX-HN7

Shangyingxiang 上迎香 EX-HN8

Fig. 98 Extraordinary acupoints on the head and face

图98 头面部奇穴图

Indications: Headache, vertigo, insomnia, amnesia and epilepsy.

【主治】 头痛,眩晕;失眠,健忘,癫痫。

2.3.1.2 Yintang (EX-HN 3)

Location: This acupoint is located midway between the medial ends of the two eyebrows (see Fig. 98).

Indications: Headache, vertigo, epistaxis, nasosinusitis, infantile convulsion, insomnia and sunstroke.

2. 印堂 EX-HN3

【位置与取法】 在额部,当两眉头之中间(见图98)。

【主治】 头痛,眩晕;鼻衄,鼻渊;小儿惊风,失眠,中暑。

2.3.1.3 Taiyang (EX-HN 5)

Location: This acupoint is located between the lateral end of the eyebrow and the outer canthus and in the depression about one finger-breadth posterior (see Fig. 99).

3. 太阳 EX-HN5

【位置与取法】 在颞部，当眉梢与目外眦之间，向后约一横指的凹陷处(见图99)。

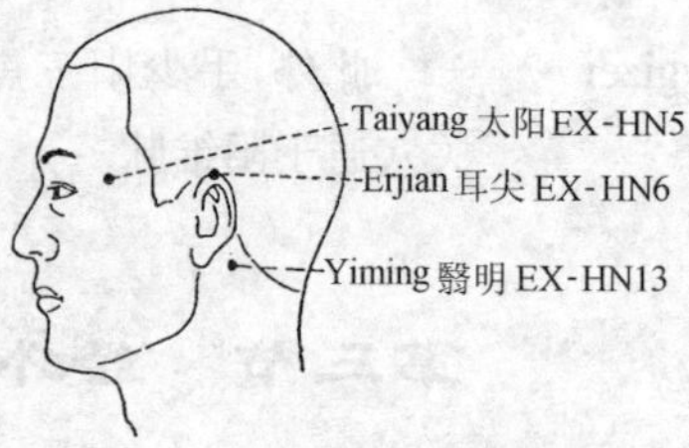

Taiyang 太阳 EX-HN5
Erjian 耳尖 EX-HN6
Yiming 翳明 EX-HN13

Fig. 99 Extraordinary acupoints on the head and neck

图99 头颈部奇穴图

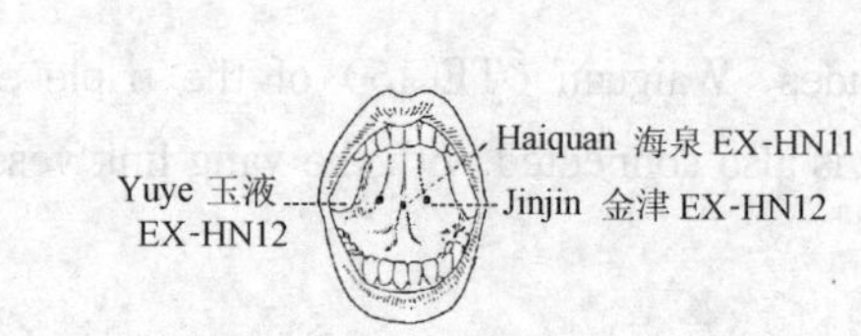

Fig. 100 Extraordinary acupoints below the tongue

图100 舌底部奇穴图

Indications: Migraine, headache and eye disorders.

【主治】 偏正头痛，目疾。

2.3.1.4 Jinjin, Yuye (EX-HN 12)

Location: This acupoint is located on the veins on both sides of the frenulum of the tongue (see Fig. 100).

Indications: Oral sore, tongue swelling, vomiting and diabetes.

4. 金津 玉液 EX-HN12

【位置与取法】 在口腔内，当舌下系带左侧、右侧的静脉上(见图100)。

【主治】 口疮；舌肿；呕吐；消渴。

2.3.1.5 Yiming (EX-HN 13)

Location: This acupoint is located 1 cun posterior to Yifeng (TE 17) (see Fig. 99).

Indications: Eye disorders, tinnitus and insomnia.

5. 翳明 EX-HN13

【位置与取法】 在项部，当翳风后1寸(见图99)。

【主治】 目疾；耳鸣；失眠。

2.3.2 Acupoints on the chest and abdomen

二、胸腹部穴

Zigong (EX-CA 1)

Location: This acupoint is located on the lower abdomen, 4 cun directly below the umbilicus and 3 cun lateral to Zhongji (CV 3) (see Fig. 102).

子宫 EX-CA1

【位置与取法】 在下腹部，当脐中下4寸，中极旁开3寸(见图102)。

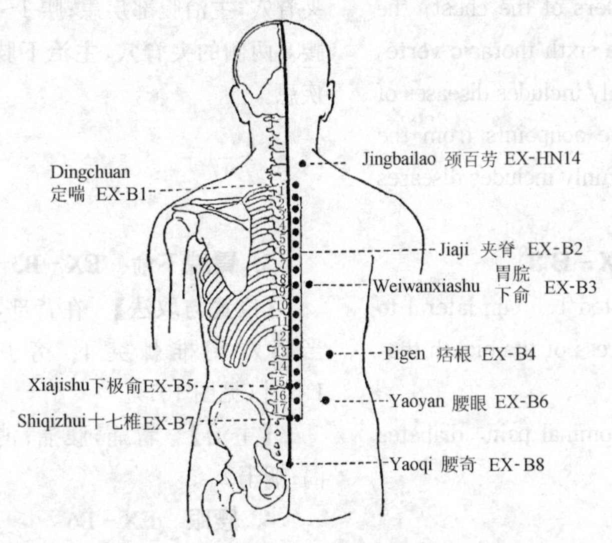

Fig. 101 Extraordinary acupoints on the back

图 101 背腰部奇穴图

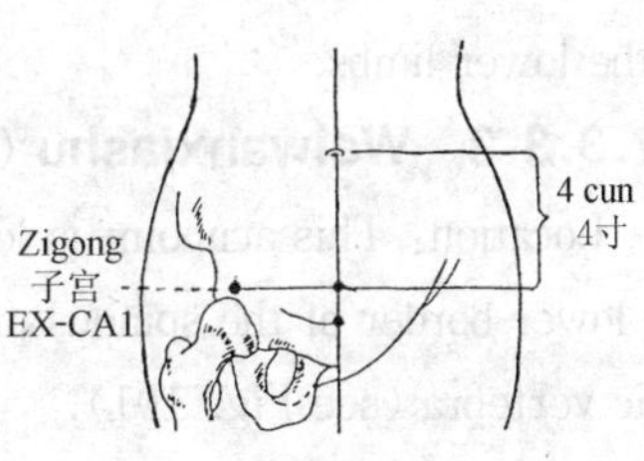

Fig. 102 Extraordinary acupoints on the abdomen

图 102 腹部奇穴图

Indications: Prolapse of uterus, irregular menstruation and sterility.

【主治】 阴挺,月经不调,不孕。

2.3.3 Acupoints on the back

三、背部穴

2.3.3.1 Dingchuan (EX - B 1)

Location: This acupoint is located below the spinous process of the seventh cervical vertebra and 0.5 lateral to the posterior midline (see Fig. 101).

Indications: Asthma and cough.

1. 定喘 EX - B1

【位置与取法】 在背部,当第七颈椎棘突下,旁开0.5寸(见图101)。

【主治】 气喘,咳嗽。

2.3.3.2 Jiaji (EX - B 2)

Location: A group of 34 acupoints on both sides of the spinal column, 0.5 cun lateral to the lower border of each spinous process from the first thoracic vertebra to the fifth lumbar vertebra (see Fig. 101).

Indications: The indication for the acupoints from the first to the third thoracic vertebrae on both sides mainly includes disease of the upper limbs; the indication for the acupoints from the first to the eighth thoracic vertebrae

2. 夹脊 EX - B2

【位置与取法】 在背腰部,当第一胸椎至第五腰椎棘突下两侧,后正中线旁开0.5寸,一侧17个穴(见图101)。

【主治】 胸1～胸3两侧的夹脊穴,主治上肢疾患;胸1～胸8两侧的夹脊穴,主治胸部疾患;胸6～腰5两侧的

on both sides mainly includes disorders of the chest; the indication for the acupoints from the sixth thoracic vertebra to the fifth lumbar vertebra mainly includes diseases of the abdomen; the indication for the acupoints from the first to the fifth lumbar vertebrae mainly includes diseases of the lower limbs.

夹脊穴,主治腹部疾患;腰 1～腰 5 两侧的夹脊穴,主治下肢疾患。

2.3.3.3 Weiwanxiashu (EX-B 3)

Location: This acupoint is located 1.5 cun lateral to the lower border of the spinous process of the eighth thoracic vertebra (see Fig. 101).

Indications: Stomachache, abdominal pain, diabetes and dry throat.

3. 胃脘下俞 EX-B3

【位置与取法】 在背部,当第八胸椎棘突下,旁开 1.5 寸(见图 101)。

【主治】 胃痛,腹痛;消渴;咽干。

2.3.3.4 Yaoyan (EX-B 6)

Location: This acupoint is located below the spinous process of the fourth lumbar vertebra and in the depression 3.5 cun lateral to the spinous process of the fourth lumbar vertebra (see Fig. 101).

Indications: Lumbago, irregular menstruation and leukorrhagia.

4. 腰眼 EX-B6

【位置与取法】 在腰部,当第四腰椎棘突下,旁开约 3.5 寸凹陷中(见图 101)。

【主治】 腰痛,月经不调,带下。

2.3.3.5 Shiqizhui (EX-B 7)

Location: This acupoint is located on the posterior midline and below the spinous process of the fifth lumbar vertebra (see Fig. 101).

Indications: Pain in the waist and leg, paralysis of the lower limbs, metrorrhagia and metrostaxis, irregular menstruation and dysuria in pregnancy.

5. 十七椎 EX-B7

【位置与取法】 在腰部,当后正中线上,第五腰椎棘突下(见图 101)。

【主治】 腰腿痛,下肢瘫痪,崩漏,月经不调,转胞。

2.3.3.6 Yaoqi (EX-B 8)

Location: This acupoint is located 2 cun directly above the coccyx (see Fig. 101).

Indications: Epilepsy, headache, insomnia and constipation.

6. 腰奇 EX-B8

【位置与取法】 在骶部,当尾骨端直上 2 寸,骶角之间凹陷中(见图 101)。

【主治】 癫痫,头痛,失眠,便秘。

2.3.4 Acupoints on the upper limbs

2.3.4.1 Yaotongdian (EX - UE 7)

Location: This acupoint is located on the dorsum of the hand, midway between the transverse wrist crease and metacarpophalangeal joint, between the second and third metacarpal bones, and between the fourth and fifth metacarpal bones, four acupoints in all on both hands. (see Fig. 103)

四、上肢部穴

1. 腰痛点 EX - UE 7

【位置与取法】 在手背侧,当第二三掌骨及第四五掌骨之间,当腕横纹与掌指关节中点处,一侧2穴(见图103)。

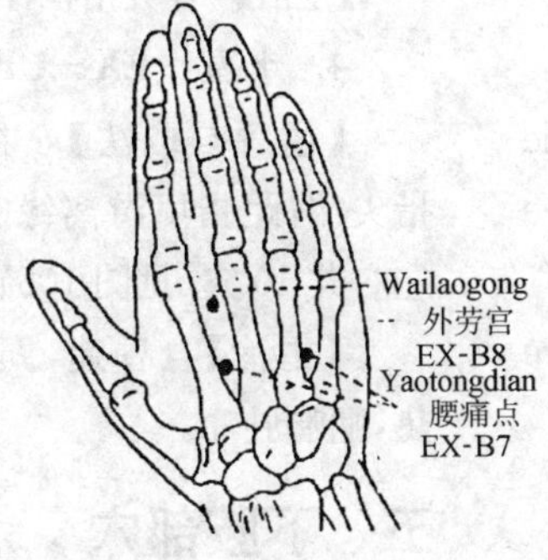

Fig. 103 Extraordinary acupoints on the dorsum of hand

图103 手背部奇穴图

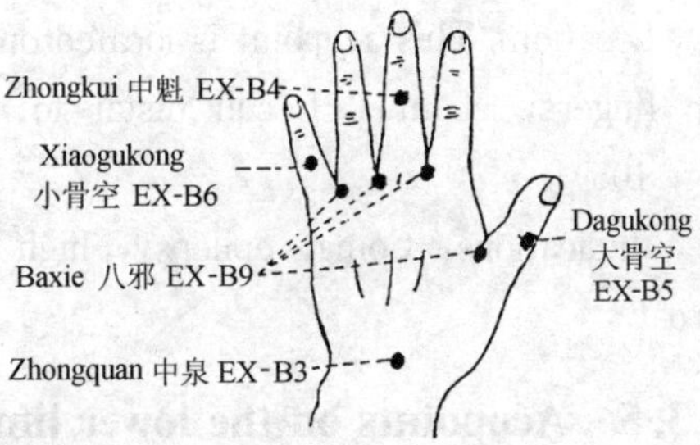

Fig. 104 Extraordinary acupoints on the dorsum of hand

图104 手背部奇穴图

Indications: Acute sprain of waist.

2.3.4.2 Baxie (EX - UE 9)

Location: This acupoint is located on the dorsum of the hand, at the junction of the white and red skin of the hands webs, eight in all, making a loose fist to locate the acupoints (see Fig. 104).

Indications: Fever with dysphoria, pain of eyes, swelling and pain of arms due to snake bite.

2.3.4.3 Sifeng (EX - UE 10)

Location: This acupoint is located on the palmar surface, in the midpoint of the transverse creases of the proximal interphalangeal joints. There are four acupoints on each hand (see Fig. 105).

【主治】 急性腰扭伤。

2. 八邪 EX - UE 9

【位置与取法】 在手背侧,微握拳,第一至第五指间,指蹼缘后方赤白肉际处,左右共8穴(见图104)。

【主治】 烦热,目痛,毒蛇咬伤手臂肿痛。

3. 四缝 EX - UE10

【位置与取法】 在第二至第五指掌侧,近端指关节的中央,一侧4穴(见图105)。

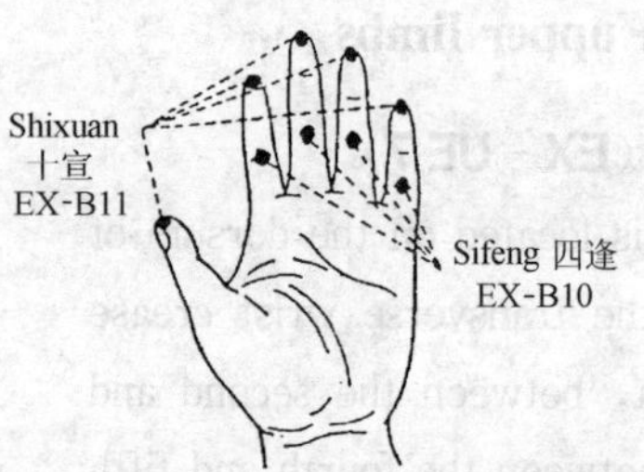

Fig. 105　Extraordinary acupoints on the palm

图 105　手掌部奇穴图

Indications: Infantile malnutrition and whooping cough.

【主治】 小儿疳积,百日咳。

2.3.4.4　Shixuan (EX－UE 11)

4. 十宣　EX－UE11

Location: This acupoint is located on the tips of the ten fingers, about 0.1 cun distal to the nails (see Fig. 105).

【位置与取法】 在手十指尖端,距指甲游离缘0.1寸,左右共10穴(见图105)。

Indications: Coma, epilepsy, high fever and sore throat.

【主治】 昏迷,癫痫,高热,咽喉肿痛。

2.3.5　Acupoints on the lower limbs

五、下肢部穴

2.3.5.1　Heding (EX－LE 2)

1. 鹤顶　EX－LE2

Location: This acupoint is located on the knee and in the depression of the midpoint of the superior patellar border (see Fig. 106).

【位置与取法】 在膝上部,髌底的中点上方凹陷处(见图106)。

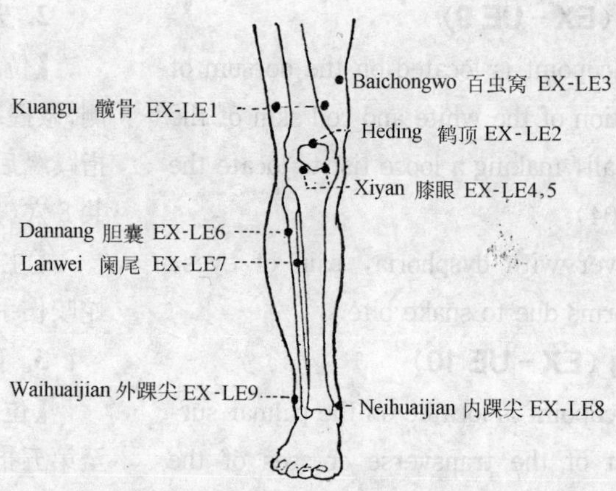

Fig. 106　Extraordinary acupoints on the lower limb

图 106　下肢部奇穴图

Indications: Knee pain, weakness of the foot and leg, and paralysis.

【主治】 膝痛，足胫无力，瘫痪。

2.3.5.2 Xiyan (EX - LE 4,5)

2. 膝眼 EX - LE4,5

Location: This acupoint is located in the two depressions medial and lateral to the patellar ligament when the knee is flexed. These two acupoints are also called medial Xiyan (EX-LE 4) and lateral Xiyan (EX-LE 5) respectively (see Fig. 106).

【位置与取法】 屈膝，在髌韧带两侧凹陷处，在内侧的称内膝眼(EX - LE4)，在外侧的称外膝眼(EX - LE5)(见图106)。

Indications: Knee pain, heaviness and pain of the leg and beriberi.

【主治】 膝痛，腿脚重痛，脚气。

2.3.5.3 Dannang (EX - LE 6)

3. 胆囊 EX - LE6

Location: This acupoint is located superior and lateral to the shank in the depression 2 cun directly below the small head of the fibia (see Fig. 106).

【位置与取法】 在小腿外侧上部，当腓骨小头前下方凹陷处(阳陵泉)直下 2 寸(见图 106)。

Indications: Acute and chronic cholecystitis, cholelithiasis, biliary ascariasis and flaccidity and obstruction syndromes of the lower limbs.

【主治】 急、慢性胆囊炎，胆石症，胆道蛔虫症，下肢痿痹。

2.3.5.4 Lanwei (EX - LE 7)

4. 阑尾 EX - LE7

Location: This acupoint is located anterior and superior to the shank, 5 cun below Dubi (ST 35) and one finger breadth lateral to the anterior border of the tibia (see Fig. 106).

【位置与取法】 在小腿前侧上部，当犊鼻下 5 寸，胫骨前缘旁开一横指(见图 106)。

Indications: Acute and chronic cholecystitis, dyspepsia and paralysis of lower limbs.

【主治】 急、慢性阑尾炎，消化不良，下肢瘫痪。

2.3.5.5 Bafeng (EX - LE 10)

5. 八风 EX - LE10

Location: This acupoint is located on the dorsum of foot, in the depressions on the webs between toes, proximal to the margins of the webs, four acupoints on each foot (see Fig. 107).

【位置与取法】 在足背侧，第一至第五趾间，趾蹼缘后方赤白际处，一侧 4 穴，左右共 8 穴(见图 107)。

Indications: Beriberi, pain of toe, swelling and pain of foot due to snake bite.

【主治】 脚气，趾痛，毒蛇咬伤足跗肿痛。

2.3.5.6 Qiduan (EX - LE 12)

6. 气端 EX - LE12

Location: This acupoint is located on the tip of ten

【位置与取法】 在足十

toes and 0.1 cun lateral to the toe nail (see Fig. 107).

趾尖端，距趾甲游离缘0.1寸，左右共10穴(见图107)。

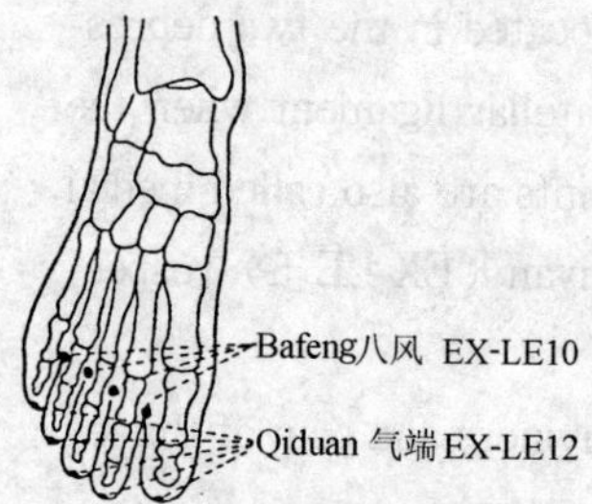

Fig. 107　Extraordinary acupoints on the foot

图107　足部奇穴图

Indications: Numbness of toes, redness, swelling and pain of dorsum of foot and emergent treament of apoplexy.

【主治】 足趾麻木，脚背红肿疼痛，中风急救。

3 Manipulating methods

第三章 针灸操作方法

3.1 Preparations prior to treatment

第一节 针灸施术前的准备

3.1.1 Explanation

一、解释

To some first visit patients, acupuncture and moxibustion therapy, especially acupuncture, may engender nervous tension. They may be afraid of stabbing pain, or needling of some important regions, such as head. The acupuncturist should pay attention to the patients' expression and explain to the patients in order to relax them and enable them to cooperate in the treatment.

一些初诊病人对针灸疗法尤其是针刺会产生紧张心理，或怕刺痛，或对重要部位如头部等的针刺存有顾虑，医者应认真观察病人神态，做适当的解释工作，使病人缓解紧张状态，消除顾虑，放松肌肉，配合施术。

3.1.2 Needles

二、针具

The filiform needles are usually used in clinical treatment. Most of them are made of stainless steel. The common filiform needles vary in length and diameter (Table 3-1, 3-2).

临床常用的针具是毫针，多由不锈钢制成，其针身的长度和直径有不同规格，主要有以下几种(见表 3-1，3-2)：

Table 3-1 Length of Different Filiform Needles

cun	0.5	1.0	1.5	2.0	2.5	3.0	3.5	4.0	4.5	5.0
mm	15	25	40	50	65	75	90	100	115	125

表 3-1 不同规格毫针长度规格对照表

寸	0.5	1.0	1.5	2.0	2.5	3.0	3.5	4.0	4.5	5.0
mm	15	25	40	50	65	75	90	100	115	125

Table 3 - 2　　Diameter of Different Filiform Needles

Gauge	26	28	30	32	34
Dia. (cm)	0.45	0.38	0.32	0.28	0.23

表 3 - 2　　不同规格毫针直径规格对照表

号　码	26	28	30	32	34
直径(mm)	0.45	0.38	0.32	0.28	0.23

Clinically the needles ranging from gauges 28 - 32 in diameter and 1 - 3 cun in length are frequently used in clinical treatment. The needles are selected according to the patient's constitution, age, condition and regions to be punctured. The needles should be carefully examined before insertion. If the needle body gets rusty, crooked, or the area combined with the handle has become loose, or the needle tip is too blunt or hook-like, it will affect insertion, cause pain or even break the needle. These kinds of needles should not be used.

其中以 28～32 号，1～3 寸长的毫针较为常用。临床上对具体针具的选择，要根据病人的体质、年龄、病情以及针刺部位等不同情况来确定。针刺前要检查针具，凡针身有锈痕、弯曲或与针柄相接处有松动，针尖过钝或有钩等，会影响进针，易致疼痛，甚或折针，不宜应用。

3.1.3　Postures

三、体位

Appropriate posture of the patient is important for correct location of acupoints, prolonged retention of the needle and prevention of bending and breaking the needle as well as fainting during acupuncture. Before needling, the patient is advised to relax himself or herself, keep a comfortable and natural posture so as to maintain the position for a longer time. The following are some of the commonly selected postures:

针刺时须要求病人采取和保持一定的体位姿势，以便于取穴、持久留针、防止针身弯曲折断和晕针。针前嘱病人尽量把身体姿势放得舒服自然，能坚持较长时间而不移动。常用的针刺体位主要有如下几种：

3.1.3.1　Lying posture

（一）卧位

Lying posture is most frequently used, especially for the aged, the patients with poor constitution or serious diseases or nervousness. Therefore lying position is significant in preventing fatigue or fainting. The following are some lying postures:

一般多取卧位，尤其是年老、体弱、病重以及精神紧张者，以防病人疲劳难支或晕针。卧位又分为：

Supination: Suitable for needling the acupoints on the head and face, chest and abdominal regions, and the limbs.

仰卧位：适用于取头面、胸腹部腧穴，以及四肢部的多数腧穴。

Lateral recumbent posture: Suitable for needling the acupoints on the posterior region of the head, neck, back, and the lateral side of the limbs.

侧卧位：适用于取头后、项、背部腧穴，以及四肢的部分腧穴。

Pronation: Suitable for needling the acupoints located on the posterior region of the head, neck, back, lumbar and buttock regions, and the posterior region of the lower limbs.

俯卧位：适用于取头后、项、背、腰、臀部腧穴，以及下肢后侧的腧穴。

3.1.3.2 Sitting position

（二）坐位

Sitting position is suitable for needling the acupoints located on the head, neck, upper extremities or the back of the patient whose illness is mild. The following are some of the sitting positions:

一般用于取穴局限在头项、上肢或背部腧穴，且病情较轻者。坐位又分为：

Sitting in pronation: Applicable to the acupoints located on the posterior region of the head, neck and back.

俯伏坐位：适用于取头后、项、背部的腧穴。

Sitting in supination: Applicable to the acupoints located on the head and face as well as the upper chest region.

仰靠坐位：适用于取头面部和上胸部的腧穴。

Sitting with inclining position: Applicable to the acupoints located on the lateral side of the head and ear areas.

侧伏坐位：适用于取侧头部、耳部的腧穴。

3.1.4 Sterilization

四、消毒

Sterilization includes sterilization of the needles, selected region for needling, and the hands of the acupuncturist.

包括针具、针刺部位以及医者双手的消毒。

3.1.4.1 Needle sterilization

（一）针具消毒

Sterilized needles, which should be used only once, are recommended. The needles for repeated use should be sterilized with autoclave. Method: The needles wrapped in gauze are sterilized in an autoclave under 15 pounds atmospheric pressure and 120℃ for 15 minutes. Boiling sterilization: The needles wrapped in gauze are boiled in

提倡使用经过消毒的一次性针具。如果是反复使用的一般针具，最好用高压消毒，方法是用纱布将针具包好，放入高压蒸汽锅内，在15磅气压、120℃高温下持续15

water for 15 - 20 minutes. Medical sterilization: The needles are soaked in 75% alcohol for 30 minutes and then taken out and cleaned with a piece of dry cloth. Twee zers, needle tray and other devices are sterilized by being soaked in 2% lysol liquid or 1 : 1,000 corrosive sublimate liquid for 1 - 2 hours.

分钟,即可达到消毒要求。也可用煮沸消毒法,用纱布包好针具,放在清水中煮沸15~20分钟即可。或者用药物消毒,用75%酒精浸泡针具30分钟,取出擦干应用。镊子和放置针具的针盘等器具的消毒,可用2%来苏溶液或1∶1 000的升汞溶液浸泡1~2小时即可。

3.1.4.2 Disinfection of the region selected for needling

The area selected for needling must be sterilized with a 75% alcohol cotton ball or with 2.5% iodine first and then with a 75% alcohol cotton ball. The selected area is sterilized from the center to the sides. After sterilization, measures should be taken to avoid recontamination.

(二)针刺部位消毒

在选取的针刺部位用75%酒精棉球擦拭;或先用2.5%碘酒棉球擦拭,再用75%酒精棉球涂擦。擦拭时,应从消毒部位的中心向外周绕圈涂擦。消毒后要注意避免消毒部位的再次污染。

3.1.4.3 Disinfection of the acupuncturist's fingers

Before needling, the acupuncturist should wash his or her hands with soapsuds or sterilize with 75% alcohol cotton balls.

(三)医者手指消毒

针刺施术前,医者的手要用肥皂水洗净,或用75%酒精棉球擦拭。

3.2 Needling methods

第二节　针刺方法

3.2.1 Traditional methods

一、传统方法

3.2.1.1 Needling with filiform needles

(一)毫针刺法

3.2.1.1.1 Insertion

1. 进针方法

The needle usually should be held with the right hand known as the puncturing hand. The left hand, known as the pressing hand, pushes firmly against the area close to the acupoint or presses the needle body from both sides to

针刺施术时,一般是右手持针(称"刺手"),进行针刺的主要操作;左手配合(称"押手"),切按所刺部位或夹持针

assist the right hand. The needle should be inserted coordinately with the help of both hands. The following are some of the commonly used methods of insertion in clinical treatment:

身，以帮助右手进针，双手协同操作将针刺入皮肤。临床上常用的进针方法有以下几种：

Nailing insertion of the needle (Inserting the needle aided by the pressure of the finger of the pressing hand): Press beside the acupoint with the nail of the thumb or the index finger of the left hand, hold the needle with the right hand and keep the needle tip closely against the nail, and then insert the needle into the acupoint (Fig. 108). This method is suitable for puncturing with short needles.

指切进针法：用左手拇指或食指的指甲切按在穴位处，右手将针紧靠左手指甲缘刺入腧穴（见图 108）。此法适用于短针的进针。

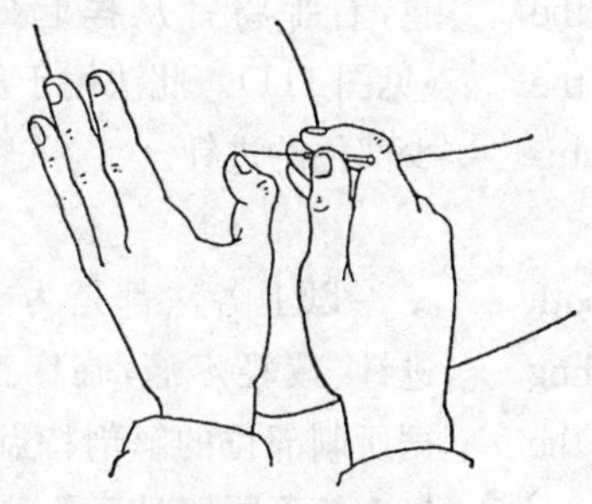

Fig. 108 Nailing insertion of the needle
图 108 指切进针法

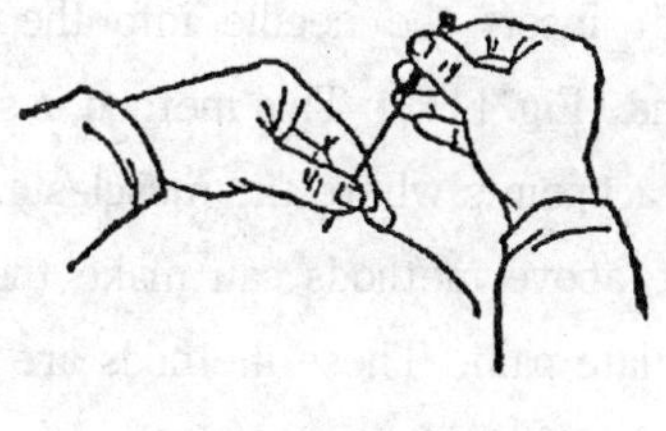

Fig. 109 Holding insertion of the needle
图 109 夹持进针法

Holding insertion of the needle (Inserting the needle with the help of the puncturing and pressing hands): Hold the needle tip with sterilized dry cotton balls held by the thumb and the index finger of the left hand, keep the needle tip on the skin surface of the acupoint. Then insert the needle into the skin with both hands (Fig. 109). This method is suitable for puncturing with long needles.

夹持进针法：用左手的拇指和食指拿消毒干棉球夹住针身的下端，将针尖轻置于穴位的皮肤表面，然后右手与左手同时用力，将针刺入皮肤（见图 109）。此法适用于长针的进针。

Relaxed insertion of the needle (Inserting the needle with the fingers stretching the skin): Stretch the skin where the acupoint is located with the thumb and the index finger of the left hand, hold the needle with the right hand and then insert it into the area between the two fingers (Fig. 110). This method is suitable for puncturing

舒张进针法：以左手的拇指和食指将穴位处的皮肤向两侧撑开而使皮肤绷紧，右手将针从两指之间刺入（见图 110）。此法用于皮肤松弛部位的进针。

the acupoints located on the regions with loose skin.

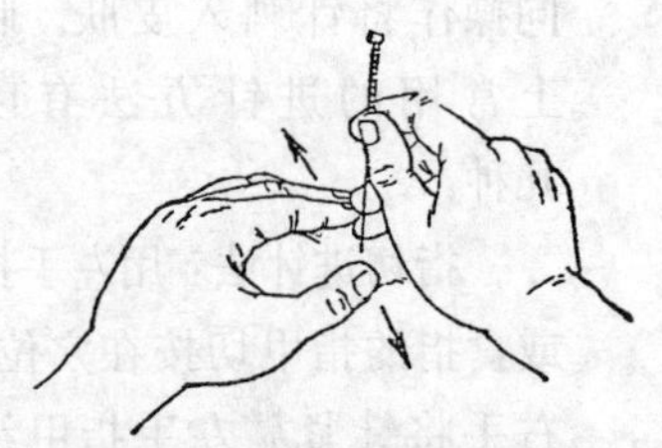

Fig. 110　Relaxed insertion of the needle

图 110　舒张进针法

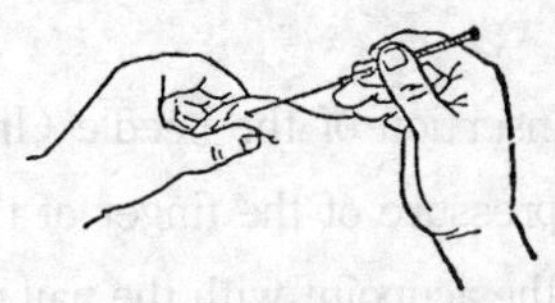

Fig. 111　Lifting and pinching insertion of the needle

图 111　提捏进针法

Lifting and pinching insertion of the needle (Inserting the needle by pinching the skin): Pinch the skin up around the acupoint with the thumb and index finger of the left hand, insert the needle into the acupoint with the right hand (Fig. 111). This method is suitable for puncturing the acupoints where the muscles are thin.

提捏进针法：用左手拇指、食指将穴位处的皮肤捏起，右手将针从捏起处刺入(见图 111)。此法用于皮薄肉少部位的进针。

The above methods can make the insertion smooth and alleviate pain. These methods are selected according to the anatomical features of the needled area and the depth of needle insertion in clinical treatment.

以上各法都是为了顺利进针、减轻疼痛，临床上应根据所刺部位的解剖特点、针刺深度等不同情况而灵活选用。

3.2.1.1.2　Angle and depth of insertion

2. 针刺的角度、深度

Different angles and depth in needling the same acupoint may puncture different tissues, produce varied needling sensation and therapeutic effects. To different acupoints, appropriate angle and depth are selected according to the location of the acupoints. Therefore, angle and depth are especially important in the process of needle insertion. Correct angle and depth are helpful in producing desired therapeutic effects and preventing needling accidents.

对同一个腧穴，如果针刺的角度、深度不同，所刺及的组织、产生的针刺感应和治疗效果会有明显的差异；对不同的腧穴，由于所在部位的解剖特点各异，针刺的角度和深度就应有所区别。所以，掌握正确的针刺角度与深度，对于获得预期的针刺治疗效果、防止意外事故的发生等，都具有重要的意义。

Angle of insertion: The angle formed by the needle and the skin surface is usually classified into three kinds (see Fig. 112):

(1) 针刺角度：指进针时针身与皮肤表面间的夹角。一般分为三种角度(见图 112)：

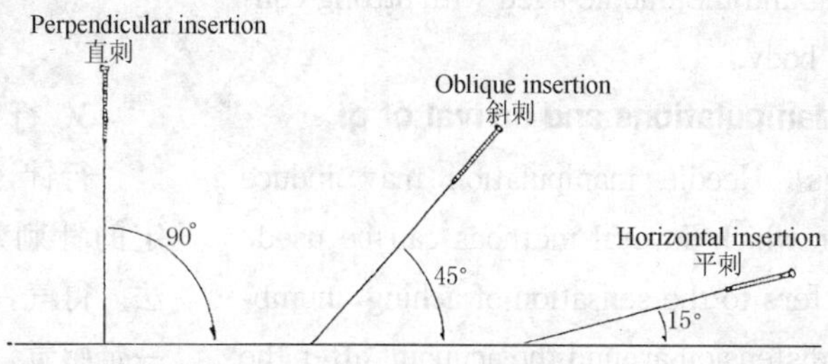

Fig. 112 Needling angles

图 112 针刺角度

Perpendicular insertion: Perpendicular insertion, in which the needle is inserted perpendicularly, means that there is an angle of 90° formed between the needle and the skin surface. This method is applicable to most acupoints on the body.

直刺：指针身与皮肤表面呈 90°角左右垂直刺入。适用于大部分腧穴。

Oblique insertion: The needle is inserted obliquely to form an angle of approximately 45° between the needle and the skin surface. This method is used for needling the acupoints close to the important viscera or tissues, or the acupoints which are not suitable for perpendicular and deep insertion.

斜刺：指针身与皮肤表面呈 45°角左右斜向刺入。适用于内有重要组织或脏器，或不宜直刺、深刺的腧穴。

Horizontal insertion: The needle is inserted transversely to form an angle of about 15° between the needle and the skin surface, also known as transverse insertion. This method is applicable to the areas where the muscle is thin.

平刺：指针身与皮肤表面呈 15°角左右沿皮刺入，又称"横刺"、"沿皮刺"。适用于皮薄肉少部位的腧穴。

Depth of needle insertion: In clinical treatment, the depth of insertion mostly depends upon the location of the acupoints, the constitution of the patient and the pathological conditions. For example, shallow insertion is applicable to the needling of such areas as the head, face, chest and abdominal region as well as such patients as infants, people with delicate constitution, or the aged. Deep insertion is applicable to the needling of the acupoints located on the limbs, buttocks and abdominal region

（2）针刺深度：指针身刺入肌肤的深浅程度。临床上主要根据腧穴部位、病人体质、疾病情况等因素决定针刺的深浅。比如头面胸腹部、小儿、瘦弱、年老者宜浅刺，四肢腹臀部、青壮年、体胖者可深刺。

as well as the young and the middle-aged with strong constitution and heavy body.

3.2.1.1.3 Manipulations and arrival of qi

Manipulations: Needle manipulation may induce needling effect, for which several methods can be used. The arrival of qi refers to the sensation of aching, numbness, heaviness or distension around the acupoint after the needle is inserted. At the same time the acupuncturist may feel heaviness and tension beneath the needle.

The arrival of qi is directly related to the therapeutic effect. Generally speaking, obvious and quick arrival of qi suggests good therapeutic effects, while unclear and slow arrival of qi shows poor therapeutic effects. Many factors may influence the arrival of qi, such as the constitution of the patient, pathological conditions, the acupoints selected, and the needling method used. Clinically the patient with abundant yang-qi may experience quick needling sensation, while the patient with abundant yin-qi may feel slow arrival of qi. Accurate location of acupoints on thick muscles is easy to induce needling sensation while inaccurate location of acupoints on these areas is difficult to induce the arrival of qi. Proper and skillful manipulation promotes the arrival of qi. Therefore, correct manipulations are prerequisite to better therapeutic effects.

Manipulations can be divided into basic manipulation techniques and supplementary ones:

Basic manipulation techniques:

Twirling-rotating: After the needle is inserted to the desired depth, the needle is twirled and rotated backward and forward with the thumb, index and middle fingers of the right hand.

Lifting-thrusting: After the needle is inserted to a certain depth, the needle is lifted and thrusted perpendi-

3. 行针与得气

行针，指进针后为产生一定的针刺效应而施用针刺手法。得气，是指针刺时产生的一定感觉，患者会由针刺部位产生酸、麻、重、胀等的感觉，医者会觉得指下的针有沉紧感。

得气与针刺治疗的效果有直接关系，一般是得气明显、迅速时疗效较好，得气不明显或缓慢时疗效较差。影响得气的因素较多，主要与病人的体质、病情，选取的腧穴，施用的针刺手法等因素有关。临床上，若病人属阳盛体质者则易于得气，阴盛体质者则不易得气；取穴准确、肌肉丰厚处易于得气，反之则不易得气；使用适当的针刺手法、且手法熟练者，可促使得气。因此，掌握正确的行针方法是提高疗效的重要环节。

行针手法可分为基本手法和辅助手法两类：

(1) 基本手法

捻转法：进针至一定深度后，(以右手的拇指和食、中二指持针柄)来回捻转针柄。

提插法：进针至一定深度后，将针身在肌肉中进行上

cularly and continuously.

提、下插的反复操作。

Twirling-rotating and lifting-thrusting are the two basic manipulations and can be used individually or in combination. The amplitude of twirling and the scope of lifting-thrusting as well as the frequency and duration of manipulation depend upon the patient's constitution, pathological conditions and the acupoints to be needled.

捻转法和提插法，是构成针刺手法的基本操作方法，两者既可单独使用，也可结合运用。捻转的角度、提插的幅度，以及操作的频率、持续时间等量度，要根据病人的体质、病情和所刺部位而定。

The supplementary manipulation techniques: Under certain conditions, the supplementary manipulations are employed after insertion. The following are the commonly used techniques:

(2) 辅助手法：指进针后在某种情况下施行的辅助行针方法。常用的有以下几种：

Pressing: Slightly rub, knead and press the skin along the route of the meridian or around the acupoint to promote the flow of qi and blood. This method is used to promote the arrival of qi.

循法：在所刺腧穴的四周或经脉的循行路径，以手指轻柔地按压揉摩，促使气血运行。属催气的方法。

Scraping: Scrap the needle handle with the nail of the thumb, or the index or middle finger downward and upward, or vice versa. This method can be used to strengthen the needling sensation.

刮法：以拇指或食指或中指的指甲，由下而上或由上向下地频频刮动针柄。此法可加强得气感。

Plucking: Pluck the needle handle lightly to make the needle body shake slightly. It is often used to strengthen the stimulation in order to obtain qi.

弹法：用手指轻弹针柄，使针身产生轻微的振动。常用以加强得气感。

Shaking: Shaking the needle handle slightly with the hand can strengthen the needling sensation. If the needle is inserted obliquely or horizontally, shaking the needle handle can make the needling sensation transmit toward a certain direction.

摇法：手持针柄轻微摇动，以加强得气感。如果是斜刺或平刺而摇动，可使针感向一定方向传导。

3.2.1.1.4 Retention and withdrawal of the needle

4. 留针和出针

Retention: Retention means to hold the needle in the acupoint after the use of needling manipulations. For patients with a slow and weak needling sensation, retention of the needle may strengthen needling effect and

(1) 留针：即在施用针刺手法后，将针留置于腧穴内。留针能加强针刺的作用，对得气较慢较弱者还可起到候气

induce needling sensation. Whether the needles should be retained or not and the duration of retention depend on the patients' conditions. For common diseases, the needles can be withdrawn or be retained for 10 - 20 minutes after the application of needling manipulations. But for some special diseases, the time for retaining the needle may be appropriately prolonged. At the same time, manipulations may be performed at intervals in order to improve the therapeutic effects.

的作用。留针与否、留针时间的长短，主要依病情而定。一般病证，施用一定针刺手法后即可出针，或留针 10～20 分钟；某些特殊病证，可适当延长留针时间，并在留针过程中间歇行针，以增强疗效。

Withdrawal: For the withdrawal of the needle, press the skin around the acupoint slightly with sterilized dry cotton balls held by the left hand, rotate the needle handle gently and lift it slowly to the subcutaneous level with the right hand, then withdraw it quickly and press the punctured acupoint with sterilized dry cotton balls to prevent bleeding. After the treatment, the acupuncturist should count the number of the needles to make sure that all the needles are withdrawn.

（2）出针：出针时，左手用消毒干棉球轻轻压住针孔周围的皮肤，右手微捻针柄，慢慢将针上提至皮下，而后迅速拔出，随即用消毒干棉球按住针孔，以防出血。最后，医者应检查针数，以防遗漏。

3.2.1.1.5 Reinforcing and reducing methods

Reinforcing and reducing methods refer to specific needling manipulations used to treat asthenia and sthenia syndromes. They can be used to regulate the asthenia and sthenia states of the body. In terms of manipulations, the reinforcing and reducing manipulations in each kind of reinforcing-reducing method are in relation to each other. The following are some of the commonly used methods in clinical treatment:

Reinforcing and reducing manipulation by twirling and rotating the needle: When qi is obtained after insertion of the needle, rotating the needle gently and slowly with small amplitude is known as the reinforcing manipulation, while rotating the needle rapidly with large amplitude is known as the reducing manipulation. Rotating the needle forward with the thumb and backward with the

5．针刺补泻手法

针刺补泻手法是一类用于虚证和实证的有特定操作方式的针刺方法。补泻针法具有调整机体虚实状态的作用。在操作方法上，每种针刺补泻手法的补法与泻法都是相互对应的。临床常用的有以下几种：

（1）捻转补泻法：进针得气后，进行小角度的缓慢捻转为补法；大角度的较快捻转为泻法。或以拇指向前、食指向后的左转为补法；拇指向后、食指向前的右转为泻法。

index finger means reinforcing, while rotate the needle backward with the thumb and forward with the index finger means reducing.

Reinforcing and reducing manipulation by lifting and thrusting the needle: After the needling sensation has been achieved, the reinforcing effect is obtained by repeatedly thrusting the needle heavily and rapidly and then lifting the needle gently and slowly. The reducing effect is achieved by repeatedly lifting the needle forcefully and rapidly and then thrusting the needle gently and slowly.

（2）提插补泻法：进针得气后，将针由浅层快速下插，而后缓慢上提，反复操作，为补法；由深层快速上提，而后缓慢下插，反复操作，为泻法。

Reinforcing and reducing manipulation by rapid and slow insertion and withdrawal of the needle: After the needle is inserted into the subcutaneous level, inserting the needle slowly and withdrawing it rapidly means reinforcing, while inserting the needle rapidly and withdrawing it slowly means reducing.

（3）徐疾补泻法：刺入表皮后，由浅入深缓慢进针，出针时速度快为补法；由浅入深快速进针，慢速出针为泻法。

Reinforcing and reducing manipulation by keeping the needled acupoint open or close: Pressing the acupoint quickly to close it after the withdrawal of the needle means reinforcing, while shaking it to enlarge the needled hole means reducing.

（4）开阖补泻法：出针后迅速按闭针孔为补法；出针时，摇针以扩大针孔，不按闭针孔为泻法。

Reinforcing and reducing manipulation by the direction of the needle tip toward which the tip of the needle points: The needle tip pointing to the direction following the flowing route of the meridian means reinforcing while the needle tip pointing to the direction against the flowing route of the meridian means reducing.

（5）迎随补泻法：针尖顺着经脉循行方向刺入为补法；针尖逆着经脉循行方向刺入为泻法。

Reinforcing and reducing manipulation by means of respiration: The reinforcing is achieved by inserting the needle when the patient breathes out and withdrawing the needle when the patient breathes in. The opposite way of practice means reducing.

（6）呼吸补泻法：待病人呼气时进针、吸气时出针为补法；吸气时进针、呼气时出针为泻法。

The above reinforcing and reducing methods can be used individually or in combination.

以上各种补泻手法，既可单独应用，也可数种综合运用。

In addition, for treatment of diseases without typical sthenia or asthenia syndrome, mild reinforcing and reducing method can be used. Mild reinforcing and reducing method means to lift and thrust as well as twirl and rotate the needle evenly and gently at moderate speed when the needle is inserted into the acupoint.

此外，对虚实不甚明显的病证，可用"平补平泻法"，方法是进针得气后，均匀地、速度适中地行提插、捻转操作。

3.2.1.1.6 Cautions

6. 注意事项

It is advisable to delay giving acupuncture treatment to the patients who are very nervous, or over-fatigued.

(1) 对精神过度紧张、过于疲劳者，不宜立即针刺。

It is inadvisable to give acupuncture treatment to women during pregnancy, or women with menstruation. Acupoints on the vertex of infants should not be needled when the fontanel is not closed. Acupoints on the areas with infection, ulcer, scar or tumor should not be needled. Patients with disturbance of blood coagulation and hemorrhagic tendency should not be punctured.

(2) 孕妇、妇女月经期不宜针刺；小儿囟门未合时，头顶部不宜针刺；皮肤有感染、溃疡、瘢痕及肿瘤部位，不宜针刺；凝血机能障碍，有出血倾向者，不宜针刺。

Acupoints on the ocular area, neck, or close to the vital organs or large blood vessels should be carefully needled (see Section 3.5).

(3) 眼区、颈项部、靠近重要脏器和大血管处的腧穴慎刺(详见第五节"各部常用腧穴的针刺方法")。

The selection of needling methods should be made according to the tolerance of patients. For the patients who are very nervous or weak, mild manipulation can be used.

(4) 针刺手法的轻重应以病人能够耐受为度，对体质虚弱、精神过度紧张者手法宜轻。

3.2.1.1.7 Management of possible accidents

7. 异常情况的处理

Fainting: This is caused by nervousness, delicate constitution, over-fatigue, improper position or forceful manipulation. During acupuncture treatment, there may display such manifestations as dizziness, vertigo, pallor, palpitation, chest distress, nausea, vomiting and cold limbs. In severe cases, sudden syncope may be caused. When fainting has occurred, the needle should be withdrawn immediately. The acupuncturist should soothe the patient, help the patient lie down and offer him or her

(1) 晕针：由于病人精神过度紧张、体质虚弱、过于疲劳、体位不当或针刺手法过重等原因，病人在针刺过程中突然出现头晕目眩、面色苍白、心慌胸闷、恶心欲呕、四肢发冷，甚或突然昏倒。此时应立即出针，同时安慰病人，使其平卧，轻者经饮温开水、休息

some warm boiled water. The patient's condition will be improved after a short rest. In severe cases, acupoints like Shuigou (GV26), Suliao (GV25) and Neiguan (PC6) can be needled and Baihui (GV20), Guanyuan (CV4) can be moxibusted to resuscitate the patient. If the patient does not respond to the treatment, other emergency measures should be taken.

片刻后，就可恢复；重者还要针刺水沟、素髎、内关、灸百会、关元等穴，以促苏醒。如仍不省人事，应采取其他急救措施。

Stuck needle: When stuck needle happens, the acupuncturist may feel tense and unsmooth beneath the needle and difficult to twirl, rotate, lift or thrust the needle; the patient feels unbearably painful. Then the needle should not be twirled and rotated again. The methods used to cope with such accidents vary according to the conditions of the patient. If stuck needle is caused by nervousness and excessive contraction of the local muscles, the acupuncturist should soothe the patient first, appropriately prolong the retention of the needle, or press the local region gently, or insert another needle near the stuck needle. If it is caused by excessive rotation to one direction, then rotation of the needle to the opposite direction with slight lifting and thrusting will solve the problem.

(2) 滞针：是指医者感觉针下非常紧涩，难以进行捻转和提插等操作，病人也感觉疼痛难忍。处理方法须视不同原因而定，如果是由于病人紧张致局部肌肉过度收缩者，应安慰病人，适当延长留针时间，或在局部轻柔按压，或在邻近处再刺一针；如果是因医者单向捻针所致者，应反方向捻针，再轻轻提插，即可消除滞针。

Bent needle: When the needle is bent, twirling and rotating manipulation should in no case be applied. The needle may be removed and withdrawn slowly by following the direction of bending. The following methods can be taken to avoid bending the needle: During needling, the patient should not change his or her position; the acupuncturist should manipulate the needle gently, avoiding forceful manipulation. And during the retention period, the needle handle shall in no case be impacted or pressed by external force.

(3) 弯针：如果在针刺后出现针身弯曲，不可再行捻转等操作，应将针顺着弯曲方向缓缓退出。针刺前应嘱病人不要变更体位；医者针刺操作要轻柔，不可用力过猛；留针时针柄不得受外物碰撞和压迫，以避免发生弯针。

Broken needle: When the needle is broken, the acupuncturist should keep calm, ask the patient not to change his or her position to prevent the broken needle from

(4) 断针：若出现针身断于体内的情况，医者须镇静，令病人不要变动体位，以防断

getting deeper into the body. If the broken part protrudes over the skin, it should be removed with forceps. If the broken part is kept at the same level of the skin or a little depressed, the skin around the needle is pressed perpendicularly with the thumb and the index finger of the left hand in order to expose the broken end which is then removed with forceps. If it is completely sunken into the skin, surgical treatment should be resorted to. The following methods can be taken to prevent breaking of the needle: The quality of the needle is inspected carefully prior to the treatment; the patient is advised not to change the position; manipulation should be performed gently and slightly, avoiding forceful manipulation lest the needle be broken.

针陷入深部。如果针身尚有部分露于体外，可用镊子取出；如果断端与皮肤相平或稍陷，可用左手拇、食两指在针旁垂直向下按压皮肤，以使针体露出，右手用镊子将针取出；如果针体已进入深部，应手术取出。针刺前要做好预防工作，应认真检查针具；嘱病人不要变更体位；医者针刺操作要轻柔，不可用力过猛等，以防断针。

Hematoma: Hematoma refers to swelling pain caused by subcutaneous hemorrhage around the area needled. If the local region is cyanotic or painful after the withdrawal of the needle, the needled region should be immediately sterilized with dry cotton balls for a while to stop bleeding. If hematoma is mild, it will disappear automatically. If the local swelling and pain is serious and the area with cyanosis is large, cold compress can be used to stop immediate bleeding. After bleeding is stopped, hot compress or pressure is performed slightly and gently to help disperse the hematoma.

(5) 血肿：是指针刺部位出现皮下出血而致肿痛。如果出针后局部青紫或疼痛，应立即用消毒干棉球按压针孔片刻，即能止血；若是微量的皮下出血所致局部小块青紫可自行消退；若局部肿胀疼痛较剧，青紫面积大，须即时冷敷止血，待血止后改用热敷或轻轻揉按以助消散。

Pneumatothorax: On puncturing the acupoints located on the supraclavicular fossa, chest, back, axilla, and hypochondriac region, deep insertion may lead to pneumothorax due to the injury of the pleura and lung. The manifestations are sudden chest distress, pectoralgia, and short breath. In severe cases, there may exhibit dyspnea, cyanosis of the lips and nails, sweating and drop of blood pressure. Physical examination may find hyperresonance in percussing the chest, attenuation or disappearance of

(6) 气胸：在针刺缺盆胸、背、腋、胁等部位的腧穴时，如果直刺过深，刺伤胸膜和肺脏，则使空气进入胸腔而致气胸。表现为病人突感胸闷、胸痛、气短；甚则呼吸困难，唇甲发绀、出汗、血压下降等。体检时胸部叩诊过度反响，肺泡呼吸音减弱或消失

vesicular respiration, or shift of the trachea to the healthy side. X-ray can diagnose the degree of pneumothorax. If it is mild, the patient may rest in half-lying position and take some antitussive and antiseptic. The patient should be treated under careful inspection. In severe cases, emergency measures should be employed at once.

甚者气管向健侧移位。X线胸部透视可确诊气胸的程度。对轻者可取半卧位休息,给予镇咳、抗菌药物等对症处理,并严密观察;重者应立即采取抢救措施。

3.2.1.2 Needling methods of the three-edged needles

(二)三棱针刺法

The three-edged needle is the needle shaped with a triangular head and a sharp tip, known as "Lance needle" in the ancient times. It is used to prick superficial vein for bloodletting.

三棱针是一种针身呈三棱形、针尖锋利的针具,古代称"锋针"。用于刺络放血。

3.2.1.2.1 Scope of application

1. 适用范围

Pricking superficial vein for bloodletting with three-edged needle can dredge the meridians and collaterals, promote blood circulation to remove blood stasis, resuscitate the patient and expel heat. It is often used to treat sthenia syndrome and heat syndrome as well as acute and chronic diseases due to qi and blood stagnation in the meridians and collaterals, blood stasis and exuberance of pathogenic factors, such as high fever, loss of consciousness, convulsion and syncope, blood stasis in local region and pain syndrome.

以三棱针刺络放血,可起到疏通经络、活血祛瘀、开窍泄热的作用。多用于经络气血壅滞、血脉瘀阻、邪气盛实的实证、热证、急症以及某些慢性病,如高热、昏迷、惊厥、局部瘀血、痛证等。

3.2.1.2.2 Manipulations

2. 操作方法

Spot pricking: Hold the three-edged needle with the right hand, prick swiftly about 2 - 3 mm in depth for bloodletting. The needle is withdrawn immediately following bleeding. Or squeeze the punctured hole slightly to let out several drops of blood, then press the hole with a sterilized dry cotton ball until the bleeding stops.

(1) *点刺法*:右手持三棱针,对准要放血的部位迅速刺入约2~3毫米深,随之立即出针,以出血为度;也可用手轻轻挤压针孔周围,使之出血数滴即可,然后用消毒干棉球按压针孔止血。

Clumpy pricking: Prick around an affected small area, squeeze slightly with the hand or use cupping to drive the decayed blood out. This method can remove pathogenic

(2) *散刺法*:在患处的周围散在性地点刺出血,可以用手轻轻挤压或加拔火罐,使恶

factors and stop pain. It is usually used for treating carbuncles and obstructive syndrome, etc.

血尽出，有消毒止痛的作用。多用于外科痈肿、痹证等。

Pricking: Find the reaction point of disease first for pricking, pinch up the local skin with the left hand, prick about 2 mm in depth into the reaction point with a three-edged needle and push the needle up swiftly for bloodletting.

(3) 挑刺法：先在皮肤上寻找出要挑刺的疾病反应点，以左手捏起该处皮肤，用三棱针刺入反应点的表皮约 2 毫米深，迅速向上一挑，即可挑破出血。

3.2.1.2.3 Cautions

3. 注意事项

It is advisable to make necessary explanations for the patient.

Sterilization of the area for operation must be done strictly.

The pricking should be slight, shallow and swift; it is inadvisable to induce excessive bleeding; cares should be taken to avoid pricking the large blood vessels.

It is inadvisable to apply this method to the treatment of the patients with poor constitution or pregnant women or the patients with susceptibility to bleeding.

(1) 宜先对病人做好解释工作。

(2) 施术部位必须严格消毒。

(3) 针刺操作要轻、浅、快，出血不宜过多，切勿刺伤深部大动脉。

(4) 体弱、孕妇慎用，有出血倾向者不宜使用。

3.2.2 Modern methods

二、现代方法

3.2.2.1 Electro-acupuncture

(一) 电针

Electro-acupuncture is a kind of therapy by which the needle is attached to a trace pulse current after it is inserted to the selected acupoint for the purpose of producing synthetic effect of electric and needling stimulation. Different kinds of electric instruments are used. Most of them are composed of semiconductor elements and adopt oscillators. They generate low-frequency impulse current which is close to bioelectric current in the human body.

电针是在刺入人体的(毫)针上通以微量的脉冲电流，利用针、电两种刺激的综合作用治疗疾病的一种疗法。

应用器材主要是电针器，种类较多，多以半导体元件装制，采用振荡发生器，输出接近人体生物电的低频脉冲电流。

3.2.2.1.1 Manipulations

1. 操作方法

After the needle is inserted into a certain acupoint and the needling sensation is felt, adjust the output

毫针刺入穴位得气后，将电针器上的输出电位器调至

potential instrument of the electro-acupuncture stimulator to zero, then connect the two output wires with the two needle handles, select the required waveform and frequency, and then gradually amplify the output current to the tolerance of the patient. One to two minutes later, the human body will be adaptive to the stimulation and feel that the stimulation is getting weaker. At the time, increase the output current appropriately. The stimulation continues for 10 - 20 minutes or longer according to the pathological conditions of the patient. When the treatment is finished, the output potential instrument is adjusted back to zero, the electricity supply is cut off, the wires are taken away and then the needles are withdrawn.

"0"度，然后把两根输出导线分别接在两根针的针柄上，开启电源，选择所需波型和频率，再将输出电流逐渐调大至病人能耐受的程度。经1～2分钟的电刺激后，人体会产生适应而感觉刺激在变弱，此时可适当加大输出电流。通电时间一般为10～20分钟，也可根据病情需要适当延长通电时间。当结束电针治疗时，要在出针前将输出电位器调回到"0"度，然后关闭电源，取下导线，最后出针。

3.2.2.1.2 Scope of application

Generally speaking, it can be used to treat any disease within the indication of acupuncture, especially pain syndromes, obstructive syndromes, flaccidity syndromes. It can also be used for acupuncture anaesthesia.

2. 适用范围

凡针刺治疗的适应证，一般都可适用。多用于各种痛证、痹证、痿证，也常用于针刺麻醉。

3.2.2.1.3 Cautions

Before using the electro-acupuncture stimulator, careful examination mustbe made to make sure that it is in good condition and that the switches are off.

The current should be reinforced gradually in adjustment. Sudden increase should be avoided lest spasm of the muscles and breaking of the needles be caused.

If the highest output voltage of the electro-acupuncture stimulator is over 40 volts, the strongest output current should be controlled within 1 mA to prevent electric shock.

For the patients with cardiopathy, the current return circuit through the heart should be avoided. For the patients with weak physique, it is inadvisable to adopt strong

3. 注意事项

(1) 使用前须先检查电针器是否良好，各开关应处于关闭状态。

(2) 调节电流量时，应逐渐由小到大，不可突然增强，以防引起肌肉强烈收缩而致弯针、断针。

(3) 电针器最大输出电压在40伏以上者，其最大输出电流应控制在1毫安内，以免发生触电事故。

(4) 心脏病患者，应避免电流回路通过心脏。体弱者，电流不宜过大，以防晕针。

current in order to avoid fainting.

It is inadvisable to select the needles that were used for heated needling, because their handle surface is oxidized and cannot conduct electricity.

（5）温针灸用过的毫针，针柄因火烧而使表面氧化不导电，不宜使用。

3.2.2.2 Acupoint injection

（二）穴位注射

Acupoint injection, also known as "water-needling", is a therapy used to inject the medicated solution into an acupoint or a point with positive reaction to produce a synthetic effect of acupuncture and medicaments.

穴位注射也称"水针"，是将药液注入穴位或阳性反应点，通过针刺和药物的双重作用治疗疾病的一种疗法。

3.2.2.2.1 Manipulations

1. 操作方法

The medicated solution is drawn with a suitable injector and a syringe needle, inserted quickly to the subcutaneous region of an acupoint and pushed it slowly to a certain depth. When the needling sensation (such as aching and distention) is induced, the syringe needle is withdrawn a little and the medicated solution is injected if there is no blood drawn into the injector. For the patients with deficiency syndrome or poor constitution, the speed of injection should be slow; while for the patients with excessive syndrome or good constitution, the injection can be quickened appropriately.

以适当的注射器及针头吸取药液，快速刺入穴位处的皮下，然后慢慢刺达一定深度，待病人有酸、胀等得气感后，将针头回抽一下，如无回血，即可注入药液。虚证、体弱者，注入速度宜慢；实证、体强者，注入速度应适当加快。

The injection dose for each acupoint depends on the location of the acupoint, pathological conditions of the patient and the concentration of the medicated solution. Generally speaking, the injection dose for the acupoints located on the head and face is 0.3 - 0.5 ml, for those located on the chest and back region is 0.5 - 1 ml, and for those located on thick muscles of the limbs, waist and buttocks is 2 - 5 ml. For injection with small dose, the dose is 1/10 - 1/2 of the original dose of medicated solution. Usually the injection can be given once a day or once every other day. Six to eight times make up one course of treatment. For the treatment of emergent syndromes, the injection is given once or twice a day.

每个穴位的注射剂量，要根据部位、病情、药物浓度等酌情而定。一般情况下，头面部注射 0.3～0.5 毫升，胸背部注射 0.5～1 毫升，四肢及腰臀等肌肉丰厚处可注射 2～5 毫升。作小剂量注射时，可用原药物剂量的 1/10～1/2。一般每日或隔日注射 1 次，6～8次为 1 个疗程；急症每日 1～2次。

3.2.2.2.2 Scope of application

Acupoint injection can be used to treat most of the diseases in all clinical departments and often be applied to obstructive syndrome, stomachache, chronic bronchitis, asthma, and hypertension.

2. 适用范围

穴位注射可用于临床各科的大部分病症，常用于痹证、胃痛、慢性支气管炎、哮喘、高血压病等。

3.2.2.2.3 Cautions

Strict sterilization is needed to avoid infection; attention should be paid to the properties, pharmacological action, dosage, contraindication of compatibility, term of validity, side effect and allergic reactions of the drugs. As to the drugs which can induce allergic reaction, hypersensitive test should be done first. The vessels, articular cavity, and spinal column should in no case be injected with drugs. When the needle tip touches the trunk of the nerve and the patient feels like electricity shock, the needle must be withdrawn, the angle of insertion must be changed and the drugs are injected after the trunk of nerve is avoided. This therapy should be used with great care to treat the aged, patients with poor constitution, pregnant women and infants.

3. 注意事项

严格消毒，以防感染；注意药物的性能、药理作用、剂量、配伍禁忌、有效期、副作用和过敏反应等，凡能引起过敏反应的药物，须先作过敏试验；切勿将药物注入血管、关节腔、脊髓腔；若针尖触及神经干，患者有触电感，须退针、改变角度，避开神经干后方可注入药物；年老体弱者、孕妇、小儿等慎用。

3.2.2.3 Scalp acupuncture

Scalp acupuncture, also known as "head acupuncture", is a therapeutic method to puncture specific stimulating zone on the scalp, which is mainly used to treat encephalopathy.

(三) 头皮针

头皮针又称"头针"，是针刺头皮上的特定刺激区域以治疗疾病的一种方法。主要适用于脑源性疾病。

3.2.2.3.1 Location of stimulating zone and indication

Two standard lines must be decided first for dividing the stimulating zones (see Fig. 113).

Anterior-posterior midline: It refers to the line from the midpoint between the eyebrows (the anterior point of the midline) to the inferior border of the external occipital protuberance (the posterior point of the midline).

Brow-occipital line: It refers to the cephalic lateral

1. 刺激区部位和主治

先确定划分刺激区的两条标准定位线(见图 113)：

前后正中线：从两眉间中点(为正中线的前点)至枕外粗隆尖端下缘(为正中线的后点)的经过头顶的连线。

眉枕线：从眉中点上缘和

side line from the midpoint of the superior border of eyebrow to the tip of the external occipital protuberance.

枕外粗隆尖端的头侧面连线。

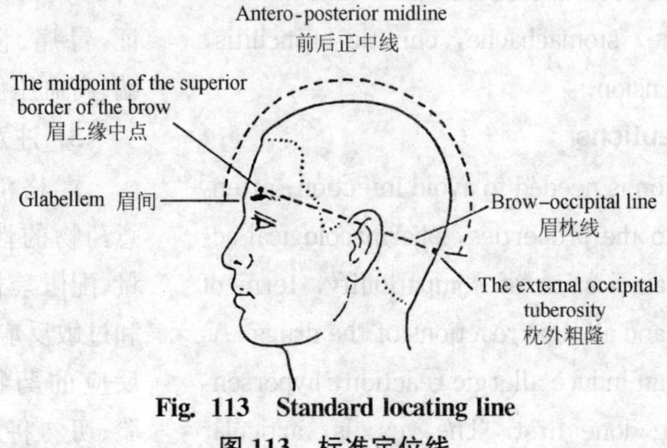

Fig. 113　Standard locating line

图 113　标准定位线

Motor zone:

Location: The superior point is located 0.5 cm posterior to the midpoint of the anterior-posterior midline, the inferior point at the junction of the brow-occipital line and the anterior border of temporal hairline. The line connecting the two points is the motor zone. The line is divided into five equal parts: the upper 1/5 is the motor zone of the lower limbs and trunk; the middle 2/5 is the motor zone of the upper limbs; the lower 2/5 is the motor zone of the face, also called the first lingual zone (see Fig. 114).

(1) 运动区:

部位：上点在前后正中线中点向后 0.5 厘米处，下点在眉枕线和鬓角发际前缘相交处，上下两点的连线即是运动区。将连线分作五等分，连线的上 1/5 段，为下肢、躯干运动区；中 2/5 段，为上肢运动区；下 2/5 段，为面运动区，也称言语一区(见图 114)。

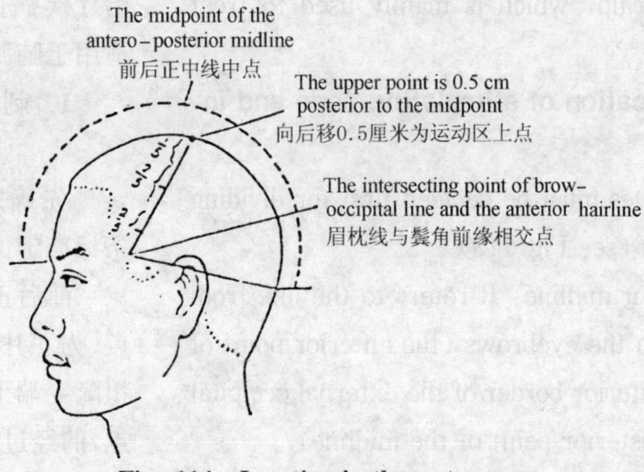

Fig. 114　Location in the motor zone

图 114　运动区定位

Indications: The upper 1/5 is for the treatment of contralateral paralysis of the lower limb; the middle 2/5 is for the treatment of contralateral superior paraplegia of the upper limb; the lower 2/5 is for the treatment of contralateral central facial paralysis, aphemia, drooling and dysphonia.

主治：上段主治对侧下肢瘫痪；中段主治对侧上肢瘫痪；下段主治对侧中枢性面瘫，运动性失语，流涎，发音障碍。

Sensory zone:

(2) 感觉区：

Location: It refers to the horizontal line 1.5 cm posterior to the motor zone. It is divide into five equal parts: the upper 1/5 is the sensory zone of the lower limbs, head and trunk; the middle 2/5 is the sensory zone of the upper limbs; the lower 2/5 is the sensory zone of the face (see Fig. 115).

部位：由运动区向后 1.5 厘米的平行线即是。将全线也分作五等分，上 1/5 段，为下肢、头、躯干感觉区；中 2/5 段，为上肢感觉区；下 2/5 段，为面感觉区(见图 115)。

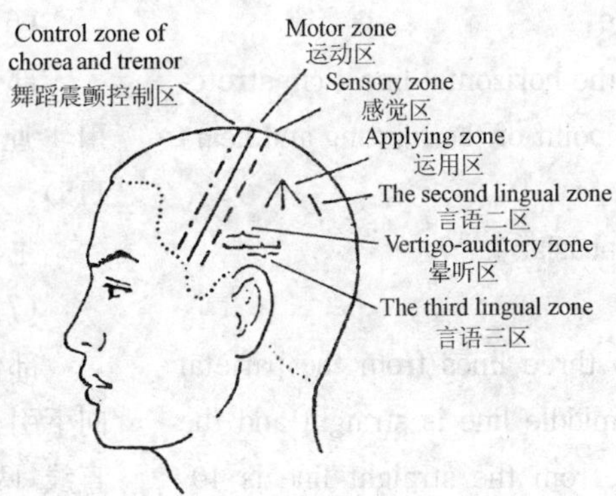

Fig. 115 Lateral stimulating zone

图 115 侧面刺激区

Indications: the upper 1/5 for contralateral lumbocrural pain, numbness, paresthesia, occiput pain, neck pain, vertigo, tinnitus; the middle 2/5 for contralateral upper limb pain, numbness, paresthesia; the low 2/5 for contralateral facial numbness, migraine, temporomandibular arthritis.

主治：上段主治对侧腰腿痛、麻木、感觉异常，后头、颈项部疼痛，头晕、耳鸣；中段主治对侧上肢疼痛、麻木、感觉异常；下段主治对侧面部麻木，偏头痛，颞颌关节炎等。

Control zone of chorea and tremor:

(3) 舞蹈震颤控制区：

Location: It refers to the horizontal line 1.5 cm anterior to the motor zone (see Fig. 115).

部位：自运动区向前 1.5 厘米的平行线即是(见图 115)。

Indications: Chorea, paralysis agitans.

Vertigo-auditory zone:

Location: It refers to the horizontal line 1.5 cm directly from above the tip of the ear, stretching 2 cm to the face and occiput respectively (see Fig. 115).

Indications: Vertigo, tinnitus, hypoacusis.

The second lingual zone:

Location: It refers to the straight line 2 cm postero-inferior to the parietal tubercule and parallel to the anteroposterior midline, stretching 3 cm straightly and downwards (see Fig. 115).

Indications: Anomic aphasia.

The third lingual zone:

Location: It refers to the horizontal line 4 cm stretching backward from the midpoint of the fainting and hearing zone (see Fig. 115).

Indications: Sensory aphasia.

Applying zone:

Location: It refers to three lines from the parietal tubercule downward. The middle line is straight and the angle of the bilateral lines from the straight line is 40° respectively. All the three lines are 3 cm in length (see Fig. 115).

Indications: Apraxia.

The zone of pedal movement and sensation:

Location: It refers to two straight lines 3 cm stretching back 1 cm from both sides of the midpoint of the anteroposterior median line and parallel to the midline (see Fig. 116).

Indication: Paralysis, pain and numbness of the contralateral lower limb, acute lumbar sprain, nocturia, cortical diuresis and hysteroptosis.

主治：舞蹈病，震颤麻痹。

(4) 晕听区：

部位：从耳尖直上1.5厘米处，向前、后各引2厘米的水平线即是(见图115)。

主治：眩晕，耳鸣、听力减退。

(5) 言语二区：

部位：从顶骨结节后下方2厘米处引一平行于前后正中线的直线，向下取3厘米长直线(见图115)。

主治：命名性失语。

(6) 言语三区：

部位：在晕听区中点向后引4厘米长的水平线(见图115)。

主治：感觉性失语。

(7) 运用区：

部位：以顶骨结节为起点向下引三条线，中间的为一垂直线，两侧的线分别与中线呈40°夹角，长度均为3厘米(见图115)。

主治：失用症。

(8) 足运感区：

部位：在前后正中线的中点旁开左右各1厘米，向后引3厘米长的平行于正中线的直线(见图116)。

主治：对侧下肢瘫痪、疼痛、麻木，急性腰扭伤，夜尿，皮质性多尿，子宫脱垂等。

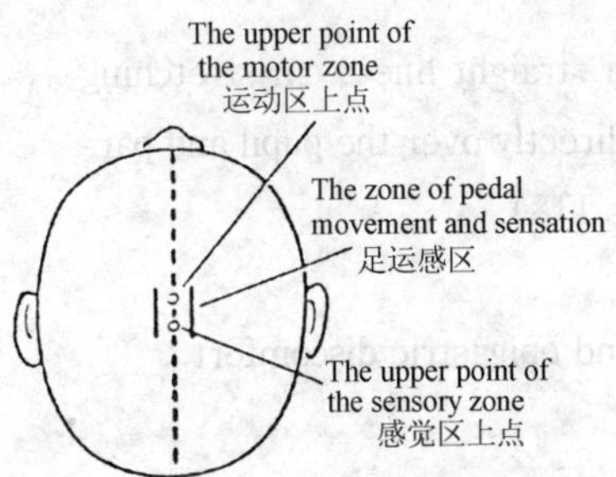

Fig. 116 Vertex stimulating zone
图 116 顶面刺激区

Visual zone:

Location: It refers to a straight line 4 cm stretching upwards 1 cm from both sides of the posterior point of the anteroposterior midline and parallel to the midline (see Fig. 117).

(9) 视区:

部位:在前后正中线的后点旁开左右 1 厘米处,向上引 4 厘米长的平行于前后正中线的直线(见图 117)。

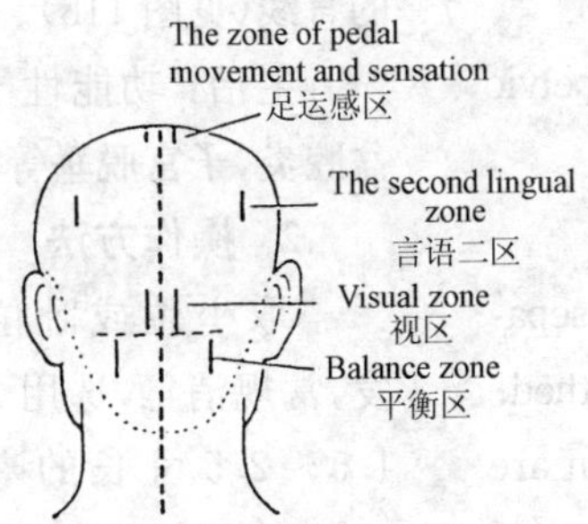

Fig. 117 Posterior stimulating zone
图 117 后面刺激区

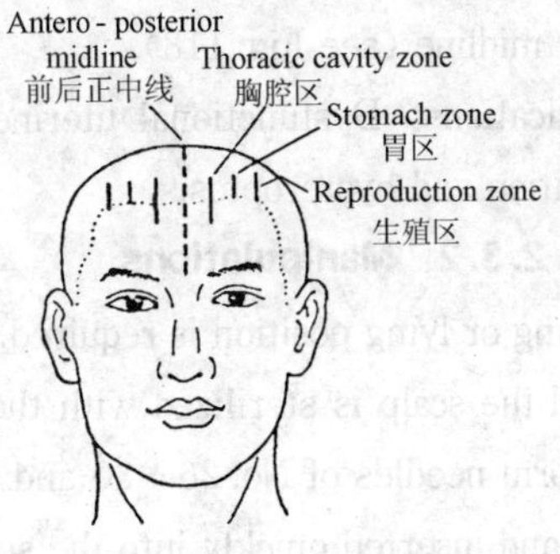

Fig. 118 Anterior stimulating zone
图 118 前面刺激区

Indications: Cortical visual disturbance.

主治:皮质性视力障碍。

Balance zone:

Location: It refers to a straight line 4 cm stretching downwards and 3.5 cm from both sides of the posterior point of the anteroposterior midline and parallel to the midline (see Fig. 117).

Indications: Ataxia due to cerebellar diseases and paraequilibrium.

(10) 平衡区:

部位:在前后正中线的后点旁开左右 3.5 厘米处,向下引 4 厘米长的平行于前后正中线的直线(见图 117)。

主治:小脑疾病引起的共济失调,平衡障碍。

Stomach zone:

Location: It refers to a straight line 2 cm stretching upwards from the hair line directly over the pupil and parallel to the midline (see Fig. 118).

Indications: Gastritis and epigastric discomfort.

Thoracic cavity zone:

Location: Between the stomach zone and the anteroposterior midline, two straight lines 2 cm stretching from the hairline upwards and downwards respectively and parallel to the midline (see Fig. 118).

Indications: Asthma and thoracic discomfort.

Reproduction zone:

Location: It refers to a straight line 2 cm stretching upwards from the frontal angle and parallel to the anterioposterior midline (see Fig. 118).

Indications: Dysfunctional uterine bleeding, pelvic inflammation and hysteroptosis.

3.2.2.3.2 Manipulations

Sitting or lying position is required. The hair is separated and the scalp is sterilized with the routine method. The filiform needles of No. 26 - 30 and 1.5 - 2.5 cun are selected and inserted quickly into the subcutaneous region or the muscular layer with an angle of about 30° and along the stimulating area to a corresponding depth followed by rapid twirling and rotation. Method: The index finger in semi-flexion, the palmar surface of the thumb and the radial surface of the index finger hold the needle handle, twirl and rotate the handle quickly at the speed of approximately 200 times per minute for 1 - 2 minutes (or use electro-acupuncture to replace twirling and rotation of the needle), retain the needle for 5 - 10 minutes, repeatedly manipulate the needles for twice or 3 times and then

(11) 胃区：

部位：以瞳孔直上的发际处为起点，向上引 2 厘米长的平行于前后正中线的直线(见图 118)。

主治：胃痛、上腹部不适等症。

(12) 胸腔区：

部位：在胃区与前后正中线之间，从发际向上、下各引 2 厘米长的平行于前后正中线的直线(见图 118)。

主治：哮喘，胸部不适等症。

(13) 生殖区：

部位：从额角处向上引 2 厘米长的平行于前后正中线的直线(见图 118)。

主治：功能性子宫出血，盆腔炎，子宫脱垂等。

2. 操作方法

取坐位或卧位，分开头发，常规消毒，选用 26～30 号 1.5～2.5 寸长的毫针，以约 30°角快速刺入头皮下或肌层，沿刺激区进针到相应的深(长)度后，进行快速捻转。方法是食指呈半屈曲状，用拇指掌侧面与食指的桡侧面捏住针柄，并快速搓捻针柄，约 200 次/分钟左右，持续约 1～2 分钟(也可以电针代替手捻)，留针 5～10 分钟，再反复操作 2～3次，即可出针。留针期间可让病人活动患肢(或作被动

withdraw the needle. During the retention of the needles, the patient is advised to exercise the affected limb (or doing passive movement) to strengthen functional exercise. This treatment is given once a day or once every other day and 10 - 15 times make up one course of treatment. There is an interval of one week between two courses of treatment.

活动),以加强功能锻炼。一般每日或隔日治疗1次,10～15次为1个疗程,疗程之间休息1周。

3.2.2.3.3 Cautions

Sterilize strictly to avoid infection. When withdrawing the needle, press the punctured point with disinfected dry cotton balls to prevent bleeding. For the patients with cerebral hemorrhage, it is advisable to treat them with scalp acupuncture after the pathological condition and blood pressure are stable.

3. 注意事项

严格消毒,以防感染。出针时用消毒干棉球按压针孔,防止出血。对脑出血患者,宜在病情及血压稳定后再进行头皮针治疗。

3.2.2.4 Ear acupuncture

Ear acupuncture is a therapy to treat and prevent diseases by stimulating certain points on the auricle with needles. The scope of indication is wide. It is a commonly used therapy in clinical acupuncture treatment.

(四)耳针

耳针是用针刺等方法刺激耳郭上的特定部位来防治疾病的一种方法。其治病范围广,为针灸临床常用的疗法。

3.2.2.4.1 Terminology for the anatomical regions of the auricular surface (see Fig.119)

1. 耳郭表面解剖名称(见图119)

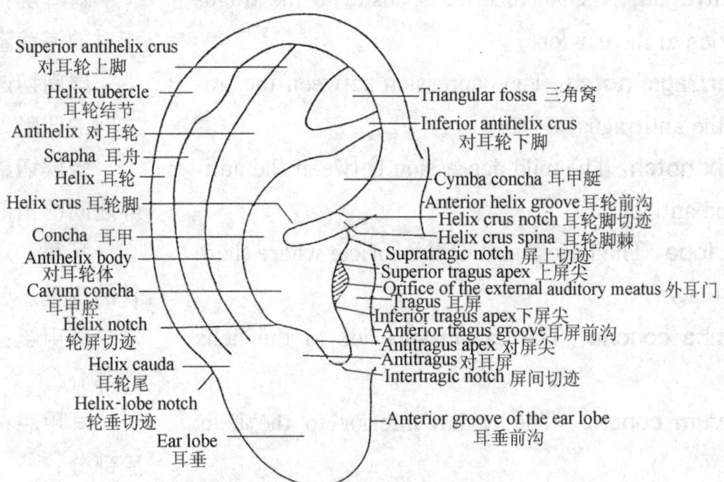

Fig. 119 Superficial anatomy of auricle

图119 耳郭表面解剖

Helix: The prominent rim of the auricle. A transverse ridge of helix extending into the ear cavity is called "**helix crus**"; a small tubercle at the posterior-inferior side of the helix is called "**helix tubercle**"; the junction of the inferior part of the helix and the lobule is called "**helix cauda**".

耳轮：耳郭最外缘的卷曲部分。耳轮深入至耳腔的横行突起部分称"**耳轮脚**"；耳轮后上方稍突起处称"**耳轮结节**"；耳轮末端与耳垂的交界处称"**耳轮尾**"。

Antihelix: An elevated ridge anterior and parallel to the helix at the medial side of the helix, also called "**the principal part of antihelix**". The superior branch of the bifurcation of the antihelix is called "**superior antihelix crus**", and the inferior branch is called "**inferior antihelix crus**".

对耳轮：位于耳轮的内侧，是与耳轮相对的、上部有分叉的隆起部分，又称"**对耳轮体**"。其分叉的上支称"**对耳轮上脚**"，下支称"**对耳轮下脚**"。

Triangular fossa: The triangular depression between the two crura of the antihelix.

三角窝：指对耳轮上脚、下脚之间的三角形凹陷。

Scapha: The curved depression between the helix and antihelix.

耳舟：是耳轮与对耳轮之间的凹沟。

Tragus: A curved flap in front of the auricle.

耳屏：耳郭前面的瓣状突起部。

Supratragic notch: The depression between the helix crus and the upper border of the tragus.

屏上切迹：耳屏上缘与耳轮脚之间的凹陷。

Antitragus: A small tubercle opposite to the tragus and inferior to the ear lobe.

对耳屏：耳垂上部与耳屏相对的瓣状隆起。

Intertragic notch: The depression between the tragus and the antitragus.

屏间切迹：耳屏与对耳屏之间的凹陷。

Helix notch: The mild depression between the antitragus and antihelix.

轮屏切迹：对耳轮与对耳屏之间的稍凹陷处。

Ear lobe: The lowest part of the auricle where there is no cartilage.

耳垂：耳郭最下部，无软骨的皮垂。

Cymba concha: The cavum superior to the helix crus.

耳甲艇：耳轮脚以上的耳腔部分。

Cavum concha: The cavum inferior to the helix crus.

耳甲腔：耳轮脚以下的耳腔部分。

Orifice of the external auditory meatus: The orifice anterior to the cavum concha.

外耳门：耳甲腔前方的孔窍。

3.2.2.4.2 Distribution of auricular acupoints

In view of the corresponding relationship between auricular acupoints and each part of the human body, the distribution of auricular acupoints is just like an inverted fetus (see Fig. 120). The acupoints located in the lower part of the ear (ear lobe) are related to the head and face, those in the upper part of the ear (including scapha and superior antihelix crus) to the limbs, those in the middle part of the ear (including cymba concha and cavum concha) to the internal organs, and those mainly in the middle part of the ear (the principal part of antihelix) to the trunk.

2. 耳穴的分布规律

从耳穴与人体各部的对应关系来看,耳穴在耳郭上的分布,像一个倒置的胎儿(见图 120),与头面相应的穴位在耳的下部(耳垂),与四肢相应的穴位在耳的上部(耳舟、对耳轮上脚),与内脏相应的穴位在耳的中部(耳甲艇、耳甲腔),与躯干相应的穴位也大体在耳的中部(对耳轮体)。

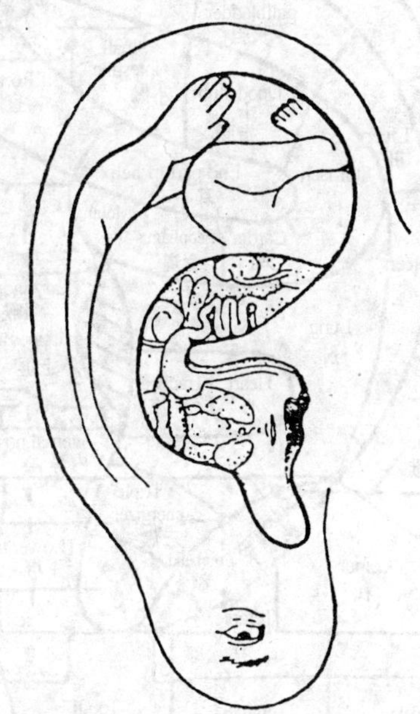

Fig. 120 Image distribution of the ear
图 120 耳穴的形象分布

3.2.2.4.3 Name, location and indication of the commonly used ear acupoints (see Fig. 121 and 122)

Helix:

Middle Ear HX$_1$—On the helix crus, also called HX$_1$. Indications: Hiccup, urticaria, cutaneous pruritus, infantile enuresis and hemoptysis.

3. 常用耳穴的名称、部位和主治(见图 121、图 122)

耳轮部:

耳中 HX$_1$——在耳轮脚上,即耳轮 1 区。主治呃逆,荨麻疹,皮肤瘙痒,小儿遗尿,咯血。

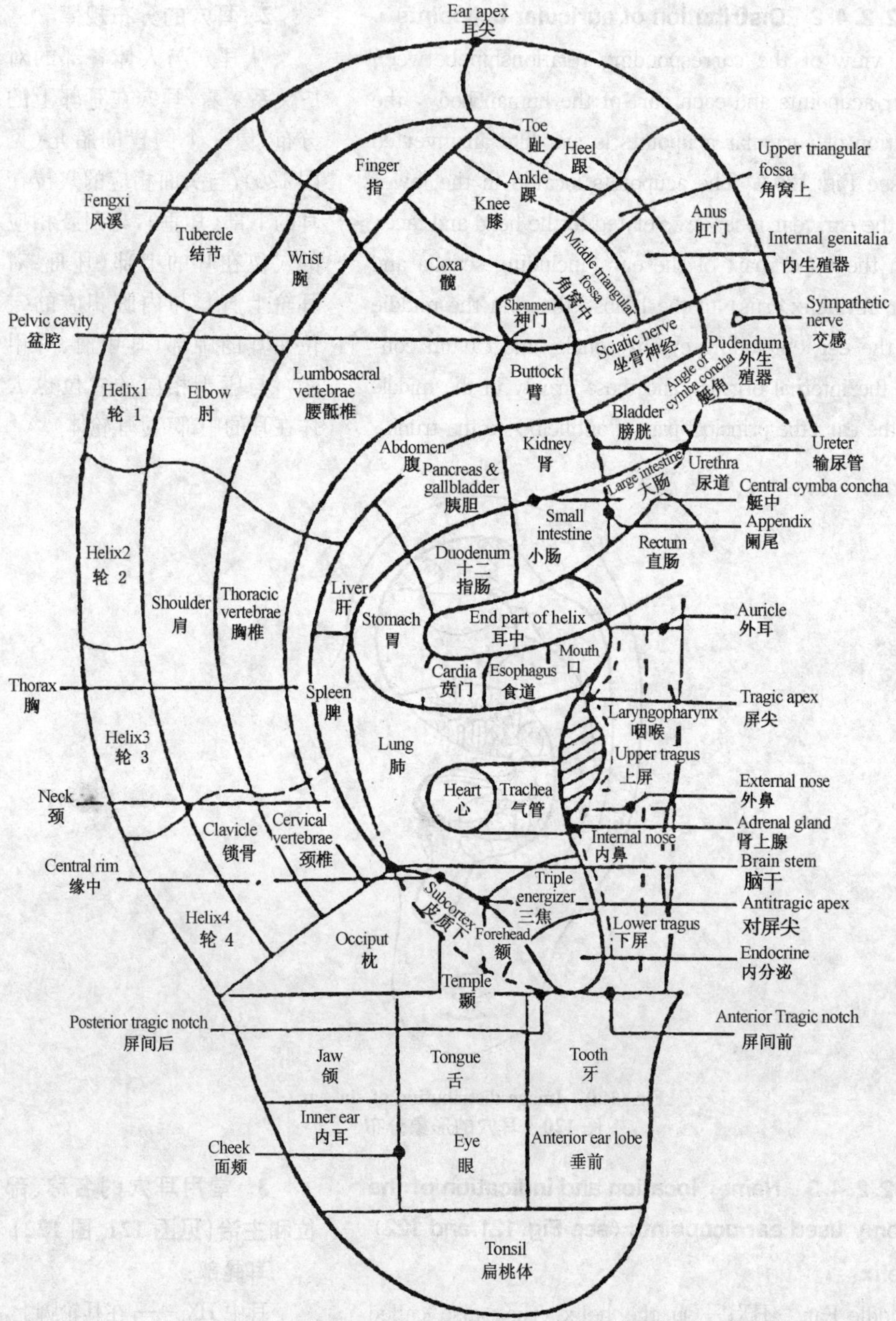

Fig. 121 Location of the ear (front)

图 121 耳穴定位（正面）

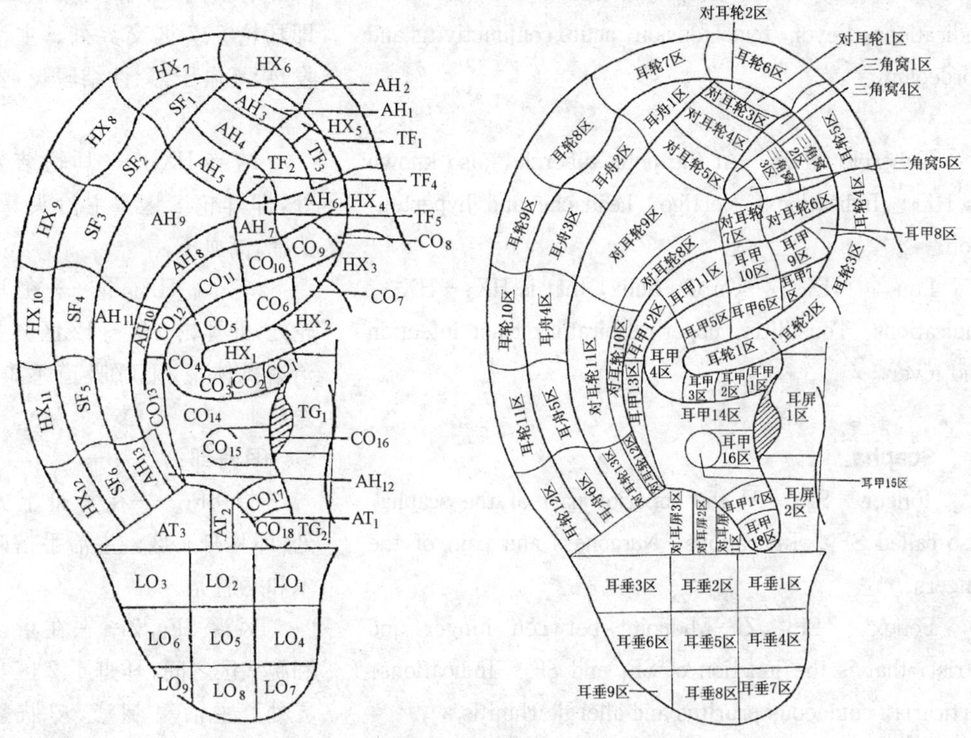

Fig. 122 Divisions of the auricle (front)

图 122 耳郭分区(正面)

Rectum HX_2—On the helix near the supratragic notch, also called HX_2. Indications: Constipation, diarrhea, anus prolapse and hemorrhoids.

直肠 HX_2——在近屏上切迹的耳轮处,即耳轮 2 区。主治便秘,腹泻,脱肛,痔疮。

Urethra HX_3—On the helix superior to Rectum, also called HX_3. Indications: Frequent, urgent and painful urination as well as retention of urine.

尿道 HX_3——在直肠上方的耳轮处,即耳轮 3 区。主治尿频,尿急,尿痛,尿潴留。

External Genitalia HX_4—On the helix at level with the upper border of inferior antihelix crus, also called HX_4. Indications: Orchitis, epididymidis and pruritus of vulva.

外生殖器 HX_4——在与对耳轮下脚上缘相平的耳轮处,即耳轮 4 区。主治睾丸炎,附睾炎,外阴瘙痒症。

Anus HX_5—On the helix at level with the anterior border of superior antihelix crus, also known as HX_5. Indications: Hemorrhoid and anal fissure.

肛门 HX_5——在与对耳轮上脚前缘相对的耳轮处,即耳轮 5 区。主治痔疮,肛裂。

Ear Apex $HX_{6,7}$—At the tip of auricle when folded

耳尖 $HX_{6,7}$——将耳轮向

towards tragus, that is at the junction of HX_6 and HX_7. Indications: Fever, hypertension, acute conjunctivitis and hordeolum.

耳屏对折时,耳郭上尖端处,即耳轮6、7区交界处。主治发热,高血压,急性结膜炎,麦粒肿。

Tubercle HX_8—At the helix tubercle, also known as HX_8. Indications: Vertigo, headache and hypertension.

结节 HX_8——耳轮结节处,即耳轮8区。主治头晕,头痛,高血压。

Lun$_{1-4}$ HX_{9-12}—On the helix, that is HX_9 - HX_{12}. Indications: Tonsillitis, upper respiratory tract infection and fever.

轮$_{1\sim4}$ $HX_{9\sim12}$——在耳轮处,即耳轮9区～12区。主治扁桃体炎,上呼吸道感染,发热。

Scapha:

耳舟部:

Finger SF_1—At the superior part of the scapha, also called SF_1. Indications: Numbness and pain of the fingers.

指 SF_1——在耳舟上方处,即耳舟1区。主治手指麻木和疼痛等。

Fengxi SF_1, Zi—Midpoint between Finger and Wrist, that is the junction of SF_1 and SF_2. Indications: Urticaria, cutaneous pruritus and allergic rhinitis.

风溪 SF_1,Zi——在指区和腕穴区之间,耳舟1、2区交界处。主治荨麻疹,皮肤瘙痒,过敏性鼻炎。

Wrist SF_2—The point inferior to Finger, also known as SF_2. Indication: Pain of the wrist.

腕 SF_2——在指区下方,即耳舟2区。主治腕部疼痛。

Elbow SF_3—The point inferior to Wrist, also called SF_3. Indications: External humeral epicondylitis and pain of the wrist.

肘 SF_3——在腕区下方,即耳舟3区。主治肱骨外上髁炎,肘部疼痛。

Shoulder $SF_{4,5}$—The point inferior to Elbow, also known as SF_4, SF_5. Indication: Scapulohumeral periarthritis.

肩 $SF_{4,5}$——在肘区下方,即耳舟4、5区。主治肩关节周围炎。

Clavicle SF_6—The point inferior to Shoulder, also called SF_6. Indication: Scapulohumeral periarthritis.

锁骨 SF_6——在肩区下方,即耳舟6区。主治肩关节周围炎。

Antihelix:

对耳轮部:

Heel AH_1—Superior and medial of superior antihelix crus, near Triangular fossa, also called AH_1. Indication: Heel pain.

跟 AH_1——在对耳轮上脚的前上方,近三角窝上部,即对耳轮1区。主治足跟痛。

Toe AH_2—Superior and lateral of superior antihelix crus, also called AH_2. Indication: Toe pain.

趾 AH_2——在对耳轮上脚的后上方，即对耳轮 2 区。主治足趾疼痛。

Ankle AH_3—Midway between Heel and Knee, also called AH_3. Indication: Ankle sprain.

踝 AH_3——在跟、膝两穴区之间，即对耳轮 3 区。主治踝关节扭伤。

Knee AH_4—At middle 1/3 portion of superior antihelix crus, also called AH_4. Indication: Swelling and pain of the knee joint.

膝 AH_4——在对耳轮上脚的中 1/3 处，即对耳轮 4 区。主治膝关节肿痛。

Hip AH_5—At lower 1/3 portion of superior antihelix crus, also called AH_5. Indications: Pain of hip and sciatica.

髋 AH_5——在对耳轮上脚的下 1/3 处，即对耳轮 5 区。主治髋关节疼痛，坐骨神经痛。

Sciatic Nerve AH_6—At the anterior 2/3 of the inferior antihelix crus, also called AH_6. Indication: Sciatica.

坐骨神经 AH_6——在对耳轮下脚的前 2/3 处，即对耳轮 6 区。主治坐骨神经痛。

Sympathetic Nerve AH_{6a}—At the junction of the terminal of the inferior antihelix crus and helix, that is the anterior part of AH_6. Indications: Gastrointestinal spasm, angina pectoris, biliary colic, ureterolith and functional disorder of autonomous nerve system.

交感 AH_{6a}——在对耳轮下脚末端与耳轮交界处，即对耳轮 6 区前端。主治胃肠痉挛，心绞痛，胆绞痛，输尿管结石，自主神经功能紊乱。

Buttocks AH_7—At lateral 1/3 of the inferior antihelix crus, also called AH_7. Indications: Sciatica and gluteal fascitis.

臀 AH_7——在对耳轮下脚的后 1/3 处，即对耳轮 7 区。主治坐骨神经痛，臀筋膜炎。

Abdomen AH_8—At medial 2/5 of the principal part of antihelix, also known as AH_8. Indications: Abdominal pain and distension, diarrhea and acute lumbar sprain.

腹 AH_8——在对耳轮体前部上 2/5 处，即对耳轮 8 区。主治腹痛，腹胀，腹泻；急性腰扭伤。

Lumbosacral Vertebrae AH_9—At lateral of Abdomen, also called AH_9. Indication: Pain of lumbosacral region.

腰骶椎 AH_9——在腹区后方，即对耳轮 9 区。主治腰骶部疼痛。

Chest AH_{10}—At middle 2/5 of the anterior principal part of antihelix, also known as AH_{10}. Indications: Hypochondriac pain and mastadentitis.

胸 AH_{10}——在对耳轮体前部中 2/5 处，即对耳轮 10 区。主治胸胁痛，乳腺炎。

Thoracic Vertebrae　AH_{11}—Posterior to Chest，also called AH_{11}. Indications：Distending pain of breast，mastadentitis and hypogalactia after delivery.

胸椎 AH_{11}——在胸区后方，即对耳轮 11 区。主治胸痛，经前乳房胀痛，乳腺炎，产后缺乳。

Neck　AH_{12}—At lower 1/5 of the anterior principal part of antihelix，also called AH_{12}. Indications：Stiffness and swelling pain in the neck.

颈 AH_{12}——在对耳轮体前部下 1/5 处，即对耳轮 12 区。为颈椎穴区前侧。主治落枕，颈项肿痛。

Cervical Vertebrae　AH_{13}—Posterior to Neck，also called AH_{13}. Indications：Stiff neck and cervical vertebrae syndrome.

颈椎 AH_{13}——在颈区后方，即对耳轮 13 区。主治落枕，颈椎综合征。

Triangular Fossa：

三角窝部：

Upper Triangular Fossa　TF_1—At the upper part of anterior 1/3 of the fossa. Indication：Hypertension.

角窝上 TF_1——在三角窝前 1/3 的上部。主治高血压。

Internal Genitalia　TF_2—At the lower part of anterior 1/3 of the fossa. Indications：Dysmenorrhea，irregular menstruation，leukorrhea，dysfunctional uterine bleeding，seminal emission and prospermia.

内生殖器 TF_2——在三角窝前 1/3 的下部。主治痛经，月经不调，白带过多，功能性子宫出血，遗精，早泄。

Middle Triangular Fossa　TF_3—At middle 1/3 of the fossa. Indication：Asthma.

角窝中 TF_3——在三角窝中 1/3 处。主治哮喘。

Shenmen　TF_4—At the upper part of posterior 1/3 of the fossa. Indications：Insomnia，dream disturbed sleep and pain syndrome.

神门 TF_4——在三角窝后 1/3 的上部。主治失眠，多梦，痛证。

Pelvic Cavity　TF_5—At the lower part of posterior 1/3 of the fossa. Indication：Pelvic inflammation.

盆腔 TF_5——在三角窝后 1/3 的下部。主治盆腔炎。

Tragus：

耳屏部：

Upper Tragus　TG_1—At the upper 1/2 of the external tragus. Indications：Laryngopharyngitis and rhinitis.

上屏 TG_1——在耳屏外侧面上 1/2 处。主治咽炎，鼻炎。

Lower Tragus　TG_2—At the lower 1/2 of the external tragus. Indications：Rhinitis and stuffy nose.

下屏 TG_2——在耳屏外侧面下 1/2 处。主治鼻炎，鼻塞。

External Ear　TG_{10}—Anterior to supratragic notch and near helix. Indications：Inflammation of external

外耳 TG_{10}——在屏上切迹前方近耳轮部。主治外耳

auditory canal, tympanitis and tinnitus.

Tragic Apex TG_{1p}—At the tip of upper free border of tragus. Indications: Fever and toothache.

External Nose $TG_{1,2i}$—Midpoint of the lateral side of tragus. Indications: Nasal vestibulitis and rhinitis.

Adrenal Gland TG_{2p}—At the tip of lower free border of tragus. Indications: Hypotension, rheumatic arthritis and parotitis.

Throat TG_3—At upper 1/2 of the medial side of tragus. Indications: Hoarseness, laryngopharyngitis and tonsillitis.

Internal Nose TG_4—At lower 1/2 of the medial side of tragus. Indications: Rhinitis, paranasal sinusitis and epistaxis.

Anterior Intertragus TG_{21}—Anterior to the intertragic notch, the lowest part of tragus. Indications: Stomatitis, maxillary sinusitis and nasopharyngitis.

Antitragus:

Forehead AT_1—At anterior part of the lateral side of antitragus. Indications: Vertigo, headache, insomnia and dreaminess.

Posterior Intertragus AT_{11}—Posterior to the intertragic notch and anterior-inferior to the antitragus. Indication: Maxillary sinusitis.

Temple AT_2—At the middle part of the lateral side of antitragus. Indication: Migraine.

Occiput AT_3—At the posterior part of the lateral side of antitragus. Indications: Vertigo, headache, asthma, epilepsy and neurosism.

Subcortex AT_4—At the medial side of Antitragus. Indications: Pain syndrome, neurosism and pseudomyopia.

道炎,中耳炎,耳鸣。

屏尖 TG_{1p}——在耳屏游离缘上部尖端。主治发热,牙痛。

外鼻 $TG_{1,2i}$——在耳屏外侧面的中部。主治鼻前庭炎,鼻炎。

肾上腺 TG_{2p}——在耳屏游离缘下部尖端。主治低血压,风湿性关节炎,腮腺炎。

咽喉 TG_3——在耳屏内侧面的上 1/2 处。主治声音嘶哑,咽喉炎,扁桃体炎。

内鼻 TG_4——在耳屏内侧面的下 1/2 处。主治鼻炎,副鼻窦炎,鼻衄。

屏间前 TG_{21}——在屏间切迹前方耳屏最下部。主治口腔炎,上颌炎,鼻咽炎。

对耳屏部:

额 AT_1——在对耳屏外侧面的前部。主治头晕,头痛,失眠,多梦。

屏间后 AT_{11}——在屏间切迹后方对耳屏前下部。主治颌窦炎。

颞 AT_2——在对耳屏外侧面的中部。主治偏头痛。

枕 AT_3——在对耳屏外侧面的后部。主治头晕,头痛,哮喘,癫痫,神经衰弱。

皮质下 AT_4——在对耳屏的内侧面。主治痛证,神经衰弱,假性近视。

Antitragic Apex　$AT_{1,2,4i}$—At the tip of antitragus. Indications: Asthma, parotitis, itching skin, orchitis and epididymidis.

对屏尖 $AT_{1,2,4i}$——在对耳屏的尖端。主治哮喘，腮腺炎，皮肤瘙痒，睾丸炎，附睾炎。

Middle Border　$AT_{2,3,4i}$—Midpoint between antitragic apex and helixtragic notch. Indications: Enuresis and auditory vertigo.

缘中 $AT_{2,3,4i}$——在对屏尖与轮屏切迹之中点处。主治遗尿，内耳眩晕症。

Brain Stem　$AT_{3,4i}$—At the helixtragic notch. Indications: Occipital headache, vertigo and pseudomyopia.

脑干 $AT_{3,4i}$——在轮屏切迹处。主治后头痛，眩晕，假性近视。

Concha:

耳甲部：

Mouth　CO_1—At anterior 1/3 of the inferior helix crus. Indications: Facial paralysis, stomatitis, cholecystitis and cholelithiasis.

口 CO_1——在耳轮脚下方前1/3处。主治面瘫，口腔炎，胆囊炎，胆石症。

Esophagus　CO_2—At middle 1/3 of the inferior helix crus. Indications: Esophgitis and esophagismus.

食道 CO_2——在耳轮脚下方中1/3处。主治食管炎，食管痉挛。

Cardia　CO_3—At posterior 1/3 of the inferior helix crus. Indications: Cardiospasm and neurogenic vomiting.

贲门 CO_3——在耳轮脚下方后1/3处。主治贲门痉挛，神经性呕吐。

Stomach　CO_4—At area where the helix crus terminates. Indications: Gastrospasm, gastric ulcer, gastritis, insomnia, toothache and indigestion.

胃 CO_4——在耳轮脚消失处。主治胃痉挛，胃炎，胃溃疡，失眠，牙痛，消化不良。

Duodenum　CO_5—At the posterior 1/3 between the helix crus, part of helix and AB line. Indications: Duodenal ulcer, cholepathy and pylorospasm.

十二指肠 CO_5——在耳轮脚及部分耳轮与AB线之间的后1/3处。主治十二指肠溃疡，胆管疾病，幽门痉挛。

Small Intestine　CO_6—At middle 1/3 between the helix crus, part of helix and AB line. Indications: Indigestion and palpitation.

小肠 CO_6——在耳轮脚及部分耳轮与AB线之间的中1/3处。主治消化不良，心悸。

Large Intestine　CO_7—At medial 1/3 between the helix crus, part of helix and AB line. Indications: Diarrhea, constipation, cough and acne.

大肠 CO_7——在耳轮脚及部分耳轮与AB线之间的前1/3处。主治腹泻，便秘，咳嗽，痤疮。

Appendix $CO_{6,7i}$—Between Small Intestine and Large Intestine. Indications: Appendicitis and diarrhea.

阑尾 $CO_{6,7i}$——在小肠区与大肠区之间。主治单纯性阑尾炎,腹泻。

Angle of Cymba Concha CO_8—At medial inferior part of inferior antitragus crus. Indications: Prostatitis and urethritis.

艇角 CO_8——在对耳轮下脚下方前部。主治前列腺炎,尿道炎。

Bladder CO_9—At middle inferior part of inferior antitragus crus. Indications: Cystitis, enuresis, anuresis, lumbago, sciatica and occipital headache.

膀胱 CO_9——在对耳轮下脚下方中部。主治膀胱炎,遗尿,尿闭,腰痛,坐骨神经痛,后头痛。

Kidney CO_{10}—At the lateral inferior part of inferior antitragus crus. Indications: Lumbago, tinnitus, insomnia, vertigo, irregular menstruation, seminal emission, prospermia and asthma.

肾 CO_{10}——在对耳轮下脚下方后部。主治腰痛,耳鸣,失眠,眩晕,月经不调,遗精,早泄,遗尿,哮喘等。

Ureter $CO_{9,10i}$—Between Bladder and Kidney. Indications: Stone and colic pain of ureter.

输尿管 $CO_{9,10i}$——在肾区与膀胱穴区之间。主治输尿管结石绞痛。

Pancrease and gallbladder CO_{11}—At the lateral superior part of the cymba concha. Indications: Cholepathy, migraine, herpes zoster, otitis media, tinnitus and acute pancreatitis.

胰胆 CO_{11}——在耳甲艇的后上部。主治胆管疾病,偏头痛,带状疱疹,中耳炎,耳鸣,急性胰腺炎。

Liver CO_{12}—At the lateral inferior part of the cymba concha. Indications: Hypochondriac pain, vertigo, eye diseases, premenstrual tension, irregular menstruation, menopausal syndrome and hypertension.

肝 CO_{12}——在耳甲艇的后下部。主治胁痛,眩晕,眼病,经前期紧张症,月经不调,更年期综合征,高血压等。

Middle Cymba Concha $CO_{6,10i}$—Between the Small Intestine and Kidney. Indications: Abdominal pain and distension, ascariasis of biliary tract and parotitis.

艇中 $CO_{6,10i}$——在小肠区与肾区之间。主治腹痛,腹胀,胆管蛔虫症,腮腺炎。

Spleen CO_{13}—Below the BD line, at lateral and superior part of cavum concha. Indications: Abdominal distension, diarrhea, constipation, anorexia, dysfunctional uterine bleeding, leukorrhea and auditory vertigo.

脾 CO_{13}——在 BD 线下方,耳甲腔的后上部。主治腹胀,腹泻,便秘,食欲不振,功能性子宫出血,白带过多,内耳眩晕症。

Heart CO_{15}—In the central depression of cavum

心 CO_{15}——在耳甲腔中

concha. Indications: Diseases of cardiovascular system, neurosism, hysteria and stomatoglossitis.

央。主治心血管系统疾病，神经衰弱，癔病，口舌生疮。

Trachea CO_{16}—Midpoint of Heart and External Ear. Indication: Asthma.

气管 CO_{16}——在心穴区与外耳门之间。主治咳喘。

Lung CO_{14}—Around Heart and Trachea. Indications: Cough and asthma, chest distress, acne, flat wart, itching skin and constipation.

肺 CO_{14}——在心、气管穴区周围处。主治咳喘，胸闷，痤疮，扁平疣，皮肤瘙痒症，便秘。

Triple Energizer CO_{17}—Lateral and inferior to the orifice of external auditory meatus and between Lung and Endocrine. Indications: Constipation, abdominal distension and pain of lateral side of the upper limbs.

三焦 CO_{17}——在外耳门后下，肺与内分泌区之间。主治便秘，腹胀，上肢外侧痛。

Endocrine CO_{18}—In the intertragic notch, at the medial inferior part of the cavum concha. Indications: Dysmenorrhea, irregular menstruation, menopausal syndrome and acne.

内分泌 CO_{18}——在屏间切迹内，耳甲腔的前下部。主治痛经，月经不调，更年期综合征，痤疮。

Ear Lobule:

耳垂部:

Tooth LO_1—On the medial upper part of the front side of ear lobule. Indications: Toothache, periodontitis and hypotension.

牙 LO_1——在耳垂正面前上部。主治牙痛，牙周炎，低血压。

Tongue LO_2—On the middle upper part of the front side of ear lobule. Indications: Glossitis and stomatitis.

舌 LO_2——在耳垂正面中上部。主治舌炎，口腔炎。

Jaw LO_3—On the lateral upper part of the front side of ear lobule. Indications: Toothache and disorder of temporomandibular joint.

颌 LO_3——在耳垂正面后上部。主治牙痛，颞颌关节功能紊乱。

Frontal Ear Lobe LO_4—On the medial middle part of the front side of ear lobule. Indications: Neurosism and toothache.

垂前 LO_4——在耳垂正面前中部。主治神经衰弱，牙痛。

Eye LO_5—In the center of the front side of ear lobule. Indication: Pseudomyopa.

眼 LO_5——在耳垂正面中央部。主治假性近视。

Internal Ear LO_6—On the lateral middle part of the front side of ear lobule. Indications: Auditory vertigo, tinnitus and impaired hearing.

内耳 LO_6——在耳垂正面后中部。主治内耳眩晕症，耳鸣，听力减退。

Cheek $LO_{5,6i}$—On the ear lobe, between Eye and

面颊 $LO_{5,6i}$——在耳垂正

Internal Ear. Indications: Peripheral facial paralysis, prosopalgia, acne and flat wart.

面眼区与内耳区之间。主治周围性面瘫,三叉神经痛,痤疮,扁平疣。

Tonsil $LO_{7,8,9}$—On the lower part of the front side of the ear lobe. Indications: Tonsillitis and pharyngitis.

扁桃体 $LO_{7,8,9}$——在耳垂正面下部。主治扁桃体炎,咽炎。

Back Auricle:

耳背部:

Groove on the Back Auricle PS—In the Y-shaped depression on the back auricle. Indications: Hypertension and itching skin (see Fig. 123).

耳背沟 PS——在耳郭背面呈"Y"形的凹沟中(见图 123)。主治高血压,皮肤瘙痒。

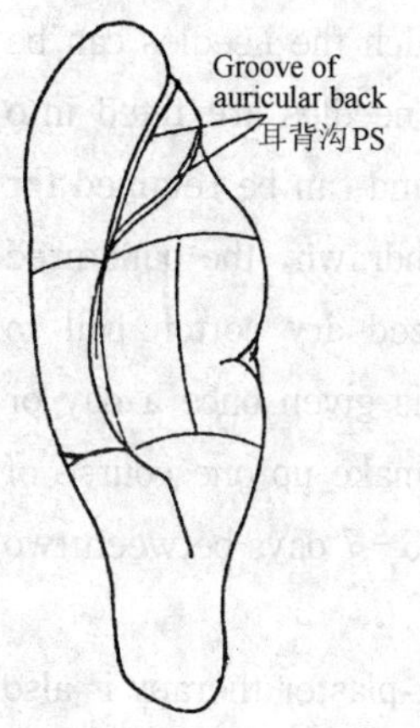

Fig. 123 Location of the ear (back)

图 123 耳穴定位(背面)

3.2.2.4.4 Detection of Ear Acupoints

4. 耳穴探查

When pathological changes have taken place in the human body, usually "positive reaction point" can be detected at the corresponding areas of the auricle, such as tenderness, discoloration and pigmentation, morphological changes (upheaval, depression and cords), desquamation, pimples, low electrical resistance, and so on. These points are used not only for clinical diagnosis, but also for treating diseases. Therefore when the prescription based on the symptoms is formulated, reaction points should be detected through careful observation, pressure with the

机体发生病变时,常会在耳郭的相应部位出现"阳性反应点",如压痛、变色、变形(隆起、凹陷、条索)、脱屑、丘疹、电阻低等。这些反应点,既是诊断的参考,又是耳针的治疗点。因此,临证时,在根据病症拟定耳穴处方后,还应通过仔细观察、利用针柄等物按压或测定皮肤电阻等方法,认真

needle handle, or determination with the electrical resistance of the skin for strengthening the curative effect.

寻找这些穴区内的反应点,以提高疗效。

3.2.2.4.5 Manipulations

The ear acupoints are sterilized routinely with 2% iodine and 75% alcohol. The acupuncturist holds the auricle with the left hand and swiftly inserts the filiform needle of 0.5 cun or pin-like needle with the right hand into the depth of the cartilage, avoiding penetration through the ear. The usual sensations are pain, or distension or burning. The needles are usually retained for 20 - 30 minutes. But chronic diseases, the needles may be retained for a longer period, and during which the needles can be manipulated at intervals. Pin-like needles are fixed into the acupoints with adhesive tapes and can be retained for 2 - 3 days. After the needle is withdrawn, the punctured acupoint is pressed with a sterilized dry cotton ball to avoid bleeding. Such a treatment is given once a day or once every other day. Ten times make up one course of treatment. There is an interval of 5 - 7 days between two courses of treatment.

Apart from needling, auricular-plaster therapy is also a commonly used therapy in clinical treatment. Method: The skin is sterilized routinely. Small granular drugs, such as Wangbuliuxingzi (Semen Vaccariae), is fixed onto the ear acupoints with adhesive tape. The patient is advised to press the acupoints several times a day and about 1 minute for each point. It is changed once every 3 - 5 days. Five to ten times make up one course of treatment.

5. 操作方法

用2%碘酒和75%酒精常规消毒后,左手固定耳郭,右手持 0.5 寸毫针或图钉形揿针刺入,深度以刺入软骨而不透过对侧皮肤为度。患者多有局部疼痛或胀或热的感觉。留针一般 20～30 分钟,慢性病可适当延长,留针期间可间断行针。揿针用胶布固定,可留针 2～3 日。出针后,用消毒干棉球按压针孔片刻,以防出血。每日治疗 1 次或隔日 1 次,10 次为 1 个疗程。休息 5～7日后再开始下 1 个疗程。

除针刺外,临床还常用压籽的方法,常规消毒后,将王不留行籽等物用胶布固定于耳穴上,嘱病人每天自行按压数次,每穴约 1 分钟,3～5 日更换。5～10 次为 1 个疗程。

3.2.2.4.6 Cautions

Sterilization must be strict to avoid infection. Needling should not be used if inflammation or chilblain is present on the auricle. For slight inflammation, 2.5% alcohol should be applied timely to it.

Ear acupuncture is inapplicable to gravida with the

6. 注意事项

(1) 严格消毒,以防感染。耳郭有炎症或冻疮的部位禁针。轻度感染时,应及时涂擦2%碘酒。

(2) 有习惯性流产史的孕

history of miscarriage. It is inadvisable to be used to treat the aged and patients with weak constitution and overstrain.

妇禁用耳针；年老体弱、过度疲劳者慎用。

3.3 Moxibustion methods

第三节 艾灸方法

Moxibustion is a therapy used to treat and prevent diseases by applying burning moxa to stimulate the human body. The material used for moxibustion is mainly Chinese mugwort leaf which is fragrant and easy to be ignited. It is processed into mugwort wool for clinical use.

灸法，是利用灸火刺激人体以防治疾病的一种疗法，为针灸疗法的重要组成部分。施灸的材料多用艾叶，其味香而易燃，临床所用是由干燥艾叶加工制成的艾绒。

3.3.1 Moxibustion with moxa cone

一、艾炷灸

Moxa cone is a cone-shaped mugwort wool, the size of which varies from the size of wheat grain to the size of a Chinese date (see Fig. 124). The measurement unit of moxibustion is called "Zhuang". The burning out of one moxa cone is called one Zhuang. The moxa cone is placed on the acupoint selected in performing moxibustion. Moxibustion with moxa cones is either direct or indirect, depending on whether there is something between the moxa cone and the skin.

将艾绒制成圆锥形的艾团，称为艾炷，大小不一，可小如麦粒，大如大枣（见图 124）。施灸的计量单位为"壮"，每燃一个艾炷称一壮。治疗时将艾炷置于所灸部位，根据艾炷与皮肤之间是否放置间隔物，又分为直接灸和间接灸两类。

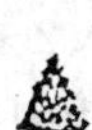
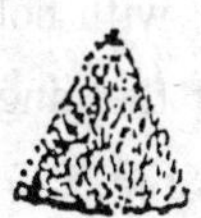
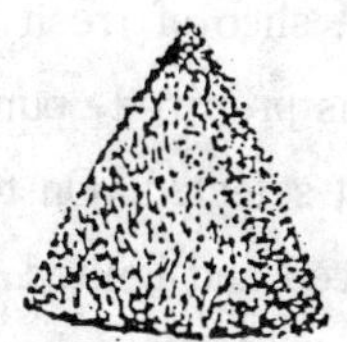

Fig. 124 Moxa cone (small, middle and large)

图 124 艾炷（小、中、大）

3.3.1.1 Direct moxibustion

（一）直接灸

Direct moxibustion means that the moxa cone is placed directly on the acupoint and ignited. Prior to moxibustion, some garlic juice or vaseline can be applied to the

即艾炷直接放在皮肤上施灸。灸前可先在施灸部位涂以蒜汁或少量凡士林，使艾

site in order to increase the adhesion of the moxa cone to the skin. This type of moxibustion is either scarring or non-scarring according to the degree of burning over the skin.

炷易于粘附。根据用灸火烧灼皮肤程度的不同，又分为无瘢痕灸和瘢痕灸。

Non-scarring moxibustion: When 2/5 of a moxa cone is burnt, or when the patient feels a burning pain, the cone is replaced by a new one. The moxibustion continues until the local skin becomes reddish but without blisters. Usually each acupoint can be moxibusted for 3 - 7 cones without suppuration and scar formation. So this method of moxibustion is easy to be accepted by the patient and is usually used to treat asthenia-cold syndrome.

无瘢痕灸：当艾炷燃剩至约2/5，病人感到灼痛时，即更换艾炷再灸，灸至局部皮肤发红而不起泡为度。一般每穴灸3～7壮。这种方法灸后不化脓，不留瘢痕，病人易于接受。常用于虚寒性病证。

Scarring moxibustion: When the moxa cone completely burns out, it is replaced by a new one. This procedure continues until blisters are formed. About one week later after moxibustion, suppuration is formed at the local region. And about 5 - 6 weeks later, the wound heals automatically, the scab exfoliates and scar is formed. It is often used to treat certain chronic diseases, such as asthma and pulmonary tuberculosis.

瘢痕灸：在艾炷燃尽后，才换炷再灸，直到燃完规定壮数为止。灸至局部皮肤起泡。灸后1周左右局部化脓，约5～6周后自行痊愈，结痂脱落，留有瘢痕。用于哮喘、肺痨等慢性疾病。

3.3.1.2 Indirect moxibustion

（二）间接灸

The ignited moxa cone is isolated from the skin by some materials, such as ginger and garlic, in order to avoid burning the skin. A slice of fresh ginger or garlic about 0.2 - 0.3 cm thick is prepared, punched with holes and placed on the acupoint selected. On top of the ginger slice, a moxa cone is placed and ignited (see Fig. 125). After the moxa cone completely burns out, it is replaced by a new one. This procedure is repeated until the local skin turns reddish but without blisters formed. This method is always used to treat obstructive syndrome due to pathogenic wind-cold, abdominal pain and diarrhea due to cold.

即施灸时在艾炷与皮肤之间放置某种物品，常用生姜、蒜等，以防止烫伤皮肤。先将新鲜的姜或大蒜切成0.2～0.3厘米的薄片，并在其中间用针刺数孔，置于施术部位，上置艾炷施灸(见图125)。待艾炷燃尽后，更换艾炷再灸。灸至局部皮肤发红而不起泡为度。常用于风寒痹痛，寒性腹痛、腹泻等。

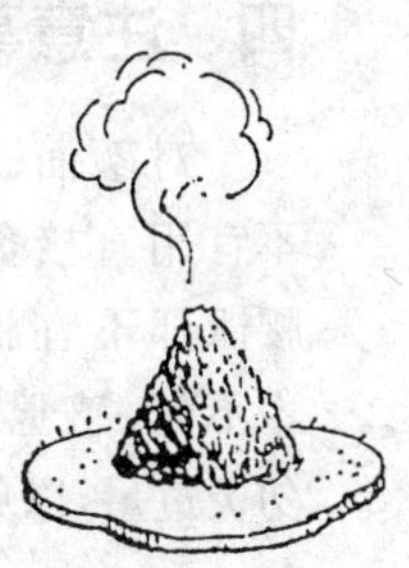

Fig. 125 Ginger-isolated moxibustion

图 125 隔姜灸

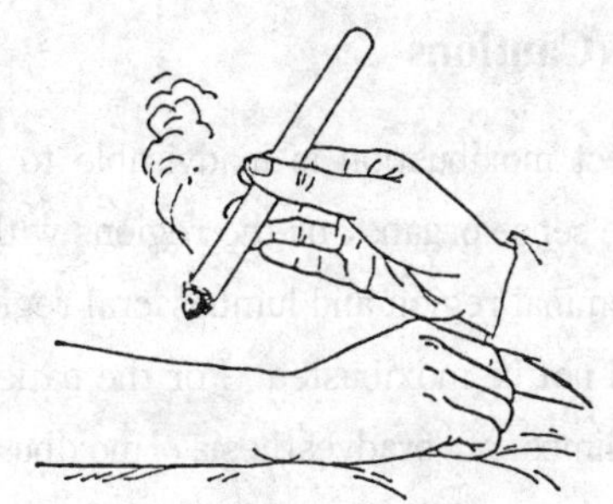

Fig. 126 Moxibustion with moxa roll

图 126 艾条灸

3.3.2 Moxibustion with moxa roll

Moxa roll is prepared by wrapping mugwort wool (other herbal medicines may be mixed in it) with a piece of paper. It is cylinder-shaped, 1.5 cm in diameter and 20 cm in length. A lighted moxa roll is pointed 3 cm to the region selected and moved upwards and downwards, to the left and right or around. The patient feels warm but no scorching. Usually each acupoint can be moxibusted for 5 - 7 minutes. This method can be used to treat many kinds of diseases and syndromes (see Fig. 126).

二、艾条灸

艾条由纸包裹艾绒卷制而成，一般为直径 1.5 厘米、长 20 厘米的圆筒形。也可在艾绒中加入药末制成药艾条。施灸时，将一端点燃，对准施灸部位薰烤，距皮肤约 3 厘米，或作上下、左右、回旋等方式的移动，以病人有热感而无灼痛为宜。一般每穴灸 5～7 分钟。可用于多种病症的治疗(见图 126)。

3.3.3 Moxibustion with warmed needles

Moxibustion with warmed needle is a method of acupuncture combined with moxibustion. During the retention of the needle, the needle handle is wrapped with some moxa or coated with one section of a moxa roll about 2 cm in length to be burned. The needle is withdrawn after the moxa completely burns out and the ash is cleared. Moxibustion with warmed needle can be used to treat various common diseases.

三、温针灸

这是一种将针刺与艾灸合并使用的方法。在针刺留针时，将一团艾绒捏在针柄上，或截下一段长约 2 厘米的艾条插套在针柄上点燃，待燃尽后除去灰烬，再出针。用于各种常见病的治疗。

3.3.4 Cautions

Direct moxibustion is inadvisable to perform on the face, five sense organs, or the regions with large vessels. The abdominal region and lumbosacral region of the gravida should not be moxibusted. For the patients with numbness of limbs or bradyesthesia, moxibustion should be moderate lest scald be caused.

四、注意事项

对颜面、五官、大血管处不宜用直接灸;孕妇的腹部、腰骶部不宜施灸。对肢体麻木不仁、感觉迟钝者,应注意勿灸过量,以免烫伤。

3.4 Cupping methods

Cupping is a therapy in which a jar is attached to the skin surface to cause local congestion through the negative pressure created by heat produced by ignited material in the jar. There are a great variety of jars, but the commonly used ones are bamboo jars, glass jars and pottery jars. The latter two are more powerful in suction.

第四节　拔罐方法

拔罐疗法是以罐杯为工具,用燃烧等方法造成罐内负压而吸附于皮肤上,引起局部充血的一种疗法。火罐的种类很多,常用的有竹罐、玻璃罐、陶罐等,后两种吸力较大。

3.4.1 Manipulations

A cotton ball with 95% alcohol held by forceps is ignited, put into the cup, moved inside the cup for one circle and then taken out. When the burning cotton ball is taken out, the cup is immediately covered on the selected region. This method is called fire-flashing method (see Fig. 127). Or an ignited alcohol cotton ball or a piece of burning paper is thrown into the cup, the cup is immediately covered on the selected region. Usually the cup is sucked in place for about 10 minutes. For the withdrawal of the cup, the skin around the rim of the cup is pressed with the index finger to let air in, then the cup is removed slowly.

In addition, cupping may be used together with acupuncture. Method: During the retention of the needle, a cup is sucked over the needling area. The needle is withdrawn when the cup is removed. Or a three-edged

一、操作方法

用镊子夹住一个95%的酒精棉球,点燃后在罐内绕一圈即退出,迅速将火罐扣在施术部位,称闪火法(见图127)。也可将点燃的酒精棉球或纸片投入罐内,然后速将火罐扣在皮肤上。一般留置10分钟左右。起罐时,以食指在罐口旁的皮肤上略加按压,使空气进入罐内,便可取下火罐。

拔罐还可与针刺结合使用,方法是:在留针时,将罐吸拔在以针为中心的部位,起罐后再起针。或是在三棱针点

needle is used to prick for bloodletting and then a cup is sucked over the pricked area for strengthening the curative effect.

刺出血后，再于该处拔罐，以加强刺血的治疗作用。

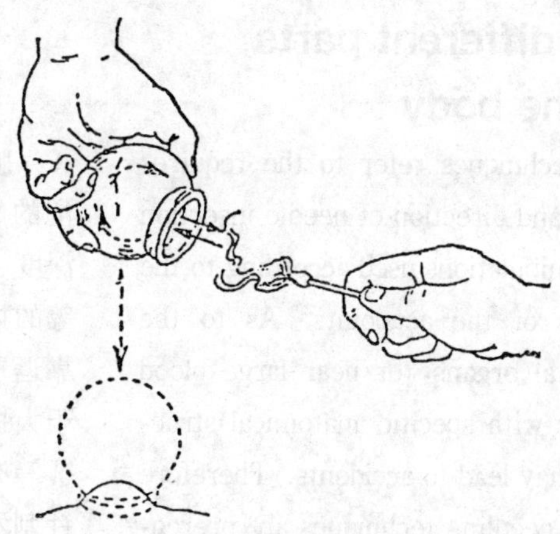

Fig. 127 Performance of cupping (fire-flashing method)

图 127 拔罐操作(闪火法)

3.4.2 Indications

This method is often used to treat wind-dampness syndrome, obstructive syndrome, numbness of the limbs, acute sprain, common cold, cough, stomachache, abdominal pain, diarrhea, and some external diseases.

二、适用范围

多用于治疗风湿痹痛、肢体麻木；急性扭伤；感冒、咳嗽；胃痛、腹痛、腹泻；某些外科病证。

3.4.3 Cautions

3.4.3.1 It should not be used in patients with high fever and convulsion, edema as well as areas with large blood vessels, allergic skin or skin ulcer and the abdominal and lumbosacral regions of the gravida.

3.4.3.2 Cares should be taken to avoid burning or scorching the skin; retention of the cup should not be too long lest impairment of the skin be caused.

3.4.3.3 If the local congestion is severe after the removal of the cup, it is forbidden to perform cupping on the region again.

三、注意事项

1. 高热抽搐、水肿、孕妇的腹部和腰骶部、大血管处、皮肤过敏或有溃破者，不宜拔罐。

2. 注意防止烫伤或灼伤皮肤；留罐时间不宜过长，以免损伤皮肤。

3. 拔罐后如局部瘀血严重者，不宜在原位再行拔罐。

3.5 Needling methods for the commonly used acupoints located on different parts of the body

第五节 各部常用腧穴的针刺方法

Acupoint needling techniques refer to the requirement of the depth, angle and direction of needle insertion as well as posture and manipulations used according to the anatomical characteristics of the acupoints. As to the acupoints close to the vital organs, or near large blood vessels, nerves, or joints with specific anatomical structure, improper needling may lead to accidents. Therefore the basic requirements of needling techniques are prerequisite to the safety of needling and curative effect. Generally speaking, the needling method for the acupoints near each other is the same or similar because their anatomical structure is the same or similar. But the needling requirements and methods for the acupoints located on different areas are different, because their anatomical structure is different.

腧穴刺灸方法，指根据穴位的解剖特点所规定的针刺深度、角度、方向、体位及手法等的操作要求和方法。穴位靠近重要的内脏、器官，或位于大血管、神经附近，或在关节等有特殊解剖结构之处，若针刺不当则易发生意外。所以，穴位的基本针刺操作要求和方法，是安全针刺、产生治疗效应的基本前提。一般来说，部位邻近的腧穴，由于解剖结构相同或相近，其针刺方法相似；不同部位的腧穴，解剖结构也有所不同，针刺的要求和方法就有区别。

3.5.1 Acupoints on the head, face and neck

一、头面颈项部腧穴

3.5.1.1 Acupoints on the head

(一) 头部腧穴

The subcutaneous tissue of the head is thin and blood vessels are rich, so the acupoints on the area covered with hair (except the neck) are usually needled horizontally 0.5-0.8 cun. The needles can be gently and slightly twirled and rotated. After the withdrawal of the needles, the punctured acupoints are pressed to avoid bleeding.

头部皮下组织薄少，血管丰富，所以在头发覆盖部位(项部除外)的腧穴，一般平刺0.5～0.8寸，可以捻转，操作宜轻；出针后按压针孔，以防出血。

Baihui (GV 20)—It is needled horizontally forward or backward, or is needled to the left or to the right horizontally according to the pathological conditions.

百会——一般向前或向后平刺，也可依病情需要向左或右平刺。

Xinhui (GV 22)—It should not be needled when the fontanel of infant is not closed.

囟会——小儿囟门未闭时禁刺。

3.5.1.2 Acupoints on the face

（二）面颊部腧穴

Acupoints on the cheek are usually needled perpendicularly or obliquely or horizontally 0.3－0.8 cun.

一般直刺或斜刺或平刺0.3～0.8寸。

Yintang (EX-HN 3)—It is needled horizontally downwards 0.3－0.5 cun when the skin is pinched. It should not be needled deeply downwards to the bilateral sides lest the eye ball be impaired.

印堂——捏起皮肤，向下平刺0.3～0.5寸。不可向下方两侧深刺，以免伤及眼球。

Sibai (ST 2)—It is needled 0.2－0.3 cun perpendicularly or 0.3－0.5 cun obliquely downwards. It should not be needled deep lest the blood vessels and nerves be pricked because it is in the infraorbital foramen. After the withdrawal of the needle, the punctured acupoint is pressed to avoid bleeding.

四白——直刺0.2～0.3寸或向下斜刺0.3～0.5寸。此穴在眶下孔处，不可深刺，以防刺伤血管、神经。出针后按压针孔，以防止出血。

Yingxiang (LI 20)—It is needled obliquely and medially upwards 0.3－0.5 cun.

迎香——向内上方斜刺0.3～0.5寸。

Shuigou (GV 26), Suliao (GV 25)—They are generally needled obliquely upwards.

水沟、素髎——一般向上斜刺。

Dicang (ST 4)—It is often needled 0.5－1 cun horizontally towards Jiache (ST 6).

地仓——常向颊车方向平刺0.5～1寸。

Taiyang (EX-HN 4)—It is needled 0.3－0.5 cun perpendicularly or obliquely backwards, or is pricked for bloodletting.

太阳——直刺或向后斜刺0.3～0.5寸。可点刺出血。

Jiache (ST 6)—It is needled 0.3－0.5 cun perpendicularly or 0.5－1 cun horizontally towards Dicang (ST 4).

颊车——直刺0.3～0.5寸，或向地仓方向平刺0.5～1寸。

Acupoints on the ocular area:

眼区腧穴：

Jingming (BL 1)—There are rich blood vessels and loose tissues in the subcutaneous region. So it is easy to cause bleeding. If it is needled deep, optic nerve may be impaired. In the treatment, the patient is asked to close the eyes and the eyeball is pushed gently to the lateral side. It is needled slowly and perpendicularly 0.3－

睛明——其皮下组织内血管丰富，组织疏松，易于出血，深刺还可伤及视神经。嘱病人闭目，左手将眼球向外推开并固定，针沿眶骨边缘缓慢直刺0.3～0.7寸，不提插、捻

0.7 cun along the orbital wall. The needle should not be lifted and thrusted or twirled and rotated so as to avoid pricking blood vessels. The needle is withdrawn gently and slowly. Then the punctured point is pressed for 2 - 3 minutes with sterilized dry cotton balls in order to prevent bleeding.

转,以防刺伤血管。出针要轻缓,用消毒干棉球压迫针孔2~3分钟,以防止出血。

Chengqi (ST 1)—Before needling, the eyeball is pushed upwards for fixation. The other requirements are the same as those for Jingming (BL 1).

承泣——进针前将眼球向上推开并固定,其余操作要点参见睛明穴。

Cuanzhu (BL 2)—It is needled 0.3 - 0.5 cun horizontally downwards for the treatment of ocular diseases; it is needled horizontally and externally to Yuyao (EX-HN 4) for the treatment of facial paralysis.

攒竹——治疗眼病可向下平刺0.3~0.5寸;治疗面瘫则向外平刺透鱼腰。

Sizhukong (TE 23), Tongziliao (GB 1)—They are usually needled horizontally backward.

丝竹空、瞳子髎——一般向后平刺。

Acupoints on the ear area:

耳区腧穴:

Ermen (TE 21), Tinggong (SI 19), Tinghui (GB 2)—They are needled 0.5 - 1 cun perpendicularly when the mouth is open. When the needles are retained, the mouth is slowly closed.

耳门、听宫、听会——针刺时均须张口,直刺0.5~1寸,留针时再将口慢慢闭上。

Yifeng (TE 17)—It is needled perpendicularly 0.8 - 1 cun, or is punctured 0.5 - 1 cun from the posterior and lateral to the medial and downward. The deeper site is the place where the facial nerve perforates the stylomastoid foramen. So the needle should not be inserted too deep lest the facial nerve be impaired. The needling manipulations should not be too forceful, especially in the treatment of facial paralysis at the primary stage.

翳风——直刺0.8~1寸或从后外向内下方刺0.5~1寸。深部正当面神经从颅骨穿出处,故进针不宜过深,以免损伤面神经。尤其是面瘫初期,针刺手法不宜过强。

3.5.1.3 Acupoints on the nape

(三) 项部腧穴

The acupoints on the nape are generally needled 0.5 - 1 cun obliquely downward. The angle and depth of needle insertion should be carefully controlled so as to prevent accidents.

一般向下方斜刺0.5~1寸。针刺时须严格掌握角度与深度,以防发生意外。

Yamen (GV 15) and Fengfu (GV 16)—Deep

哑门、风府——其深部有

insertion is inadvisable. It should not be inserted over 1 cun because there are important structures in the deep layer. The needle tip should be inserted slowly toward the mandible. But it should not be inserted upwards to avoid insertion of the needle into the great occipital foramen or impairment of the medullary bulb.

重要结构,故针刺不可过深,不能超过1寸;针尖向下颌方向,不可向上,缓缓刺入,以免误入枕骨大孔,损伤延髓。

Fengchi (GB 20)—It is needled slowly with the needle tip pointing toward the tip of the nose. It should not be inserted over 1 cun lest the medullary bulb be impaired.

风池——针尖向鼻尖方向缓慢刺入,不得超过1寸,以防伤及延髓。

Tianzhu (BL 10)—It is needled perpendicularly or obliquely 0.5-0.8 cun. But it cannot be inserted deep obliquely upward lest the medullary bulb be impaired.

天柱——直刺或斜刺0.5～0.8寸,不得向上方深刺,以免损伤延髓。

3.5.1.4 Acupoints on the neck

(四)颈部腧穴

These acupoints should be inserted slowly 0.3-0.8 cun, avoiding the carotid artery.

一般避开颈动脉缓慢刺入0.3～0.8寸。

Renying (ST 9)—It is needled slowly and perpendicularly 0.2-0.5 cun in depth, avoiding the common carotid artery. Cares should be taken to avoid deep insertion, or lateral insertion, or strong manipulations.

人迎——进针时避开颈总动脉,缓慢直刺0.2～0.5寸。注意不可偏外、过深,以及手法过重。

Lianquan (CV 23)—It is needled obliquely 0.3-0.5 cun towards the root of the tongue.

廉泉——向舌根斜刺0.3～0.5寸。

3.5.2 Acupoints on the chest and abdomen

二、胸腹部腧穴

3.5.2.1 Acupoints on the chest

(一)胸部腧穴

Since the lung and heart are in the chest, these acupoints are usually punctured obliquely or horizontally 0.5-0.8 cun. The acupoints on the conception vessel are needled horizontally. Those on the intercostal space are usually needled laterally along the ribs.

内有心、肺等脏器,一般斜刺或平刺0.5～0.8寸。任脉经上的腧穴宜平刺。位于肋间隙中的腧穴,一般沿肋骨向外刺。

Tiantu (CV 22)—The trachea is in the deeper layer, and the aortic arch and its branches are located posterior to the manubrium of the sternum. The needle is inserted perpendicularly 0.2-0.3 cun and then the needle tip is pushed 0.5-1 cun slowly downward along the posterior

天突——深部为气管,胸骨柄后方有主动脉弓及其分支。针刺时应先直刺0.2～0.3寸,再将针尖转向下方,沿胸骨柄后缘、气管前缘缓慢刺

aspect of the manubrium of the sternum and the anterior aspect of the trachea. The needle should not be inserted too deep, avoiding pricking blood vessels or trachea. It is also forbidden to puncture too deep and obliquely to the lateral side lest the lung be impaired.

入 0.5～1 寸。针刺勿过深，以防刺伤气管、血管；也不可向左右斜刺过深，以免刺中肺脏。

Tanzhong (CV 17)—It is usually needled horizontally downwards and laterally for the treatment of mammary diseases.

膻中——一般向下平刺，治疗乳疾时则向外平刺。

Ruzhong (ST 17)—Acupuncture and moxibustion are forbidden to perform on this acupoint. It only serves as a landmark for locating acupoints.

乳中——不针不灸，仅作定位标志。

Rugen (ST 18)—It is needled horizontally or obliquely.

乳根——平刺或斜刺。

3.5.2.2 Acupoints on the hypochondriac region

（二）季胁部腧穴

The liver and spleen are in this region. Acupoints on this region are usually needled obliquely. It should not be needled perpendicularly or deeply.

内有肝、脾等脏器。一般斜刺，不宜直刺、深刺。

Zhangmen (LR 13) and Jingmen (GB 25)—They are needled obliquely downward 0.5 - 0.8 cun. Oblique upward needling should be avoided, especially for the treatment of the patients with hepatosplenomegaly.

章门、京门——向下斜刺 0.5～0.8 寸，不可向上斜刺，肝脾肿大者更应注意。

3.5.2.3 Acupoints on the abdomen

（三）腹部腧穴

Acupoints on the upper abdomen are usually needled perpendicularly 0.5 - 1.5 cun, but those near the chest should not be needled deeply. Those on the lower abdomen can be needled perpendicularly 1 - 2 cun; but they should not be needled in the gravida. Those on the lower abdomen should be needled after urination to avoid pricking the bladder.

上腹部一般直刺 0.5～1.5 寸，近胸部不宜深刺。下腹部腧穴，可直刺 1～2 寸；孕妇禁用或慎用；小腹部腧穴，应排尿后针刺，以防刺中膀胱。

Zhongwan (CV 12)—It is needled perpendicularly 1 - 1.5 cun. The needle should not be inserted obliquely toward the left and right to avoid puncturing the internal organs.

中脘——直刺 1～1.5 寸，不可向左右侧斜上方斜刺，以防刺伤内脏。

Shenque (CV 8)—It should not be needled. Moxibustion with the cushion of salt or ginger is applicable to this acupoint.

神阙——不宜针刺。多隔盐或隔姜灸。

3. 5. 3 Acupoints on the back and lumbosacral region

三、背腰骶部腧穴

3. 5. 3. 1 Acupoints on the governor vessel

（一）督脉诸穴

The depth of insertion is 0. 5 – 1 cun. Deep needling is avoided lest the spinal cord be impaired. The angle of insertion depends upon the angle of the spinous process. The spinous processes of the thoracic vertebrae are downbearing, so the acupoints below them should be needled obliquely upward; while the spinous processes of the lumbar vertebrae protrude almost posteriorly and horizontally, so the acupoints below them can be needled perpendicularly; the acupoints on the caudal-sacral region are needled obliquely upward.

针刺深度 0.5～1 寸，勿刺过深，以防损伤脊髓。针刺角度，根据脊椎的棘突角度而异，胸椎棘突向下，所以胸椎棘突下的腧穴应向上斜刺；腰椎棘突几乎水平地凸向后方，可直刺；尾骶部向上斜刺。

Dazhui (GV 14)—It is needled perpendicularly or obliquely 0. 5 – 1 cun. The needle is inserted slowly to a proper depth. Deep insertion should be avoided lest the vertebral canal be punctured and the spinal cord be impaired.

大椎——直刺或斜刺 0.5～1 寸。进针宜缓，不可过深，以免刺入椎管，伤及脊髓。

Changqiang (GV 1)—The needle should be parallel to the coccyx and inserted between the rectum and coccyx. Otherwise the rectum may be impaired.

长强——针刺时针须与尾骨平行，在直肠与尾骨之间刺入，否则易伤直肠。

3. 5. 3. 2 Acupoints above the spinous process of the twelfth thoracic vertebra

（二）背部第十二胸椎棘突水平线以上诸穴

As to the angle of insertion, the needle is usually inserted obliquely toward the spine or horizontally from the upper to the lower . It is inadvisable to puncture perpendicularly or obliquely and laterally. The depth of insertion is 0. 5 – 0. 8 cun. Deep insertion may puncture the pleural cavity and cause pneumatothorax.

针刺角度，一般向脊柱斜刺或从上向下平刺，不宜直刺或向外斜刺。针刺深度 0.5～0.8 寸，不可过深，以防刺入胸膜腔而致气胸。

Jianjing (GB 21)—It is needled perpendicularly about

肩井——直刺 0.5 寸左

0.5 cun. Deep insertion may impair the internal organs.

右，不可过深，以免伤及内脏。

3.5.3.3 Acupoints on the lumbar region

The acupoints on the lumbar region are needled perpendicularly 0.5 - 1cun.

（三）腰部诸穴

直刺 0.5～1 寸。

3.5.3.4 Shangliao (BL 31), Ciliao (BL 32), Zhongliao (BL 33) and Xialiao (BL 34) on the sacral region

These acupoints are needled perpendicularly 1 - 1.5 cun. On puncturing Shangliao (BL 31), the needle tip slightly points to the pubic symphysis in order to puncture into the first posterior sacral foramen.

（四）骶部的上、次、中、下髎穴

直刺 1～1.5 寸。刺上髎穴时，针尖应稍向内下，即向耻骨联合方向，方可刺中第一骶后孔。

3.5.4 Acupoints on the limbs

In needling all the acupoints on the arteries, the arteries should be avoided.

四、四肢部腧穴

所有动脉处的腧穴均应避开动脉针刺。

3.5.4.1 Acupoints on the upper arm

The acupoints are needled perpendicularly or obliquely 0.5 - 1.5 cun.

Jugu (LI 16)—It is needled obliquely and posteriorly downward 0.5 - 1 cun.

Jianyu (LI 15)—It is needled perpendicularly or obliquely downward 0.5 - 1.5 cun.

Binao (LI 14)—It is needled perpendicularly or obliquely upward 0.5 - 1.5 cun.

Jianliao (TE 14)—It is needled perpendicularly to the shoulder 1 - 1.5 cun.

Jiquan (HT 1)—It is needled perpendicularly about 0.5 cun, avoiding the arteries.

（一）上臂部腧穴

直刺或斜刺，一般 0.5～1.5 寸。

巨骨——向后下方斜刺 0.5～1 寸。

肩髃——直刺或向下斜刺 0.5～1.5 寸。

臂臑——直刺或向上斜刺 0.5～1.5 寸。

肩髎——向肩关节直刺 1～1.5 寸。

极泉——避开动脉，直刺约 0.5 寸。

3.5.4.2 Acupoints on the forearm

These acupoints are usually needled perpendicularly or obliquely 0.5 - 1.2 cun. The acupoints near the wrist are usually needled perpendicularly 0.3 - 0.5 cun.

The median nerve is in the deeper layer of the pericardium meridian of hand-jueyin. The electric shock-

（二）前臂部腧穴

一般直刺或斜刺 0.5～1.2 寸。腕关节附近腧穴，一般直刺 0.3～0.5 寸。

手厥阴心包经腧穴，其深部有正中神经，针刺时如有触

like sensation transmitting to the finger tips indicates the median nerve is punctured, the needle must be withdrawn immediately lest the median nerve be impaired. The occurrence of such electric shock-like sensation must be dealt with in time.

Quchi (LI 11)—It is needled perpendicularly 1 - 1.5 cun.

Lieque (LU 7)—It is needled obliquely towards the elbow 0.3 - 0.5 cun.

Pianli (LI 6) and Yanglao (SI 6)—They are needled perpendicularly or obliquely 0.5 - 0.8 cun.

3.5.4.3 Acupoints on the thigh

These acupoints are usually needled perpendicularly 1 -2 cun. Those on the buttocks can be needled 2 - 3 cun.

Huantiao (GB 30)—It is needled perpendicularly 2 -3 cun. If the sciatic nerve is punctured, there appears electric shock-like sensation transmitting to the heel.

3.5.4.4 Acupoints on the leg

These acupoints are usually needled perpendicularly 0.5 - 2 cun. Those near the ankle are needled perpendicularly 0.5 - 1 cun.

Xiyan (EX-LE 5)—It is needled 0.5 - 1 cun obliquely towards the knee.

Weizhong (BL 40)—It is needled perpendicularly 0.5 -1 cun or pricked for bloodletting.

Zusanli (ST 36)—It is needled perpendicularly 1 -2 cun.

Sanyinjiao (SP 6)—It is needled 1 - 1.5 cun perpendicularly and slightly posteriorly.

3.5.4.5 Acupoints on the hand and foot

These acupoints are needled perpendicularly or obliquely; the depth of insertion is usually 0.3 -1 cun; the depth for the acupoints on the tip of the fingers or toes is about 0.1 cun.

电样感觉向指端放散，是刺中神经，应立即退针，改变角度再刺，以免损伤正中神经。凡有上述触电样感觉时，均应如上处理。

曲池——直刺 1～1.5寸。

列缺——向肘部斜刺 0.3～0.5 寸。

偏历、养老——直刺或斜刺 0.5～0.8 寸。

（三）大腿部腧穴

一般直刺 1～2 寸，臀部可达 2～3 寸。

环跳——直刺 2～3 寸。刺及坐骨神经时，可有触电样感觉向下放射至足跟。

（四）小腿部腧穴

一般直刺 0.5～2 寸。踝关节附近腧穴，直刺 0.5～1 寸。

膝眼——向膝中斜刺 0.5～1 寸。

委中——直刺 0.5～1 寸，或点刺出血。

足三里——直刺 1～2 寸。

三阴交——直刺，略向后，1～1.5 寸。

（五）手、足部腧穴

直刺或斜刺；针刺深度一般 0.3～1 寸，指、趾端腧穴约 0.1 寸。

Hegu (LI 4)—It is needled perpendicularly 0.5 - 1 cun.

合 谷——直 刺 0.5 ～1寸。

Laogong (PC 8)—It is needled perpendicularly 0.3 - 0.5 cun.

劳 宫——直 刺 0.3 ～0.5寸。

Taichong (LR 3)—It is needled 0.5 - 1 cun perpendicularly or obliquely upwards.

太冲——直刺或向上斜刺0.5～1寸。

The needling sensation of the above three acupoints is strong, so the manipulations should not be too forceful.

以上3穴的针刺感应都较强,所以手法不宜过重。

Chongyang (ST 42)—It is needled perpendicularly 0.3 -0.5 cun, avoiding the arteries.

冲阳——避开动脉,直刺0.3～0.5寸。

In addition, Hegu (LI 4), Sanyinjiao (SP 6), Jianjing (GB 21), Kunlun (BL 60), Zhiyin (BL 67) are effective in promoting blood circulation and menstrual flow when needled. So these acupoints should not be needled in the gravida.

此外,合谷、三阴交、肩井、昆仑、至阴等穴,有活血通经作用,孕妇禁用。

4 General introduction to treatment

第四章 治疗总论

4.1 Examination and syndrome differentiation

第一节 诊察和辨证

The treatment of diseases with acupuncture and moxibustion is performed under the guidance of TCM theory, based on the diagnosis made by means of the four diagnostic methods (inspection, auscultation and olfaction, inquiry as well as palpation) and according to the syndrome differentiation (including syndrome differentiation of the eight principles, zang-fu organs, qi and blood as well as meridians and collaterals). The theory of meridians and collaterals is the core of the science of acupuncture and moxibustion. It is also the important basis for the examination and syndrome differentiation in the clinical practice of acupuncture and moxibustion. Therefore apart from the general methods for diagnosis and syndrome differentiation in TCM, the examination of meridians, collaterals and acupoints as well as syndrome differentiation of meridians and collaterals are specially significant in the clinical practice of acupuncture and moxibustion.

运用针灸方法治疗疾病，是在中医理论的指导下，先以望、闻、问、切的四诊方法诊察了解病情，对诊察所得的有关疾病情况进行辨证分析（包括八纲辨证、脏腑辨证、气血辨证、经络辨证等），然后才能根据辨证结果制定相应的针灸治疗方法。经络学说是针灸学的核心理论，也是针灸临床进行诊察和辨证的重要依据。所以，在针灸临床上，除了运用中医的一般诊察和辨证方法外，经络腧穴诊察、经络辨证，对于针灸临床具有特殊的重要意义。

4.1.1 Examination of meridians and acupoints

一、经络腧穴诊察

The upper, lower, internal and external parts of the body are integrated into an organic whole through the system of meridians and collaterals which promotes the circulation of qi and blood through the whole body and harmonizes zang and fu organs as well as yin and yang.

经络系统将机体的上下内外连为一体，运行气血到达周身，协调脏腑阴阳。腧穴是经络脏腑气血输注之处。在病理情况下，经络腧穴又是病

The acupoints are the specific sites through which qi and the blood of the zang-fu organs and meridians is infused. Under pathological conditions, meridians, collaterals and acupoints serve as the passageways for the transmission of diseases from the exterior to the interior and from the interior to the exterior. So the pathological changes inside the body can be manifested on the surface of the body. Therefore the pathological changes of meridians, collaterals, zang-fu organs and the location of the diseases can be identified through the examination of the abnormal changes of meridians, collaterals and acupoints, providing evidence for further differentiation of syndromes.

邪由外入内、由内而外的传注通路,以及体内病变在体表的反映部位。因此,通过诊察经络腧穴的异常变化,可以了解病变的经络、脏腑,明确病位,为进一步的辨证提供依据。

4.1.1.1 Examination of the meridians and collaterals

(一) 经络诊察

The examination is made according to the circulation and distribution of the meridians and collaterals through inspection and palpation as well as observation of the pathological reactions in the distributing areas of the meridians.

主要是根据经络的循行分布,通过望诊和触诊,了解其分布区域内的病理反应。

Inspection of the meridians and collaterals: The inspection mainly concentrates on observation of the abnormal changes of the colour and shape of the skin and vessels. For example, darkish purple vessels are always the manifestations of blood stagnation; bluish vessels indicate cold or pain syndrome and reddish ones always signify heat syndrome. Pimples and blisters on the hypochondriac region indicate pathological changes of the gallbladder meridian of foot-shaoyang and the liver meridian of foot-jueyin. While skin lesions such as pimples and erythemas on the anterior-lateral side of the lower limbs are the manifestations of the pathological changes of the stomach meridian of foot-yangming.

经络望诊:主要观察经络循行部位皮肤、血络的色泽、形态等方面的异常变化,例如:观察血络的颜色,色紫暗者多为瘀血的反映,色青者多为寒证、痛证,色红赤者多是热证;在胁肋部出现丘疹、水疱等,多为足少阳胆经、足厥阴肝经的病变;在下肢外侧前缘出现丘疹、红斑等皮损,则是足阳明胃经病变的反映。

Palpation of the meridians and collaterals: The distributing areas of the meridians and collaterals are pressed and touched to examine and inspect various

经络触诊:即在经络的循行分布部位进行触摸、按压,以体察各种反应,包括:动脉

reactions, including the states of pulsation on the arteries, subcutaneous nodes, lumps and cord-like mass, or looseness and depression as well as coolness, feverishness, pain, sensitivity and numbness of the skin. The affected meridians and collaterals can be identified according to the locations of the manifestations.

搏动处的脉动盛虚,皮下有无结节、肿块、条索状物或松软、凹陷等,肌肤的凉热、疼痛、敏感、麻木等。根据出现反应的部位,判断所病的经络。

4.1.1.2 Examination of the acupoints

The acupoints and the reaction points are pressed for examining various abnormal changes, including whether there are tenderness or comfortable sensation, or aching and distention as compared with the adjacent regions, or subcutaneous nodes or code-like mass, or looseness and depression. These abnormal changes mainly appear on some special acupoints. For example, tenderness or comfortable sensation will be felt on Feishu (BL 13) when the lung is in disorder. Pathological reactions on Front-Mu acupoint Juque (CV 14) and Back-Shu acupoint Xinshu (BL 15) often indicate heart disease. Tenderness felt on the He-Sea acuppoint Zusanli (ST 36) and Shangjuxu (ST 37) or the area between them usually indicate the disorders of the hand- and foot-yangming meridians. Tenderness felt on the crossing-point Sanyinjiao (SP 6) suggests the disorder of the foot triple yin meridians.

(二) 腧穴诊察

主要是在腧穴部位和病痛反应点进行按压,以了解各种异常反应,包括:有无压痛或舒适感,或与邻近部位相比有明显的酸胀等感觉,皮下组织有否结节、条索状物或松软、凹陷等。这些异常反应一般在特定穴处较为明显。例如:肺脏有病,常常在背部的肺俞处有压痛或舒适感;募穴巨阙、背俞心俞有病理反应,多提示病在心脏;在合穴足三里、上巨虚处或两穴之间出现压痛等病理反应,多为病在手、足阳明经;交会穴三阴交有压痛,提示病在足三阴经,等等。

In clinical practice apart from the consideration of examining the meridians, collaterals and acupoints, the four diagnostic methods of TCM should be employed at the same time to have a comprehensive understanding of the pathological conditions and make a correct diagnosis of the disease in question.

临床上,在重视进行经络腧穴诊察的同时,还应运用中医四诊方法全面了解病变情况,作出正确的判断。

4.1.2 Syndrome differentiation of meridians

The aim of syndrome differentiation of meridians and collaterals is to analyze the involvement of the meridians

二、经络辨证

经络辨证,主要是根据经脉的循行联系和经脉病候,分

and the states of asthenia, sthenia, cold and heat according to the distribution and indication of meridians for the purpose of providing evidence for selecting the needling methods.

析辨别病变的所在经脉和虚实寒热等，为制定针灸治疗方法提供依据。

4.1.2.1 Syndrome differentiation methods

（一）辨证方法

4.1.2.1.1 Identifying meridians through examining the location of diseases

1. 从病位辨经脉

Identifying meridians through examining the location of diseases means to identify the involvement of the meridians in the pathological conditions according to the distribution of the meridians where disease and pain occur. Take headache for example. The yang meridians run up to the head, but distribute differently. Yangming meridian runs up to the forehead, shaoyang merdian to the lateral side of the head, taiyang meridian to the posterior side of the head, and jueyin meridian to the vertex. Therefore headache over the forehead indicates the involvement of the yangming meridian, migraine indicates the involvement of the shaoyang meridian, and so on. Another example is toothache, the upper toothache is related to the foot-yangming meridian while the lower toothache is related to the hand-yangming meridian.

即辨别病痛部位属何经脉的循行分布区域，从而判断是何经脉的病变。例如：头痛，阳经行至于头而各有一定区域，前额属阳明经，侧头属少阳经，后头属太阳经，头顶属厥阴经，而判定前额头痛为病在阳明经，偏头痛属少阳经病证等等。牙痛，上齿痛属足阳明经，下齿痛属手阳明经。

4.1.2.1.2 Identifying meridians according to symptoms

2. 从证候辨经脉

This syndrome differentiation method is mainly based on the pathological manifestations of the twelve meridians recorded in the Chapter of *Meridian in Lingshu* (*Spiritual Pivot*). For example, the symptoms of the lung meridian are "Cough, asthmatic breathing, asthma, vexation and fullness in the chest", so cough and asthma are the symptoms of the lung meridian. The symptoms of the stomach meridian are "singing in a high place and running about without clothes", so the manifestations of mental diseases are related to the stomach meridian.

是以《灵枢・经脉》中的十二经脉病候为主要依据的辨证方法。例如：手太阴肺经病候有"咳，上气，喘喝，烦心胸满"等，所以咳嗽、气喘为手太阴经证候。足阳明胃经的病候有"上高而歌，弃衣而走"，所以见有这类精神病表现则归为足阳明经的病证。

4.1.2.1.3 Identifying meridians through the location of disease and symptoms

Some parts or zang-fu organs are connected with several meridians, or one single disease can be manifested over several meridians. Hence in the syndrome differentiation of the disease, both the location of disease and the pathological manifestations of the meridians must be taken into consideration for making accurate diagnosis. For example, the heart is connected with the heart meridian, the spleen meridian and the kidney meridian.

3. 从病位、证候辨证经脉

某些部位或脏腑器官与数条经脉有联系,或某一病候可见于数条经脉,对其病变进行辨证时,就要将病位与经脉病候二者结合考虑,才能辨证准确。例如:心,手少阴心经、足太阴脾经、足少阴肾经皆行于心。

4.1.2.1.4 Identifying meridians according to the zang-fu organs

The twelve meridians are related to the corresponding zang-fu organs respectively, so the involvement of the meridians in the pathological conditions can be identified according to the theory of zang-fu organs. Take retention of urine for example. It is a disorder of the bladder and kidney and the corresponding meridians are the bladder meridian and kidney meridian.

4. 从脏腑辨经脉

十二经脉各与相应的脏腑联系,故可以根据脏腑辨证来明确所病的经脉。如:癃闭,脏腑辨证属膀胱和肾的病变,与之相应的经脉即为足太阳膀胱经和足少阴肾经。

4.1.2.2 Syndrome differentiation of the twelve main meridians

This part is discussed in Chapter 2.

(二)十二经脉辨证

主要根据经脉的循行联系和经脉病候等来辨证。具体内容参见第二章。

4.2 Therapeutic principles

第二节 治疗原则

4.2.1 Regulating yin and yang

Yin and yang refer to qi, blood, body fluids and visceral essence in the human body. Normal physiological activities depend on the balance between yin and yang. The excess or deficiency of yin or yang will inevitably lead to dysfunction of certain organs and cause disease. The

一、调整阴阳

这里所说的阴阳,是总指一身的气血津液、脏腑精气。机体生理活动的正常,是身体阴阳保持相互协调的结果,一旦阴阳出现偏盛偏衰而失于

basic principle of acupuncture and moxibustion therapy is to regulate yin and yang and restore their coordination. That is also the therapeutic effect of acupuncture and moxibustion therapy. There are several conditions of imbalance of yin and yang. Preponderance of yin and yang, decline of yin and yang, and asthenia of both yin and yang are the basic manifestations in the disorder of yin and yang. So different therapeutic methods are used in the treatment of such pathological changes with acupuncture and moxibustion therapy. For example, heat syndrome due to yang predomination should be treated by reducing yang-heat while cold syndrome caused by yin predomination should be treated by warming and dispersing yin-cold. Asthenia-cold syndrome due to failure of yang astehnia to control yin should be treated by strengthening yang while asthenia-heat syndrome due to yin asthenia and yang sthenia should be treated by reinforcing yin. Asthenia of both yin and yang should be treated by reinforcing both yin and yang.

协调,身体的功能活动就处于紊乱状态而发病。针灸治疗的根本原则,就是调整阴阳,使其恢复协调。这也是针灸治疗的作用。阴阳失调有多种情况,阴阳偏盛、阴阳偏衰和阴阳两虚等是基本的病理变化,针灸治疗要根据不同病变采用相应的治法。例如:阳盛则热,阴盛则寒,前者要清泻阳热,后者应温散阴寒。阳虚不能制阴而成虚寒证,当补阳;阴虚不能制阳,则表现为阴虚阳亢的虚热证,应补阴。阴阳两虚,就须阴阳两补。

4.2.2 Reinforcing healthy qi and expelling pathogenic factors

The occurrence and development of a disease is the result of pathogenic factors that impair the human body and healthy qi that fails to control pathogenic factors. Therefore strengthening healthy qi and eliminating pathogenic factors is the basic therapeutic principle of acupuncture and moxibustion therapy. The basic method is to reinforce asthenia and reduce sthenia. Asthenia syndrome due to deficiency of healthy qi should be treated by strengthening healthy qi while sthenia syndrome due to excess of pathogenic factors should be treated by reducing therapy. The syndromes complicated with both asthenia and sthenia should be treated with both the reinforcing and reducing methods with modification according to the

二、扶正祛邪

疾病的发生发展,是邪气影响人体、正气不能战胜邪气的结果。所以,增强正气、祛除邪气是针灸治疗的基本原则。扶正祛邪的具体方法为补虚泻实,正气不足之虚证要用补法,邪气盛实之实证应予泻法;正虚与邪实并存的虚实兼夹证则须补泻并用,根据病情或补泻并重,或补虚为主兼以泻邪,或泻邪为主兼以补虚。

pathological conditions.

4.2.3 Concentration of treatment on the essential aspect

The causes, pathological changes and manifestations of a disease are complicated. So treatment should concentrate on the nature and main pathological changes of the disease. For example, headache due to hyperactivity of liver-yang should be treated by soothing the liver to suppress yang with the selection of acupoints on the liver and gallbladder meridians; while headache due to asthenia of qi and blood should be treated by nourishing qi and blood with the selection of acupoints on the conception and governor vessels as well as Back-Shu points.

However, for the treatment of severe urgent diseases, expectant treatment is required. For example, the treatment of syncope is to needle Shuigou (GV 26), Suliao (GV 25), Hegu (LI 4) and Zhongchong (PC 9) first. When the symptoms are alleviated, other therapeutic methods can be used to deal with the cause of the disease.

4.2.4 Selection of treatment according to the individual conditions

The therapeutic method of acupuncture and moxibustion should suit the individual conditions of patients. Due to difference in age, sex and constitution, patients differ in the conditions of qi and blood, yin and yang as well as response and tolerance to acupuncture and moxibustion stimulation. That is why the acupuncture and moxibustion methods vary according to the conditions of the patients. For example, the treatment of infants requires short and thin needles, shallow insertion, short retention or no retention of the needles; while the treatment of the aged or patients with poor constitution

三、治病求本

疾病的发生原因、病理变化以及症状表现是复杂多样的，临证时要针对病证的病变本质和主要方面进行治疗，也就是治疗其根本。例如：肝阳上亢所致的头痛，治以平肝潜阳，取足厥阴、少阳经穴为主；气血亏虚引起的头痛，则应补益气血，取任、督脉和背俞穴为主。

此外，对病势急迫者，应先针对症状治疗，即急则治其标。例如：晕厥，当先刺水沟、素髎、合谷、中冲等救治，待证情缓解后，可再针对病因继续调治。

四、因人制宜

即针灸的方法要适宜病人的自身特点。因为病人有年龄、性别、形体的不同，其体内气血阴阳的状况存在着差异，对针灸刺激的反应性和耐受性有别，所以针灸的方法就要根据病人的体质而有所区别。如小儿用针宜细，进针宜浅、留针时间宜短或不留针；年老体弱者针刺手法宜轻等等。

requires gentle and slight manipulations.

4.3 Selection of acupoints and compatibility of acupoints

The therapeutic effects of acupuncture and moxibustion are induced through stimulating the selected acupoints by means of acupuncture or moxibustion. Therefore the selection and combination of acupoints play an important role in the treatment with acupuncture and moxibustion. Correct selection and combination of acupoints are key to the curative effects of acupuncture and moxibustion therapy.

4.3.1 Methods for selecting acupoints

The main principles for selecting acupoints are to select along the meridians and according to the pathological conditions.

4.3.1.1 Selection of proximal acupoints

This is a method to select acupoints located on the adjacent area of the disease because acupoints can be needled to treat the diseases around them or near them. This method can be divided into two types: selection of local acupoints and selection of adjacent acupoints.

4.3.1.1.1 Selection of local acupoints

It means to select acupoints located in the affected area. For example, Yingxiang (LI 20) is selected to treat nasosinusitis; Dicang (ST 4) is selected to treat distortion of mouth; Tinghui (GB 2) is selected to treat tinnitus and deafness; Taiyang (EX-HN 1), Touwei (ST 8) and Baihui (GV 20) are selected to treat headache; Zhongwan (CV 12) is selected to treat stomachache; Qimen (LR 14) and Riyue (GB 24) are selected to treat hypochondriac

第三节 选穴与配穴

针灸的治疗效应是通过针刺、艾灸刺激腧穴而产生的，所以腧穴的选择及其配合运用与针灸治疗效果密切相关。正确地选穴和配穴，是达到针灸治病目的的重要环节。

一、选穴方法

选穴的主要原则和方法是循经取穴，其次是根据病情选用有针对主治作用的腧穴。

（一）近部选穴

是在靠近病变的部位选取腧穴的方法。因为腧穴都能够治疗其所在部位和邻近周围处的病证。又可分为局部选穴和邻近选穴两种：

1. 局部选穴

即在所病之处选穴。例如：鼻渊取迎香，口歪取地仓，耳鸣、耳聋取听会，头痛取太阳、头维、百会，胃痛取中脘，胁痛取期门、日月，肩部肿痛取肩髃，膝部肿痛取膝眼等等。

pain; Jianyu (LI 15) is selected to treat swelling and pain of shoulder; Xiyan (EX-LE 5) is selected to treat swelling pain of knee.

4.3.1.1.2 Selection of adjacent acupoints

It means to select acupoints located near the affected area. For example, Yintang (EX-HN 3) is selected to treat nasosinusitis; Fengchi (GB 20) is selected to treat headache; and Ciliao (BL 32) is selected to treat hemorrhoids.

2. 邻近选穴

即在病处的附近选穴。例如：鼻渊取印堂，头痛取风池，痔疮取次髎等等。

4.3.1.2 Selection of distal acupoints

It means to select acupoints distal to the affected area. The acupoints selected in this case are usually located below the elbows and knees. This method for selecting acupoints is based on the distribution of meridians and collaterals. For example, Hegu (LI 4) is selected to treat toothache; Taichong (LR 3) is selected to treat redness, swelling and pain of the eyes; Kunlun (BL 60) is selected to treat stiffness and pain of the head and neck; Lieque (LU 7) and Chize (LU 5) are selected to treat cough; Daling (PC 7) is selected to treat palpitation and angina pectoris; Neiguan (PC 6) is selected to treat nausea and vomiting; Zusanli (ST 36) is selected to treat abdominal pain; and Weizhong (BL 40) is selected to treat lumbago.

（二）远部选穴

是在距病变处的较远部位选取腧穴的方法，多是取四肢肘膝以下的腧穴。这种方法是基于经络的联系。例如：牙痛取合谷，目赤肿痛取太冲，头项强痛取昆仑，咳嗽取列缺、尺泽，心悸、心痛取大陵，恶心呕吐取内关，脘腹痛取足三里，腰痛取委中等等。

4.3.1.3 Selection of contralateral acupoints

It is a method used to select the acupoints located opposite to the affected side, known as "to select the acupoints on the right side to treat diseases on the left, and vice versa". For example, the acupoints located on the right ankle are selected to treat the sprain of the left ankle.

（三）左右选穴

或称交叉选穴，是选取与患侧相反的一侧的腧穴，所谓“左病取右，右病取左”方法。例如：左侧踝关节扭伤，可选用右侧踝部腧穴。

4.3.1.4 Selection of acupoints according to the symptoms

This method is used to select acupoints for the treatment of syndromes involving the whole body, the

（四）随证选穴

根据病证选取具有相应主治作用的腧穴。主要用于

clinical manifestations of which are not limited to a certain local area according to the indication of acupoints and the theory of syndrome differentiation. For example, Dazhui (GV 14) and Quchi (LI 11) are selected to treat high fever; Suliao (GV 25) and Shuigou (GV 26) are selected to treat syncope; Yinxi (HT 6) and Fuliu (KI 7) are selected to treat night sweating; Geshu (BL 17) is selected to treat asthenia of blood; Guanyuan (CV 4) and Qihai (CV 6) are selected to treat collapse; Zhigou (TE 6) is selected to treat constipation.

全身性病证,其临床表现不限于某一局部。根据腧穴的主治特点,以及中医辨证论治的理论方法来运用。例如:高热取大椎、曲池,昏厥取素髎、水沟,盗汗取阴郄、复溜,血虚取膈俞,虚脱取关元、气海,便秘取支沟等等。

4.3.2 Methods for the compatibility of acupoints

二、配穴组方

The prescription used in acupuncture treatment is composed of over two acupoints which are combined in the light of the syndromes. The purposes of combining acupoints are to strengthen the essential and comprehensive therapeutic effects. Therefore there are two ways to combine acupoints: one is to combine the acupoints with the same or similar indication and the other is to combine the corresponding acupoints according to pathological conditions or differentiation of syndromes.

针对病证将两个以上的腧穴配合使用,组成针灸治疗的用穴处方。配穴的目的主要有两方面:一是加强主治作用,二是具有综合、全面的治疗作用。因此,其配穴方法也就有两大类:一是将主治作用相同或相近的腧穴配合使用,二是根据病情或辨证配用有相应主治作用的腧穴。

4.3.2.1 Compatibility of acupoints according to the indications

(一)按同一主治作用配穴

It means to use the acupoints with the same curative effect together according to the pathological condition in question.

就是针对病痛,将具有同一治病作用的腧穴配合应用。

4.3.2.1.1 Proximal compatibility

1. 邻近配穴

The proximal acupoints at or near the location of the disease are combined to strengthen the therapeutic effects. For example, Cuanzhu (BL 2), Yangbai (GB 14), Yuyao (EX-HN 4), Tongziliao (GB 1) and Sizhukong (TE 23) are selected to treat facial hemiplegia

将部位邻近的腧穴配合使用,以加强其治疗作用。一般是在病变处或附近。例如:面瘫目不能合,取攒竹、阳白、鱼腰、瞳子髎、丝竹空诸穴;偏

and distorted mouth and inability to close the eyes; Taiyang (EX-HN 5), Touwei (ST 8) and Shuaigu (GB 8) are selected to treat migraine; Jianyu (LI 15), Jianliao (TE 14), Jianzhen (SI 9) and Naoshu (SI 10) are selected to treat swelling and pain of the shoulder.

头痛，取太阳、头维、率谷等穴，肩部肿痛，取肩髃、肩髎、肩贞、臑俞等。

4.3.2.1.2 Compatibility of distal-proximal acupoints

This way of combining acupoints is for strengthening the curative effect. Usually the acupoints on the same meridian or the meridians with external-internal relationship or the meridians with the same name are selected. For example, Dicang (ST 4) and Hegu (LI 4) are selected to treat distorted face; Tinghui (GB 2) and Zhongzhu (TE 3) are selected to treat tinnitus and deafness; Fengchi (GB 20) and Houxi (SI 3) as well as Kunlun (BL 60) are selected to treat stiffness and pain of the head and neck; Feishu (BL 13) and Lieque (LU 7) are selected to treat cough; Zhongwan (CV 12) and Zusanli (ST 36) are selected to treat stomachache; Tianshu (ST 25), Zusanli (ST 36) and Yinlingquan (SP 9) are selected to treat diarrhea.

2. 远近配穴

将距病变的近部和远部腧穴配合使用，以加强其治疗作用。多取同一经脉或表里经或同名经的腧穴。例如：口角歪斜，近取地仓，远取合谷；耳鸣耳聋，近取听会，远取中渚；头项强痛，近取风池，远取后溪、昆仑；咳嗽，近取肺俞，远取列缺；胃痛，近取中脘，远取足三里；泄泻，近取天枢，远取足三里、阴陵泉，等等。

4.3.2.1.3 Compatibility of anterior-posterior acupoints

The acupoints located on the chest or abdomen are combined with those on the back to strengthen the therapeutic effect. This method is mainly used to treat zang-fu syndromes. For example, Juque (CV 14) and Xinshu (BL 15) are selected to treat palpitation; Zhongwan (CV 12) and Weishu (BL 21) are selected to treat stomachache.

3. 前后配穴

将胸腹部腧穴与背腰部腧穴配合应用，以加强其治疗作用。主要用于脏腑病证。例如：心悸，前取巨阙，后取心俞；胃脘痛，前取中脘，后取胃俞。

4.3.2.2 Compatibility of acupoints according to syndrome differentiation

The acupoints are selected in the light of pathogenesis and the differentiation of syndromes. It is marked by the same combination for acupoints in the treatment of the

（二）辨证配穴

根据辨证，针对病机取用腧穴。其特点是，证相同则腧穴配伍相同，证不同则腧穴配

same syndrome and different combination of acupoints for the treatment of different disease. For example, Xingjian (LR 2) or Taichong (LR 3) is added for the treatment of headache due to hyperactivity of liver-yang; while Ganshu (BL 18), Pishu (BL 20), Shenshu (BL 23) and Zusanli (ST 36) are added for the treatment of headache due to asthenia of both qi and blood. As to the treatment of insomnia, Xinshu (BL 15), Shenshu (BL 23) and Taixi (KI 3) are selected to treat insomnia caused by disharmony between the heart and kidney; while Fengchi (GB 20), Neiguan (PC 6) and Fenglong (ST 40) are selected to treat insomnia due to disturbance of the heart by phlegm-heat. Baihui (GV 20) is selected to treat gastroptosis, hysteroptosis and proctoptosis due to qi asthenia. As to the treatment of sore throat, Shaoshang (LU 11), Hegu (LI 4) and Neiting (ST 44) are selected to treat sthenia-heat syndrome while Taixi (KI 3), Zhaohai (KI 6) and Yuji (LU 10) are selected to treat asthenia-heat syndrome.

伍不同。例如：头痛，肝阳上亢证配行间或太冲，气血两虚证配肝俞、脾俞、肾俞、足三里。失眠，心肾不交证配心俞、肾俞、太溪，痰热扰心证配风池、内关、丰隆。气虚下陷证之胃下垂、子宫下垂、脱肛，皆配用百会。咽喉肿痛，实热证以少商、合谷、内庭相配，虚热证以太溪、照海、鱼际相配。

4.3.3 Application of special acupoints

三、特定穴的应用

Most of the special acupoints are located below the elbows or knees with special names and theory. They are frequently used in clinical treatment with specific methods.

特定穴多位于四肢肘膝以下，有特定的类别名称和理论，多数有一定的应用方法，是临床上最为常用的腧穴。

4.3.3.1 The Five-Shu acupoints

（一）五输穴的应用

There are five acupoints on the twelve main meridians located below the elbows and knees, Namely Jing-Well, Ying-Spring, Shu-Stream, Jing-River and He-Sea located on every meridian respectively. Altogether there are 60 such acupoints. Clinically Jing-Well is used to treat mental diseases, febrile diseases and emergent cases; Ying-Spring, Shu-Stream, Jing-River and He-Sea are used to treat the diseases located on regions over which

五输穴指十二经脉的从肢端到肘膝的五类腧穴，依次称为井、荥、输、经、合穴，每经5个穴，共有60个穴。五输穴在临床上的运用，一般是井穴用于治疗神志病、热证和急救，荥穴、输穴、经穴及合穴用于治疗其经脉在体表循行部

the meridians run along the surface of the body. The Shu-Stream acupoints on the yin meridians are used to treat disorders of the zang organs while the He-Sea acupoints on the yang meridians are used to treat disorders of the fu organs. In addition, the selection of the Five-Shu acupoints can be made according to the combination of the Five-Shu acupoints with the five elements for the treatment of diseases in the light of the theory "reducing the Child-acupoint to treat sthenia syndrome and reinforcing the Mother-acupoint to treat asthenia syndrome" according to the inter-restraining and inter-promoting relation ships between the meridians and acupoints. The combination of yin meridians and yang meridians with the five elements is shown in Table 4 - 1 and 4 - 2.

位的病证。而阴经的输穴用于治疗脏病，阳经的合穴用于治疗腑病。此外，五输穴与五行相配而有五行属性(阴经与阳经的五行配属不同，详见表4 - 1，4 - 2)，可以根据腧穴之间、经脉之间的五行生克关系，按照"实者泻其子，虚者补其母"的方法，依病证的虚实而取五输穴治疗。

Table 4 - 1 The Five-Shu acupoints on the Yin Meridians

Meridian	Jing-Well (Wood)	Ying-Spring (Fire)	Shu-Stream (Earth)	Jing-River (Metal)	He-Sea (Water)
Lung hand-taiyin	Shaoshang (LU 11)	Yuji (LU 10)	Taiyuan (LU 9)	Jingqu (LU 8)	Chize (LU 5)
Pericardium hand-jueyin	Zhongchong (PC 9)	Laogong (PC 8)	Daling (PC 7)	Jianshi (PC 5)	Quze (PC 3)
Heart hand-shaoyin	Shaochong (HT 9)	Shaofu (HT 8)	Shenmen (HT 7)	Lingdao (HT 4)	Shaohai (HT 3)
Spleen foot-taiyin	Yinbai (SP 1)	Dadu (SP 2)	Taibai (SP 3)	Shangqiu (SP 5)	Yinlingquan (SP 9)
Liver foot-jueyin	Dadun (LR 1)	Xingjian (LR 2)	Taichong (LR 3)	Zhongfeng (LR 4)	Ququan (LR 8)
Kidney foot-shaoyin	Yongquan (KI 1)	Rangu (KI 2)	Taixi (KI 3)	Fuliu (KI 7)	Yingu (KI 10)

表 4-1 阴经五输穴表

经 脉	五 输				
	井 （木）	荥 （火）	输 （土）	经 （金）	合 （水）
手太阴肺经	少 商	鱼 际	太 渊	经 渠	尺 泽
手厥阴心包经	中 冲	劳 宫	大 陵	间 使	曲 泽
手少阴心经	少 冲	少 府	神 门	灵 道	少 海
足太阴脾经	隐 白	大 都	太 白	商 丘	阴陵泉
足厥阴肝经	大 敦	行 间	太 冲	中 封	曲 泉
足少阴肾经	涌 泉	然 谷	太 溪	复 溜	阴 谷

Table 4-2 The Five -Shu Acupoints on the Yang Meridians

Meridian	Jing-Well (Metal)	Ying-Spring (Water)	Shu-Stream (Wood)	Jing-River (Fire)	He-Sea (Earth)
Large intestine hand-yangming	Shangyang (LI 1)	Erjian (LI 2)	Sanjian (LI 3)	Yangxi (LI 5)	Quchi (LI 11)
Triple energizer hand-shaoyang	Guanchong (TE 1)	Yemen (TE 2)	Zhongzhu (TE 3)	Zhigou (TE 6)	Tianjing (TE 10)
Small intestine hand-taiyang	Shaoze (SI 1)	Qiangu (SI 2)	Houxi (SI 3)	Yanggu (SI 5)	Xiaohai (SI 8)
Stomach foot-yangming	Lidui (ST 45)	Neiting (ST 44)	Xiangu (ST 43)	Jiexi (ST 41)	Zusanli (ST 36)
Gallbladder foot-shaoyang	Zuqiaoyin (GB 44)	Xiaxi (GB 43)	Zulinqi (GB 41)	Yangfu (GB 38)	Yanglingquan (GB 34)
Bladder foot-taiyang	Zhiyin (BL 67)	Zutonggu (BL 66)	Shugu (BL 65)	Kunlun (BL 60)	Weizhong (BL 40)

表 4-2 阳经五输穴表

经 脉	五输				
	井（金）	荥（水）	输（木）	经（火）	合（土）
手阳明大肠经	商 阳	二 间	三 间	阳 溪	曲 池
手少阳三焦经	关 冲	液 门	中 渚	支 沟	天 井
手太阳小肠经	少 泽	前 谷	后 溪	阳 谷	小 海
足阳明胃经	厉 兑	内 庭	陷 谷	解 溪	足三里
足少阳胆经	足窍阴	侠 溪	足临泣	阳 辅	阳陵泉
足太阳膀胱经	至 阴	足通谷	束 骨	昆 仑	委 中

4.3.3.2 Application of Yuan-Source acupoints and Luo-Connecting acupoints

4.3.3.2.1 The Yuan-Source acupoints are located in the vicinity of the wrists and ankles. Each meridian has one Yuan-Source point. Altogether there are 12 Yuan-Source acupoints which are closely related to the zang-fu organs and are the points where visceral qi is infused via triple energizer. Therefore, the disorder of zang-fu organs can be manifested on the Yuan-Source acupoints and can be treated by needling Yuan-Source acupoints. The Yuan-Source acupoints on the yang meridians are located posterior to the Shu-Stream acupoints, but the Yuan-Source acupoints on the yin meridians are just the Shu-Stream acupoints. (see Table 4-3)

（二）原穴、络穴的应用

1. 原穴是十二经脉分布在腕踝关节附近的一类腧穴，每经1个穴，共有12个穴。原穴与脏腑的关系极为密切，脏腑之气通过三焦输注于原穴之处，所以脏腑病变可反映于原穴部位，针灸原穴能够治疗脏腑病变。阳经的原穴位于“输”穴之后，阴经的原穴即是五输穴中的“输”穴。（参见表4-3）

Table 4-3 The Yuan-Source Acupoints and Luo-Connecting Acupoints

Meridian	Yuan	Luo	Meridian	Yuan	Luo	Meridian (Viscera)	Luo
Hand-taiyin	Taiyuan (LU 9)	Lieque (LU 7)	Hand yangming	Hegu (LI 4)	Pianli (LI 6)	Conception vessel	Jiuwei (CV 15)
Hand-jueyin	Daling (PC 7)	Neiguan (PC 6)	Hand shaoyang	Yangchi (TE 4)	Waiguan (TE 5)	Governor vessel	Changqiang (GV1)

(Following table)

Meridian	Yuan	Luo	Meridian	Yuan	Luo	Meridian (Viscera)	Luo
Hand-shaoyin	Shenmen (HT 7)	Tongli (HT 5)	Hand taiyang	Wangu (SI 4)	Zhizheng (SI 7)	Spleen (Major Luo)	Dabao (SP 21)
Foot-taiyin	Taibai (SP 3)	Gongsun (SP 4)	Foot yangming	Chongyang (ST 42)	Fenglong (ST 40)		
Foot-jueyin	Taichong (LR 3)	Ligou (LR 5)	Foot shaoyang	Qiuxu (GB 40)	Guangming (GB 37)		
Foot-shaoyin	Taixi (KI 3)	Dazhong (KI 4)	Foot taiyang	Jinggu (BL 64)	Feiyang (BL 58)		

表 4-3　**原穴、络穴表**

经　脉	原　穴	络　穴	经　脉	原　穴	络　穴	经　脉（脏腑）	络　穴
手太阴经	太　渊	列　缺	手阳明经	合　谷	偏　历	任　脉	鸠　尾
手厥阴经	大　陵	内　关	手少阳经	阳　池	外　关	督　脉	长　强
手少阴经	神　门	通　里	手太阳经	腕　骨	支　正	脾（大络）	大包
足太阴经	太　白	公　孙	足阳明经	冲　阳	丰　隆		
足厥阴经	太　冲	蠡　沟	足少阳经	丘　墟	光　明		
足少阴经	太　溪	大　钟	足太阳经	京　骨	飞　扬		

4.3.3.2.2　Luo-Connecting acupoints are situated at the places where the twelve regular meridians, the conception and governor vessels are distributed. Each has one Luo-Connecting acupoint and the spleen has another major Luo-Connecting acupoint. So altogether there are 15 Luo-Connecting acupoints. The Luo-Connecting acupoints function to connect the meridians internally and externally related to each other and are used to treat disorders of such pairs of meridians. The Luo-Connecting acupoints on the conception and governor vessels as well as the major Luo-Connecting acupoint of spleen are mainly

2. 络穴是络脉从十二经脉、任脉和督脉上分出部位的腧穴，各脉有 1 个络穴，脾还另有 1 个大络，共有 15 个穴。络穴起着联络的作用。十二经脉的络穴由于联络表里两经而主治表里两经的病证。任脉、督脉的络穴以及脾之大络，主要治疗躯干部的有关病证。（参见表 4-3）

used to treat diseases of the trunk (see Table 4－3).

4.3.3.2.3 In clinical treatment, the Yuan-Source acupoints and Luo-Connecting acupoints may be used independently or in combination. The method for the combination of Yuan-Source and Luo-Connecting acupoints is to select the corresponding Yuan-Source acupoint of the viscus primarily involved and the corresponding Luo-Connecting acupoint of the viscus secondarily involved. Usually this method is to deal with the disorders involving the meridians externally and internally related to each other.

3. 临床上,原穴、络穴可以单独选用,也可配合运用。原络配穴的方法是,先病脏腑取其原穴,后病脏腑取其络穴,多用于表里两经的病证。

4.3.3.3 Application of Back-Shu and Front-Mu acupoints

(三) 俞穴、募穴的应用

4.3.3.3.1 Back-Shu acupoints are located on the back while Front-Mu acupoints are located on the chest and abdomen. Each zang organ and fu organ has one Back-Shu and one Front-Mu acupoint respectively. These acupoints are the areas where visceral qi infuses. So tenderness can be found on these areas when pathological changes have taken place in the viscera. Back-Shu and Front-Mu acupoints can be used to treat visceral diseases and Back-Shu acupoints can also be used to treat disorders of tissues and organs pertaining to the corresponding viscera. For example, Ganshu (BL 18) may be chosen to treat eye or tendon disorders. (see Table 4－4)

1. 俞穴位于背部,又称背俞穴;募穴位于胸腹部,每个脏腑各有一俞一募,是脏腑之气输注的部位,所以内脏病变时往往在俞、募穴处有压痛等反应。俞、募穴主治脏腑病证;俞穴还可以治疗相应脏腑所属组织器官的病证,如肝俞可治疗肝病和目疾、筋病等。(参见表 4－4)

Table 4－4 The Back-Shu and Front-Mu Acupoints of the Twelve Zang-fu Organs

Zang Organ	Back-Shu Acupoint	Front-Mu Acupoint	Fu Organ	Back-Shu Acupoint	Front-Mu Acupoint
Lung	Feishu (BL 13)	Zhongfu (LU 1)	Stomach	Weishu (BL 21)	Zhongwan (CV 12)
Pericardium	Jueyinshu (BL 14)	Tanzhong (CV 17)	Gallbladder	Danshu (BL 19)	Riyue (GB 24)
Heart	Xinshu (BL 15)	Juque (CV 14)	Large intestine	Dachangshu (BL 25)	Tianshu (ST 25)

(Following table)

Zang Organ	Back-Shu Acupoint	Front-Mu Acupoint	Fu Organ	Back-Shu Acupoint	Front-Mu Acupoint
Liver	Ganshu (BL 18)	Qimen (LR 14)	Small intestine	Xiaochangshu (BL 27)	Guanyuan (CV 4)
Spleen	Pishu (BL 20)	Zhangmen (LR 13)	Bladder	Pangguangshu (BL 28)	Zhongji (CV 3)
Kidney	Shenshu (BL 23)	Jingmen (GB 25)	Triple energizer	Sanjiaoshu (BL 22)	Shimen (CV 5)

表 4-4　　十二脏腑俞穴、募穴表

脏	俞穴	募穴	腑	俞穴	募穴
肺	肺俞	中府	胃	胃俞	中脘
心包	厥阴俞	膻中	胆	胆俞	日月
心	心俞	巨阙	大肠	大肠俞	天枢
肝	肝俞	期门	小肠	小肠俞	关元
脾	脾俞	章门	膀胱	膀胱俞	中极
肾	肾俞	京门	三焦	三焦俞	石门

4.3.3.3.2　The Back-Shu acupoints and the Front-Mu acupoints can be used independently or in combination. When used together, this method is called Shu-Mu compatibility.

2. 俞穴和募穴可单独选用，也可配合应用。配合应用时称俞募配穴法。

4.3.3.4　Application of the Lower He-Sea acupoints

（四）下合穴的应用

The Lower He-Sea acupoints refer to the six acupoints located on the three yang meridians of foot. The Lower He-Sea acupoints of the three yang meridians of foot are the He-Sea acupoints in the Five-Shu acupoints on the meridians proper. The Lower He-Sea acupoints are closely related to the six fu organs and are used to treat the disorders of six fu organs (see Table 4-5).

下合穴是位于足三阳经上的6个腧穴，其中足三阳经的下合穴即是其本经五输穴中的“合”穴。下合穴与六腑有极其密切的联系，主治六腑病证（参见表4-5）。

Table 4 - 5 **The Lower He-Sea Acupoints**

Six Fu-Organs	Lower He -Sea Point	Pertaining Meridian
Stomach	Zusanli (ST 36)	Stomach meridian of foot-yangming
Large intestine	Shangjuxu (ST 37)	
Small intestine	Xiajuxu (ST 39)	
Gallbladder	Yanglingquan (GB 34)	Gallbladder meridian of foot-shaoyang
Bladder	Weizhong (BL 40)	Bladder meridian of foot-taiyang
Triple energizer	Weiyang (BL 39)	

表 4 - 5 **下合穴表**

六 腑	下合穴	所属经脉
胃	足三里	足阳明胃经
大 肠	上巨虚	
小 肠	下巨虚	
胆	阳陵泉	足少阳胆经
膀 胱	委 中	足太阳膀胱经
三 焦	委 阳	

4.3.3.5 Application of the Eight Confluent acupoints

The Eight Confluent acupoints refer to the eight acupoints where the essence of zang, fu, qi, blood, tendon, vessels, bone and marrow accumulates respectively. In clinical treatment, they are selected to treat the disorders related to the essence of the corresponding organs or tissues. For example, Geshu (BL 17), the confluent acupoint of the blood, is used to treat the syndrome of blood stagnation. (see Table 4 - 6)

(五) 八会穴的应用

八会穴是指脏、腑、气、血、筋、脉、骨、髓等精气分别聚会的 8 个腧穴。临床上用于治疗辨证属相关精气病变的病证，例如：瘀血证可取血会膈俞治疗。(参见表 4 - 6)

Table 4 - 6 **The Eight Confluent Acupoints**

Eight Confluences	Eight Confluent acupoints	Pertaining Meridians
Zang Organs	Zhangmen (LR 13)	Liver meridian of foot-jueyin
Fu Organs	Zhongwan (CV 12)	Conception vessel

(Following table)

Eight Confluences	Eight confluent acupoints	Pertaining Meridians
Qi	Tanzhong (CV 17)	Conception Vessel
Blood	Geshu (BL 17)	Bladder Meridian of Foot-Taiyang
Tendon	Yanglingquan (GB 34)	Gallbladder Meridian of Foot-Shaoyang
Pulses and Vessels	Taiyuan (LU 9)	Lung Meridian of Hand-Taiyin
Bone	Dazhu (BL 11)	Bladder Meridian of Foot-Taiyang
Marrow	Xuanzhong (GB 39)	Gallbladder Meridian of Foot-Shaoyang

表 4-6　八会穴表

八 会	八会穴	所属经脉
脏 会	章 门	足厥阴肝经
腑 会	中 脘	任 脉
气 会	膻 中	任 脉
血 会	膈 俞	足太阳膀胱经
筋 会	阳陵泉	足少阳胆经
脉 会	太 渊	手太阴肺经
骨 会	大 杼	足太阳膀胱经
髓 会	悬 钟	足少阳胆经

4.3.3.6 Application of Xi-Cleft acupoints

The Xi-Cleft acupoints are those located at the sites where qi and blood in the meridians converges and accumulates. There are sixteen such points on the twelve main meridians, yin link and yang link as well as yin heel and yang heel vessels. (see Table 4-7)

(六) 郄穴的应用

郄穴是经脉气血深聚部位的腧穴，十二经脉以及阴阳维脉、阴阳蹻脉各有 1 个郄穴，共 16 个郄穴。（参见表 4-7）

Table 4-7　**The Sixteen Xi-Cleft Acupoints**

Name of the Meridians	Xi-Cleft Acupoints		Name of the Meridians
Lung meridian of hand-taiyin	Kongzui (LU 6)	Wenliu (LI 7)	Large intestine meridian of hand-yangming
Pericardium meridian of hand-jueyin	Ximen(PC 4)	Huizong(TE 7)	Triple energizer meridian of hand-shaoyang

(Following table)

Name of the Meridians	Xi-Cleft Acupoints		Name of the Meridians
Heart meridian of hand-shaoyin	Yinxi (HT 6)	Yanglao (SI 6)	Small intestine meridian of hand-taiyang
Spleen meridian of foot-taiyin	Diji (SP 8)	Liangqiu (ST 34)	Stomach meridian of foot-yangming
Liver meridian of foot-jueyin	Zhongdu (LR 6)	Waiqiu (GB 36)	Gallbladder meridian of foot-shaoyang
Kidney meridian of foot-shaoyin	Shuiquan (KI 5)	Jinmen (BL 63)	Bladder meridian of foot-taiyang
Yin link vessel	Zhubin (KI 9)	Yangjiao (GB 35)	Yang link vessel
Yin heel vessel	Jiaoxin (KI 8)	Fuyang (BL 59)	Yang heel vessel

表 4-7 **十六郄穴表**

脉 名	郄 穴		脉 名
手太阴肺经	孔 最	温 溜	手阳明大肠经
手厥阴心包经	郄 门	会 宗	手少阳三焦经
手少阴心经	阴 郄	养 老	手太阳小肠经
足太阴脾经	地 机	梁 丘	足阳明胃经
足厥阴肝经	中 都	外 丘	足少阳胆经
足少阴肾经	水 泉	金 门	足太阳膀胱经
阴 维 脉	筑 宾	阳 交	阳 维 脉
阴 蹻 脉	交 信	跗 阳	阳 蹻 脉

The Xi-Cleft acupoints are used mainly to treat acute diseases. For example, Liangqiu (ST 34), the Xi-Cleft acupoint of the stomach meridian, is selected to treat acute stomachache.

郄穴在临床上多用于治疗急性病证，如急性胃痛，可取胃经郄穴梁丘。

4.3.3.7 Application of the eight Convergent acupoints

（七）八脉交会穴的应用

The Eight Convergent acupoints are the eight acupoints usually located around the wrists or ankles through

八脉交会穴是十二经脉上与奇经八脉相关的 8 个腧

which the twelve regular meridians are connected with the eight extra vessels. These eight Convergent acupoints are divided into four groups and each group is the fixed combination of the two acupoints on the hand and foot (see Table 4-8). Their indication is broad, including the diseases on the flowing route of its own meridian and the related extra vessels.

穴,多位于腕踝关节上下。这8个腧穴分为4组,每组为固定的手足两穴配伍(参见表4-8),其治病范围广泛,包括本经及相关奇经循行联系部位的病证。

Table 4-8 The Eight Convergent Acupoints

Convergent Acupoints	Pertaining Meridian	Extra Vessels	Indications
Neiguan (PC 6) Gongsun (SP 4)	Pericardium M. Spleen M.	Yin link vessel Thoroughfare vessel	Heart, chest, stomach
Houxi (SI 3) Shenmai (BL 62)	Small intestine M. Bladder M.	Governor vessel Yang heel vessel	Inner canthus, ear, neck, shoulder, back
Waiguan (TE 5) Zulinqi (GB 41)	Triple energizer M. Gallbladder	Yang link vessel Belt vessel	Outer canthus, back ear, cheek, neck, shoulder
Lieque (LU 7) Zhaohai (KI 6)	Lung M. Kidney M.	Conception vessel Yin heel vessel	Throat, lung, chest, diaphragm

表 4-8 八脉交会穴表

穴 名	所属经脉	相应奇经	主治范围
内 关 公 孙	手厥阴心包经 足太阴脾经	阴维脉 冲 脉	心、胸、胃
后 溪 申 脉	手太阳小肠经 足太阳膀胱经	督 脉 阳蹻脉	目内眦、耳、颈项、肩背
外 关 足临泣	手少阳三焦经 足少阳胆经	阳维脉 带 脉	目外眦、耳后、颊、颈、肩
列 缺 照 海	手太阴肺经 足少阴肾经	任 脉 阴蹻脉	咽喉、肺、胸膈

4.3.3.8 Application of the crossing acupoints

The crossing acupoints refer to those located at the intersection of the two or more meridians. There are

(八)交会穴的应用

交会穴为两条以上的经脉循行经过的腧穴,大多分布

nearly 100 crossing acupoints and most of them are distributed on the trunk, head and face. Since meridians converge at the crossing acupoints, so the crossing acupoints can be used to treat disorders of the multimeridians. For example, Sanyinjiao (SP 6), a crossing acupoint of the three yin meridians of foot, can be used to treat diseases of the spleen, liver and kidney meridians and diseases related to the corresponding zang-fu organs.

于躯干和头面部，有近百个。交会穴由于有数条经脉相交会，所以能治疗多经脉的病证。例如：三阴交穴，为足三阴经交会之处，可治疗脾、肝、肾的经脉和相关脏腑病证。

4.4 Main factors affecting the curative effects of acupuncture and moxibustion

第四节 影响针灸疗效的主要因素

There are many factors which may affect the curative effect of acupuncture and moxibustion including every aspects in the procedure of treatment concerning both the acupuncturist and the patient. The acupuncturist should be careful in diagnosis, treatment and nursing; while the patient should have confidence and actively cooperate with the acupuncturist in the treatment. Among these factors, proper treatment, correct selection of acupoints and performance are the most important ones.

影响针灸疗效的因素是多方面的。广义上讲，构成针灸诊治过程的各个环节、各个部分，施治的医生和求治的患者双方，都会对针灸治疗的效果产生影响。所以，在医生方面，始终要以认真的态度对待诊察、治疗、护理等各项工作；在患者方面，则应树立信心，积极配合，才能提高针灸疗效。在诸多的影响因素中，治法选择恰当、正确用穴组方和刺灸操作等，对提高针灸疗效具有更为重要的、直接的影响。

4.4.1 Factors concerning therapeutic principles

一、治法因素

The acupuncture and moxibustion therapy includes acupuncture, moxibustion and cupping, etc. Acupuncture also includes pricking collateral for bloodletting, and moxibustion includes moxibustion with moxa cone and

针灸疗法包括针刺、艾灸和拔罐等几种治疗手段，针刺方法中还有刺络放血法，艾灸方法还分为艾炷灸、艾条灸、

moxa roll as well as needle-warming moxibustion. These methods can be used independently or in combination according to the pathological conditions. One should not simply make use of the one and neglect the rest. Only correct use of different therapeutic methods can produce satisfactory curative effect.

温针灸等，这些方法应该根据病证的治疗需要，或单独应用，或结合运用，而不应有所偏废。正确地使用不同治疗手段，才能充分发挥针灸疗法的治疗作用。

4.4.2 Factors concerning the use of acupoints

二、用穴因素

4.4.2.1 Guidance of the theory of TCM

The acupuncture and moxibustion therapy is developed on the basis of the theory of TCM with the application of the theories of yin-yang and five elements as well as meridians, viscera, qi, blood and body fluids in analyzing pathogenesis, identifying the location of disease and defin-ing yin and yang, exterior and interior, cold and heat as well as asthenia and sthenia. These aspects are prerequisite to the selection and combination of acupoints.

（一）以中医理论为指导

针灸治病方法建立在中医理论的基础上，运用中医阴阳五行学说，以经络、脏腑、气血津液等理论分析病变的机理，辨别病位，明确其阴阳、表里、寒热、虚实，形成对所治病证的正确认识，这是针灸选穴配穴的基本前提。

4.4.2.2 Combination of the differentiation of syndromes with the differentiation of diseases

Differentiation of syndromes should be emphasized in the selection and combination of acupoints according to the theory and principles of meridians and acupoints. At the same time modern medical knowledge is required to diagnose diseases and for the improvement of specificity of acupoint selection and formulation of prescription.

（二）辨证结合辨病

重视辨证，按照经络、腧穴理论和规律来用穴组方；同时，结合现代医学知识，明确疾病的诊断，了解其发展变化规律，提高选用腧穴的针对性，能使配穴处方更为完善。

4.4.3 Factors concerning the manipulation

三、操作因素

4.4.3.1 Concentration

Since acupuncture and moxibustion therapy uses needles and lighted moxa to directly stimulate the body of the patient, the acupuncturist should be very careful in all the procedure of treatment. This is not only for the prevention of accidents, but also for careful observation of the

（一）重视“治神”

即高度集中精神。针灸治疗需要医生以针具和艾火的物理刺激方法直接在病人身上施术，要求医者不得有丝毫的马虎，这不仅是为了防止

reactions of the patient to the stimulation for the purpose of timely adjustment of the treatment in order to achieve satisfactory curative effect.

针灸意外的发生，也是仔细观察、体会病人对针灸刺激的反应，适时调整针灸方式而获得最佳效应的需要。

4.4.3.2 Consideration of constitutional difference

（二）重视体质差异

The degree of acupuncture and moxibustion stimulation should be monitored according to the pathological conditions and the constitutional difference of the patient. Both excessive or insufficient stimulation will make it difficult to achieve satisfactory curative effect. The modification of the stimulating degree requires correct application of proper needling techniques as well as careful clinical practice and rich experience.

施以针灸刺激的程度，根据病证而有基本的量度要求；此外，还应视病人的体质差异而有所不同，过度和不及都达不到预期的治疗效果，对其适当程度的掌握，除了按照刺灸方法的一般要求正确操作以外，更需要在临床上细心地体会和长期的经验积累。

5 Specific discussions of treatment

5.1 Infectious diseases

5.1.1 Influenza

[**Introduction**]

Influenza refers to acute infection of respiratory tract due to influenza virus. Clinically it is marked by sudden onset, evident general poisoning symptoms, appearance of fever, headache, general aching and lassitude as well as mild symptoms of the respiratory tract. This disease is similar to "Shixing Ganmao" (Influenza) in TCM. Exogenous seasonal pathogenic factor is the main cause of this disease. Due to difference in seasons and constitution, this syndrome is manifested either as wind-cold or wind-heat with the complications of summer-heat and dampness. It may be caused by pathogenic wind, cold and dampness that block the pores, stagnate yang-qi and hinder the dispersion of pulmonary qi; or by pathogenic wind, heat, summer-heat and dryness that affect the conveyance of the muscular interstices, leading to scorching of the lung by pathogenic heat and failure of the lung to depurate.

[**Syndrome differentiation**]

1. Wind-cold syndrome

Aversion to cold, fever, no sweating, headache, heaviness and aching of the limbs, nasal itching and sneezing, running nose, throat itching and cough, thin spu-

第五章 治疗各论

第一节 传染性疾病

一、流行性感冒

【**概述**】

流行性感冒是由流感病毒引起的急性呼吸道传染病。其临床特点为起病急骤，全身中毒症状明显，出现发热、头痛、全身酸痛、乏力等症状，而呼吸道症状相对较轻。本病相当于中医的“时行感冒”。病因主要为外感时邪病毒。由于发病季节的不同及体质的差异，证候表现一般为风寒、风热两大类，并有挟暑、挟湿之兼证。若因风寒湿邪，则毛窍闭塞，阳气郁阻，肺气失宣；若因风热暑燥，则腠理疏泄失畅，邪热灼肺，肺失清肃。

【**辨证**】

1. 风寒证

恶寒发热，无汗，头痛，肢体酸重，鼻痒喷嚏，流清涕，喉痒咳嗽，痰液清稀，舌苔薄白，

tum, thin and white tongue fur, floating or floating and tense pulse.

脉浮或浮紧。

2. Wind-heat syndrome

Severe fever and slight aversion to cold, or sweating, pain and distension in the head, dry mouth, dry throat or sore throat, heavy cough, yellow and sticky sputum, nasal obstruction with thick sputum, yellow and thin tongue fur, floating and rapid pulse.

2. 风热证

发热重而恶寒轻,或有汗出,头痛昏胀,口干,咽喉干燥或疼痛,咳嗽声重,咯痰色黄而粘,鼻塞流浊涕,舌苔薄黄,脉浮数。

3. Syndrome due to seasonal pathogenic factors with dampness

Aversion to cold, fever, dull fever, unsmooth sweating, aching and heavy sensation in the body, dizzy, heavy and distending sensation in the head, fullness and oppression in the chest and epigastrium, anorexia and abdominal distension, loose stool, heavy cough, expectoration of white and sticky sputum, white and greasy or light yellow and greasy tongue fur, soft pulse.

3. 时邪挟湿证

恶寒发热,身热不扬,汗出不畅,肢体酸重,头昏重胀,胸脘痞闷,纳呆腹胀,大便溏泄,咳嗽声重,咯吐白色粘痰,舌苔白腻或淡黄腻,脉濡。

4. Syndrome due to seasonal pathogenic factors with summer-heat

Severe fever, burning sensation in the skin, non-relief after sweating, dysphoria and thirst, scanty and brown urine, cough with scanty and very sticky sputum, dry and sore throat, red tongue with yellow fur and rapid pulse.

4. 时邪挟暑证

发热较重,肌肤灼热,汗出不解,心烦口渴,小便短赤,咳嗽痰少,质粘如丝,咽干而痛,舌质红,苔黄,脉数。

[**Treatment**]

1. Body acupuncture

Prescription: Fengchi (GB 20), Lieque (LU 7), Hegu (LI 4) and Yingxiang (LI 20).

Modification: For wind-cold syndrome, Fengmen (BL 12) and Zhizheng (SI 7) are added; for wind-heat syndrome, Chize (LU 5) and Yuji (LU 10) are added; for complication of dampness, Zhongwan (CV 12), Zusanli (ST 36) and Yinlingquan (SP 9) are added; for complication of summer-heat, Dazhui (GV 14) and Quchi (LI 11)

【治疗】

1. 体针疗法

处方:风池,列缺,合谷,迎香。

随证配穴:风寒证,加风门、支正;风热证,加尺泽、鱼际;挟湿者,加中脘、足三里、阴陵泉;挟暑者,加大椎、曲池;头痛,加印堂、头维、阿是穴;咽痛,加少商、扶突。

are added; for headache, Yintang (EX-HN 3), Touwei (ST 8) and Ashi acupoints are added; for sore throat, Shaoshang (LU 11) and Futu (ST 32) are added.

Performance: Reducing needling technique is used. Shaoshang (LU 11) is pricked for bloodletting. Dazhui (GV 14) and Fengmen (BL 12) are needled with the addition of moxibustion or cupping. The needles are usually retained for 30 minutes. For the treatment of patients with high fever, the retention of needles can be prolonged. The needles are manipulated once every 5-10 minutes and the treatment is given once or twice a day.

操作：针刺用泻法。少商用点刺放血法。大椎、风门可加用灸法或拔罐。一般留针30分钟，高热病人适当延长留针时间，每隔5～10分钟行针1次。每日1～2次。

2. Ear acupuncture

2. 耳针疗法

Prescription: Lung (CO_{14}), Internal Nose (TG_4), Trachea (CO_{16}), Throat (TG_3), Forehead (AT_1) and Adrenal Gland (TG_{2p}).

处方：肺，内鼻，气管，咽喉，额，肾上腺。

Performance: Each time 2-3 acupoints are selected and needled with filiform needles with moderate stimulation. The needles are retained for 20-30 minutes each time and manipulated once every 5-10 minutes.

操作：每次选2～3穴，毫针用中等刺激，留针20～30分钟，每隔5～10分钟行针1次。

5.1.2 Mumps

二、流行性腮腺炎

[**Introduction**]

Mumps refers to acute infectious disease of respiratory tract due to mumps virus. The clinical symptoms are non-suppurative swelling of the parotid gland, pain, fever, restricted activity in chewing and involvement of various glands or viscera. Usually the prognosis is favourable. A few cases tend to develop complications like orchitis, encephalitis, meningitis, pancreatitis and ovaritis. This disease usually occurs in winter and spring among children. It is often caused by exogenous wind and warmth that stagnate shaoyang and yangming meridians. Severe attack by pathogenic factors may involve the liver meridian and lead to swelling and pain of testis. Invasion

【概述】

流行性腮腺炎是由腮腺炎病毒引起的急性呼吸道传染病。其临床特征为腮腺非化脓性肿胀、疼痛，发热，伴咀嚼受限，并有累及各种腺体组织或脏器的倾向。一般预后良好，少数有并发睾丸炎、脑炎、脑膜炎以及胰腺炎、卵巢炎的可能性。本病以冬、春季为发病高峰，主要侵犯儿童。中医称为“痄腮”。主要为外感风温邪毒，壅阻少阳、阳明

of exuberant pathogenic toxin into the pericardium may generate liver wind by extreme heat and result in deteriorated syndrome.

经脉;若感邪较重,侵犯足厥阴经,出现睾丸肿痛;若邪毒炽盛,内陷心包,热极引动肝风,而出现变证。

[Syndrome differentiation]

【辨证】

1. Stagnation of wind-heat

Parotid swelling and pain, difficulty in chewing, accompanied by aversion to cold, fever, headache, general aching sensation, thin and yellow tongue fur, and floating and rapid pulse.

1. 风热壅遏

耳下腮部漫肿、疼痛,咀嚼不便,伴恶寒,发热,头痛,全身酸痛,舌苔薄黄,脉浮数。

2. Exuberance of pathogenic toxin

Parotic swelling and unpressable pain, difficulty in chewing, sore throat, lingering high fever, restless thirst with desire to drink, headache, red tongue with yellow fur, slippery and rapid pulse. Stagnation of heat in the liver meridian may lead to swelling and pain of testis, dragging pain in the lower abdomen, or even chills and high fever. Inner sinking of virulence may result in sudden high fever, severe headache, stiff neck, or even coma, convulsion, red tongue with yellow fur, or deep-red tongue with scanty fur, large and rapid or thin and rapid pulse.

2. 邪毒炽盛

腮部肿胀,疼痛拒按,咀嚼困难,咽部红肿疼痛,壮热不退,烦渴欲饮,头痛,舌红苔黄,脉滑数。若热郁肝经则可见睾丸肿胀疼痛,小腹掣痛,甚则寒战高热;若邪毒内陷则可见突然高热,剧烈头痛,颈项强硬,甚则昏迷,痉厥,舌红苔黄,或红绛少苔,脉大而数,或细数。

[Treatment]

Body acupuncture

Prescription: Jiache (ST 6), Yifeng (TE 17), Waiguan (TE 15) and Hegu (LI 4).

Modification: For stagnation of wind-heat, Fengchi (GB 20) is added; for exuberance of pathogenic toxin, Dazhui (GV 14), Quchi (LI 11) and Guanchong (TE 1) are added; for stagnation of heat in the liver meridian, Dadun (LR 1), Ququan (LR 8) and Guilai (ST 29) are added; for inner sinking of pathogenic toxin, Shuigou (GV 26), Laogong (PC 8) and Yanglingquan (GB 34) are added.

【治疗】

体针疗法

处方:颊车,翳风,外关,合谷。

随证配穴:风热壅遏,加风池;邪毒亢盛,加大椎、曲池、关冲;热郁肝经,加大敦、曲泉、归来;邪毒内陷,加水沟、劳宫、阳陵泉。

Performance: Reducing needling technique is used. Jiache (ST 6) is needled horizontally for 0.8- 1 cun. Yifeng (TE 17) is needled obliquely downward for 0.8-1 cun. The needles are retained for 30 minutes. For the treatment of patients with high fever, the retention of needles may be prolonged. The needles are manipulated once every 5 - 10 minutes and the treatment is given once or twice a day.

操作：针用泻法。颊车穴沿面部向前平刺 0.8～1 寸。翳风穴向下斜刺 0.8～1 寸。留针 30 分钟，高热病人适当延长留针时间，每隔 5～10 分钟行针 1 次。每日 1～2 次。

5.2 Diseases of respiratory system

第二节　呼吸系统疾病

5.2.1 Acute and chronic bronchitis

一、急、慢性支气管炎

[**Introduction**]

Acute and chronic bronchitis refers to inflammation of trachea and bronchia due to various factors. The main clinical symptoms are cough, expectoration and asthma. Acute and chronic bronchitis pertains to the conceptions of cough, cough and dyspnea as well as phlegm and fluid-retention in TCM. The cause of this disease is either exogenous or endogenous. Exogenous cause refers to attack by wind, cold, heat and dryness that lead to non-conveyance of pulmonary qi, failure of body fluids to distribute and obstruction of the trachea by sputum. Endogenous cause refers to dysfunction of the lung, spleen and kidney. Lung asthenia results in failure of pulmonary qi to convey and descend; dysfunction of the spleen leads to accumulation of dampness into phlegm which attacks the lung; kidney asthenia brings about dysfunction of qi and upward adverse flow of qi; or invasion of liver fire into the lung leads to consumption of body fluid by lung heat. Acute bronchitis is usually of sthenia syndrome, while

【**概述**】

急、慢性支气管炎是由多种因素引起的气管、支气管的炎症。临床以咳嗽、咳痰、喘促等为主要症状。急、慢性支气管炎相当于中医的“咳嗽”、“咳喘”、“痰饮”等病证。本病的病因分为外感和内伤两类，外感多因风、寒、热、燥等侵袭，肺卫失宣，津液失布，痰阻气道；内伤多由于肺、脾、肾三脏功能失调，肺虚则宣降失司；脾失健运，聚湿成痰，上犯于肺；肾虚则气失摄纳，气逆于上；或肝火犯肺，肺热伤津。急性支气管炎多为实证，慢性支气管炎多见虚证或本虚标实之证。

chronic bronchitis is usually of asthenia syndrome or syndrome with asthenia in root and sthenia in branch.

[**Syndrome differentiation**]

【辨证】

1. Wind-cold encumbering lung

1. 风寒束肺

Cough with white sputum, nasal obstruction and running nose, aversion to cold and fever, headache and general aching, light-colored tongue with thin and white fur, floating and tense pulse.

咳嗽痰白,鼻塞流涕,恶寒发热,头痛,全身酸楚,舌淡,苔薄白,脉浮紧。

2. Wind-heat attacking lung

2. 风热犯肺

Cough with yellow sputum, difficulty in expectoration due to thick sputum, dry mouth and sore throat, fever and headache, tongue with red tip and margins, thin and yellow tongue fur, floating and rapid pulse.

咳嗽痰黄,质稠难咯,口干咽痛,身热头痛,舌边尖红,苔薄黄,脉浮数。

3. Dry-heat impairing lung

3. 燥热伤肺

Dry cough without sputum, or scanty and sticky sputum, or even blood in sputum, unsmooth expectoration, dry nose and throat, headache and fever, red tongue with scanty fluid, thin and yellow tongue fur, thin and rapid pulse.

干咳无痰,或痰少而粘,甚则痰中带血,咯痰不爽,鼻燥咽干,头痛发热,舌红少津,苔薄黄,脉细数。

4. Retention of phlegm and dampness in lung

4. 痰湿阻肺

Cough with profuse sputum, white and sticky sputum easy to expectorate, heavy cough, fullness and oppression in chest or dyspnea and shortness of breath, anorexia and abdominal distension, light-colored tongue with white and greasy tongue fur, soft and slippery pulse.

咳嗽痰多,痰白而粘,易于咯出,咳声重浊,胸部满闷或喘促短气,纳呆腹胀,舌淡,苔白腻,脉濡滑。

5. Liver fire scorching lung

5. 肝火灼肺

Paroxysmal cough involving the rib-side, scanty and sticky sputum difficult to expectorate, or even blood in sputum, dry and itching throat, red eyes and bitter taste in the mouth, constipation and brown urine, tongue with red tip and margins, thin and yellow tongue fur, taut and rapid pulse.

气逆咳嗽阵作,咳引胁肋作痛,痰少而粘,咯吐不易,甚则痰中带血,咽喉干痒,目赤口苦,便秘尿赤,舌边尖红,苔薄黄,脉弦数。

6. Asthenia of lung and kidney yin

6. 肺肾阴虚

Dry cough without sputum or with scanty sputum,

干咳无痰或少痰,痰粘或

sticky or bloody sputum, dry mouth and throat, feverish sensation in the palms, soles and chest, night sweating and tidal fever, emaciation, red tongue with scanty fur, thin and rapid pulse.

带血,口干咽燥,五心烦热,潮热盗汗,形体消瘦,舌红少苔,脉细数。

7. Asthenia of spleen and kidney yang

Cough and dyspnea, aggravation on exertion, thin sputum, bright white complexion, cold body and limbs, dropsy of face and limbs, dysuria, light-colored tongue, thin, white and slightly greasy tongue fur, deep and thin pulse.

7. 脾肾阳虚

咳嗽气喘,动则尤甚,痰液清稀,面色㿠白,形寒肢冷,或面浮肢肿,小便不利,舌淡,苔薄白微腻,脉沉细。

[**Treatment**]

1. Body acupuncture

Prescription: Feishu (BL 13), Lieque (LU 7), Tiantu (CV 22) and Taiyuan (LU 9).

Modification: For wind-cold encumbering the lung, Fengchi (GB 20) and Hegu (LI 4) are added; for wind-heat attacking lung, Dazhui (GV 14) and Quchi (LI 11) are added; for dry-heat impairing lung; Chize (LU 5) and Waiguan (TE 15) are added; for retention of phlegm and dampness in the lung, Zusanli (ST 36) and Fenglong (ST 40) are added; for liver fire scorching lung, Xingjian (LR 2) and Yuji (LU 10) are added; for asthenia of lung and kidney yin, Shenshu (BL 23), Gaohuang (BL 43) and Taixi (KI 3) are added; for asthenia of spleen and kidney yang, Pishu (BL 20), Shenshu (BL 23), Guanyuan (CV 4) and Zusanli (ST 36) are added; for blood in sputum, Kongzui (LU 6) is added; for night sweating, Yinxi (HT 6) is added; for dropsy of face and limbs and dysuria, Yinlingquan (SP 9) and Sanyinjiao (SP 6) are added.

Performance: Needling techniques are selected according to the nature of the syndromes. For the treatment of wind-cold encumbering the lung, retention of phlegm and dampness in the lung and asthenia of spleen and kidney yang, Back-Shu acupoint can be needled with

【**治疗**】

1. 体针疗法

处方:肺俞,列缺,天突,太渊。

随证配穴:风寒束肺,加风池、合谷;风热犯肺,加大椎、曲池;燥热伤肺,加尺泽、外关;痰湿阻肺,加足三里、丰隆;肝火灼肺,加行间、鱼际;肺肾阴虚,加肾俞、膏肓、太溪;脾肾阳虚,加脾俞、肾俞、关元、足三里;痰中带血者,加孔最;盗汗者,加阴郄;面浮肢肿,小便不利者,加阴陵泉、三阴交。

操作:根据证候虚实决定补泻手法。风寒束肺、痰湿阻肺及脾肾阳虚者,背俞可用灸或加拔火罐,关元、足三里可加灸。急性支气管炎,每日

the addition of moxibustion or cupping, Guanyuan (CV 4) and Zusanli (ST 36) can be moxibusted. For acute bronchitis, the treatment is given once or twice a day; for chronic bronchitis, the treatment is given once every 1 - 2 days.

1～2 次;慢性支气管炎者,每隔 1～2 日 1 次。

2. Ear acupuncture

Prescription: Lung (CO_{14}), Spleen (CO_{13}), Kidney (CO_{10}), Trachea (CO_{16}), Ear Shenmen (TF_4), Adrenal Gland (TG_{2p}) and Antitragic Apex ($AT_{1,2,4i}$).

Performance: Each time 2 - 3 acupoints are selected and needled with filiform needles. For acute bronchitis, the needling is done with strong stimulation; while for chronic bronchitis, the needling is done with moderate stimulation. The needles are manipulated once every 5 - 10 minutes. Or ear-pressure with Wangbuliuxingzi (Semen Vaccariae) is used.

2. 耳针疗法

处方:肺,脾,肾,气管,神门,肾上腺,对屏尖。

操作:每次选 2～3 穴,毫针刺,急性支气管炎用强刺激;慢性支气管炎用中等刺激,每隔 5～10 分钟行针 1 次。或用王不留行籽压耳法。

3. Acupoints application

Prescription: Feishu (BL 13), Gaohuang (BL 43), Dazhui (GV 14), Dazhu (BL 11), Shenzhu (BL 23), Dingchuan (EX-B 1), Tiantu (CV 22), Zhongfu (LU 1) and Tanzhong (CV 17).

Performance: This treatment is applicable to chronic bronchitis. Baijiezi (Semen Sinapis Albae), Gansui (Radix Euphordiae Kansui), Xixin (Herba Asari), Yanhusuo (Rhizoma Corydalis), Rougui (Cortex Cinnamomi) and Dannanxing (Arisaema cum Bil) are prepared into paste which is applied to 3 - 4 acupoints each time. The application is changed once every 3 days and 10 days make up one course of treatment.

3. 穴位敷贴

处方:肺俞,膏肓,大椎,大杼,身柱,定喘,天突,中府,膻中。

操作:适用于慢性支气管炎,用白芥子、甘遂、细辛、延胡索、肉桂、胆南星等制成膏药,每次敷贴 3～4 穴,每 3 日换药 1 次,10 次为 1 个疗程。

5. 2. 2 Bronchial asthma

[**Introduction**]

Bronchial asthma is a kind of paroxysmal allergic disease of the bronchia. The clinical manifestations are paroxysmal and exhaling dyspnea accompanied by wheezing.

二、支气管哮喘

【概述】

支气管哮喘是一种发作性支气管过敏反应性疾病。其临床特征为发作性、伴有哮

The patients usually have allergy and family history. This disease is similar to asthma and asthmatic cough in TCM. It is usually caused by dysfunction of the lung, spleen and kidney due to exogenous pathogenic factors, improper diet and improper caring after illness, leading to retention of endogenous phlegm in the lung. The latent phlegm is easy to be provoked by climatic changes, diet, emotional changes and overstrain, leading to ascendance of the phlegm with qi that obstructs the trachea and causes asthma. Recurrent asthma will result in simultaneous asthenia of the lung, spleen and kidney, or even involve the heart and bring about critical conditions.

鸣音、以呼气性为主的呼吸困难。病人多有过敏史或家族遗传史。本病相当于中医"哮喘"、"喘咳"等病证。主要因外邪、饮食、病后失调等因素，导致肺、脾、肾三脏功能失调，痰饮内生，伏藏于肺；此后每因气候、饮食、情志、劳累等诱因而触引内伏痰饮，痰随气升，痰气互结，壅塞气道而发为哮喘。反复发作则致肺、脾、肾三脏俱虚，甚则病及于心而出现喘脱危候。

［**Syndrome differentiation**］

【辨证】

1. Retention of cold fluid in the lung

Occurrence after cold attack, dyspnea, or sputum roaring in the throat, expectoration of thin and white sputum, usually accompanied by aversion to cold, fever, headache without sweating, light-colored tongue with white and slippery fur as well as floating and tense pulse in the early period.

1. 寒饮伏肺

遇寒触发，呼吸急促，或喉中痰鸣，咯痰稀白，初起多兼恶寒发热，头痛无汗，舌淡苔白滑，脉浮紧。

2. Retention of phlegm-heat in the lung

Dyspnea and chest oppression, sputum roaring in the throat, yellow and sticky sputum, unsmooth expectoration, or accompanied by fever, thirst, red tongue, yellow and greasy tongue fur as well as slippery and rapid pulse.

2. 痰热壅肺

喘急胸闷，喉中哮鸣，声高息涌，痰黄质稠，咯吐不爽，或伴有发热口渴，舌质红，苔黄腻，脉滑数。

3. Asthenia of spleen and lung qi

Cough, asthma and shortness of breath, aggravation on exertion, low voice in cough, thin sputum, aversion to wind and spontaneous sweating, lassitude, poor appetite and loose stool, light-colored tongue with thin and white fur, soft and thin pulse.

3. 肺脾气虚

咳喘气短，动则加剧，咳声低怯，痰液清稀，畏风自汗，神疲倦怠，食少便溏，舌淡苔薄白，脉濡细。

4. Asthenia of lung and kidney yin

Shortness of breath and dyspnea, cough with scanty

4. 肺肾阴虚

气短而喘，咳嗽痰少，头

sputum, dizziness and tinnitus, aching and weakness of loins and knees, tidal fever and night sweating, red tongue with scanty fur and thin and rapid pulse.

晕耳鸣,腰膝酸软,潮热盗汗,舌红少苔,脉细数。

5. Asthenia of heart and kidney yang

Asthma and shortness of breath, more exhalation and less inhalation, aversion to cold and cold limbs, scanty urine and edema, even dyspnea and restlessness, palpitation and low spirit, profuse cold sweating, cyanotic lips and nails, purplish tongue with ecchymoses, thin and white tongue fur, deep and thin pulse or slightly weak and slow regular intermittent pulse or slow pulse with irregular intervals.

5. 心肾阳虚

喘促短气,呼多吸少,畏寒肢冷,尿少浮肿,甚则喘急烦躁,心悸神昧,冷汗淋漓,唇甲青紫,舌质紫暗有瘀点瘀斑,苔薄白,脉沉细或微弱而结代。

[**Treatment**]

1. Body acupuncture

Prescription: Feishu (BL 13), Dingchuan (EX-B 1), Tiantu (CV 22), Zhongfu (LU 1), Tanzhong (CV 17) and Kongzui (LU 6).

Modification: For retention of cold fluid in the lung, Fengmen (BL 12) and Taiyuan (LU 9) are added; for stagnation of phlegm-heat in the lung, Dazhui (GV 14) and Fenglong (ST 40) are added; for asthenia of spleen and lung qi, Pishu (BL 20), Gaohuang (BL 43), Qihai (CV 6) and Zusanli (ST 36) are added; for asthenia of lung and kidney yin, Shenshu (BL 23), Guanyuan (CV 4), Taixi (KI 3) and Sanyinjiao (SP 6) are added; for asthenia of heart and kidney yang, Xinshu (BL 15), Shenshu (BL 23), Qihai (CV 6), Guanyuan (CV 4) and Neiguan (PC 6) are added; for tidal fever and night sweating, Yinxi (HT 6) and Fuliu (KI 7) are added; for coma, Shuigou (GV 26) and Suliao (GV 25) are added.

Performance: In the stage of attack, usually filiform needles are used with reducing techniques. For the treatment of syndrome with a mixture of asthenia and sthenia, mild reinforcing and reducing technique can be used. The

【**治疗**】

1. 体针疗法

处方:肺俞,定喘,天突,中府,膻中,孔最。

随证配穴:寒饮伏肺,加风门、太渊;痰热壅肺,加大椎、丰隆;肺脾气虚,加脾俞、膏肓、气海、足三里;肺肾阴虚,加肾俞、关元、太溪、三阴交;心肾阳虚,加心俞、肾俞、气海、关元、内关;潮热盗汗者,加阴郄、复溜;神昏者,加水沟、素髎。

操作:发作期,一般用毫针泻法,虚实夹杂证用平补平泻法,每日针刺 2 次或数次;亦可配合电针疗法,每次选用

needling is done twice or more a day. Electrical acupuncture can also be used at the same time. Each time 2 - 3 couples of acupoints are selected and dense or sparse wave can be chosen, 400 - 500 times one minute. The stimulation is monitored to the tolerance of the patient. The electricity is attached to the needles for 30 - 40 minutes. In the remission stage, reinforcing technique is used. The needling is done once every 1 - 2 days. For the treatment of cold syndrome, qi asthenia syndrome and yang asthenia syndrome, acupuncture and moxibustion can be used together; for weak and slow regular intermittent pulse and slow pulse with irregular intervals, Qihai (CV 6) and Guanyuan (CV 4) are moxibusted heavily for restoring yang and stopping prostration.

2～3 对穴，用密波或疏密波，每分钟 400～500 次，强度以病人能耐受为度，通电 30～40 分钟。缓解期多用补法，每隔 1～2 日针刺 1 次。寒证，气虚、阳虚证可针、灸并用；脉微弱而结代者，当重灸气海、关元以回阳固脱。

2. Ear acupuncture

Prescription: Antitragic Apex ($AT_{1,2,4i}$), Adrenal Gland (TG_{2p}), Trachea (CO_{16}), Lung (CO_{14}), Subcortex (AT_4) and Sympathetic (AH_{6a}).

Performance: In the stage of attack, the filiform needles are used with strong stimulation. The needles are retained for 30 minutes and manipulated once every 5 - 10 minutes. The needling is done once or twice a day. In the remission stage, needling is done with mild stimulation and twice a week.

2. 耳针疗法

处方：对屏尖，肾上腺，气管，肺，皮质下，交感。

操作：发作期毫针用强刺激，留针 30 分钟，每隔 5～10 分钟行针 1 次，每日 1～2 次；缓解期用弱刺激，每周 2 次。

3. Moxibustion in summer

Prescription: Dazhui (GV 14), Fengmen (BL 12), Feishu (BL 13), Gaohuangshu (BL 43), Pishu (BL 20), Shenshu (BL 23), Tanzhong (CV 17) and Qihai (CV 6).

Performance: The moxibustion is done in the three periods of dog days. Each time 3 - 4 acupoints are selected and moxibusted once every other day. Three times make up one course of treatment. The moxibustion in this way should continue for over three years. Such a treatment is effective in preventing bronchitis.

3. 伏灸法

处方：大椎，风门，肺俞，膏肓俞，脾俞，肾俞，膻中，气海。

操作：在夏季三伏天灸，每次选 3～4 穴，每穴 3～5 壮，隔日 1 次，3 次为 1 个疗程，需连续灸治 3 年以上。有较好的预防作用。

5.3 Diseases of circulatory system

第三节 循环系统疾病

5.3.1 Arrhythmia

一、心律失常

[Introduction]

Arrhythmia refers to abnormal frequency and rhythm of heart beating. Clinical manifestations are rapid or slow heart rate, irregular heart beating, or early heart beating, flutter, vibration, stoppage of beating and other related syndromes. Arrhythmia is usually either rapid arrhythmia or slow arrhythmia. Arrhythmia is similar to palpitation and severe palpitation in TCM. This disease is usually caused by weak constitution, emotional stimulation and invasion of pathogenic factors that lead to malnutrition of the heart due to deficiency of qi, blood, yin and yang; or by phlegm-fire attacking the heart and stagnation of heart blood. In severe cases even sudden loss of heart yang and separation of yin and yang may be caused.

【概述】

心律失常是指心脏收缩的频率或(及)节律失常。临床特征主要为心率的过快、过慢、不规则或(及)心脏过早搏动、扑动、颤动、停搏和相应的综合征表现。常可分为快速性心律失常和慢速性心律失常两类。心律失常相当于中医的"心悸"、"怔忡"等病证。本病多因体质虚弱、情志刺激、外邪入侵等因素,以致气、血、阴、阳亏损,使心失所养;或痰火扰心、心血瘀阻而引起。严重者甚至出现心阳暴脱或阴阳离决的危候。

[Syndrome differentiation]

1. Asthenia of the heart and gallbladder

Palpitation, susceptibility to fright, restlessness, insomnia and dreaminess, light-colored tongue with white fur, taut and thin pulse.

2. Interior disturbance of phlegm-fire

Palpitation and chest oppression, restlessness and susceptibility to rage, insomnia and disturbed sleep, dry stool and brown urine, red tongue with yellow and greasy fur, slippery and rapid pulse.

3. Insufficiency of heart blood

Palpitation and dizziness, lusterless complexion, lassitude, amnesia and insomnia, light-red tongue with thin

【辨证】

1. 心胆虚怯

心悸,善惊易恐,坐卧不安,少寐多梦,舌淡苔白,脉弦细等。

2. 痰火内扰

心悸胸闷,急躁易怒,夜寐难安,便干尿赤,舌质红,苔黄腻,脉滑数。

3. 心血不足

心悸头晕,面色不华,倦怠乏力,健忘失眠,舌淡红,苔

and white fur, thin and weak pulse or slow pulse with irregular intervals and slow regular intermittent pulse.

薄白,脉细弱无力或结代。

4. Stagnation of blood in collaterals

Palpitation and shortness of breath, stabbing pain in the chest, or cyanotic lips and nails, purplish tongue or tongue with ecchymoses, thin and unsmooth pulse or slow pulse with irregular intervals and slow regular intermittent pulse.

4. 瘀血阻络

心悸气短,胸痛如刺,或唇甲青紫,舌质紫暗或有瘀斑,脉细涩或结代。

5. Inactivation of heart yang

Palpitation, dizziness, cold body and limbs, chest oppression and shortness of breath, edema and scanty urine, light-colored and bulgy tongue or with purplish appearance, thin and white tongue fur, deep and slow pulse or slow pulse with irregular intervals and slow regular intermittent pulse.

5. 心阳不振

心悸,眩晕,形寒肢冷,胸闷气短,浮肿尿少,舌质淡胖或有紫气,苔薄白,脉沉迟或结代。

[**Treatment**]

【治疗】

1. Body acupuncture

Prescription: Xinshu (BL 15), Jueyinshu (BL 14), Tanzhong (CV 17), Juque (CV 14), Neiguan (PC 6), Shenmen (HT 7) and Sanyinjiao (SP 6).

Modification: For asthenia of the heart and gallbladder, Yanglingquan (GB 34) and Daling (PC 7) are added; for phlegm-fire disturbing the heart, Fenglong (ST 40) and Taiyuan (LU 9) are added; for insufficiency of heart blood, Zusanli (ST 36) and Xuehai (SP 10) are added; for stagnation of blood in the collaterals, Geshu (BL 17) and Ximen (PC 4) are added; for inactivation of heart yang, Qihai (CV 6), Guanyuan (CV 4) and Shenshu (BL 23) are added; for dizziness, Baihui (GV 20) and Fengchi (GB 20) are added; for syncope, Shuigou (GV 26) and Suliao (GV 25) are added.

Performance: The needling techniques are selected according to the manifestations of syndromes. Tanzhong (CV 17) is needled 1 cun horizontally toward the root of the left breast to direct the sensation of needling to the

1. 体针疗法

处方:心俞,厥阴俞,膻中,巨阙,内关,神门,三阴交。

随证配穴:心胆虚怯,加阳陵泉、大陵;痰火扰心,加丰隆、太渊;心血不足,加足三里、血海;瘀血阻络,加膈俞、郄门;心阳不振,加气海、关元、肾俞;头晕目眩者,加百会、风池;晕厥者,加水沟、素髎。

操作:根据证候虚实施行补泻。膻中穴向左乳根方向沿皮刺入1寸,使针感放散到心前区,再用强刺激捻转行

precordial region with strong stimulation. Back-Shu acupoints and Qihai (CV 6), Guanyuan (CV 4) and Zusanli (ST 36) can be moxibusted after needling. For mild cases, the needling is done once a day or once every other day. For severe cases, the retention of needles can be prolonged and manipulated once 3 - 5 minutes, once or twice a day.

针。背俞穴及气海、关元、足三里穴等均可加用灸法。轻者,每日或隔日 1 次;重者适当延长留针时间,每隔 3～5 分钟行针 1 次,每日 1～2 次。

2. Ear acupuncture

2. 耳针疗法

Prescription: Heart (CO_{15}), Subcortex (AT_4), Sympathetic Nerve (AH_{6a}), Adrenal Gland (TG_{2p}) and Ear Shenmen (TF_4).

处方：心,皮质下,交感,肾上腺,神门。

Performance: Each time 2 - 3 acupoints are selected and needled with filiform needles and moderate and strong stimulation. The needles are retained for 30 - 60 minutes.

操作：每次选用 2～3 穴,毫针用中强刺激,留针 30～60 分钟。

5. 3. 2　Coronary heart disease

二、冠心病

[**Introduction**]

Coronary heart disease is a kind of heart disease due to myocardial ischemia and hypoxia resulting from coronary atherosclerosis. The clinical manifestations are angina pectoris, myocardiac infarction, arrhythmia, heart failure and cardiectasis. The electrocardiogram may indicate myocardial ischemia or corresponding changes. Coronary heart disease is one of the commonly encountered heart vessel diseases among the middle aged and old people. It is similar to chest obstructive syndrome, angina pectoris and precordial pain in TCM. The occurrence of coronary heart disease is usually related to aging, weakness, improper diet and emotional factors that often lead to inactivation of chest yang, stagnation of cold and phlegm in the collaterals as well as qi stagnation and blood stasis.

【概述】

冠心病,全称为冠状动脉粥样硬化性心脏病,是指冠状动脉粥样硬化使血管腔阻塞导致心肌缺血缺氧而引起的心脏病变。临床表现以心绞痛、心肌梗死、心律不齐、心力衰竭和心脏扩大等为主,心电图可有心肌缺血型或相应的改变。是中、老年最常见的心血管疾病之一。本病相当于中医"胸痹"、"真心痛"、"厥心痛"等病证。其发生与年老、体虚、饮食、七情等密切相关,导致胸阳不振,阴寒与痰浊痹阻脉络,气滞血瘀而发病。

[**Syndrome differentiation**]

【辨证】

1. Cold coagulation in the heart vessels

1. 寒凝心脉

Attack of angina pectoris due to cold, pain in the

心痛每因受寒而突发,心

heart radiating to the back, cold sensation in the body and aversion to cold, cold sweating, palpitation and shortness of breath, light-colored tongue with thin and white fur, taut and tense pulse.

痛彻背,形寒怕冷,出冷汗,心悸气短,舌淡苔薄白,脉弦紧。

2. Obstruction of phlegm

Pain and oppression in the chest, heaviness of limbs, shortness of breath and dyspnea, obesity, profuse phlegm, light-colored tongue with thick, white and greasy fur, taut and slippery pulse.

2. 痰浊痹阻

胸中憋闷而痛,肢体沉重,气短喘促,形体肥胖,痰多,舌淡苔厚白腻,脉弦滑。

3. Stagnation of blood stasis in the collaterals

Fixed stabbing pain in the chest, aggravation of pain in the night, chest oppression and shortness of breath, palpitation, purplish tongue or tongue with ecchymoses, thin and unsmooth pulse.

3. 瘀血阻络

心胸刺痛,痛有定处,入夜更甚,胸闷气短,心悸不宁,舌质紫暗或有瘀斑,脉细涩。

4. Asthenia of both the heart and spleen

Oppression and dull pain in the chest, dizziness, amnesia and insomnia, poor appetite, lassitude, lusterless complexion, light-colored tongue with thin and white fur, thin and weak pulse or slow pulse with irregular intervals and slow regular intermittent pulse.

4. 心脾两虚

心胸憋闷或心胸隐痛,头昏目眩,健忘失眠,纳谷不香,倦怠乏力,面色无华,舌淡苔薄白,脉细弱或结代。

5. Asthenia of heart and kidney yang

Oppression in the chest, palpitation and shortness of breath, spontaneous sweating, scanty urine and edema, light-colored tongue with thin and white fur, weak and thin pulse or slow pulse with irregular intervals and slow regular intermittent pulse.

5. 心肾阳虚

心胸憋闷,心悸气短,自汗,尿少浮肿,舌淡苔薄白,脉虚细或结代。

[Treatment]

1. Body acupuncture

Prescription: Xinshu (BL 15), Juque (CV 14), Tanzhong (CV 17), Neiguan (PC 6) and Ximen (PC 4).

Modification: For coagulation of cold in the heart vessels, Guanyuan (CV 4) and Qihai (CV 6) are added; for obstruction by phlegm and turbid substance, Fenglong (ST 40) and Taiyuan (LU 9) are added; for retention of

【治疗】

1. 体针疗法

处方:心俞,巨阙,膻中,内关,郄门。

随证配穴:寒凝心脉,加关元、气海;痰浊痹阻,加丰隆、太渊;瘀血阻络,加膈俞、血海;心脾两虚,加脾俞、三阴

blood stasis in the collaterals, Geshu (BL 17) and Xuehai (SP 10) are added; for asthenia of the heart and spleen, Pishu (BL 20) and Sanyinjiao (SP 6) are added; for asthenia of heart and kidney yang, Shenshu (BL 23) and Zusanli (ST 36) are added; for cold sensation in the body, aversion to cold and cold limbs, Shenque (CV 8) is added; for susceptibility to fright, Shenmen (HT 7) is added; for scanty urine and edema, Yinlingquan (SP 9) is added.

交;心肾阳虚,加肾俞、足三里;形寒怕冷,四肢不温者,加神阙;惊恐不安者,加神门;尿少浮肿者,加阴陵泉。

Performance: Juque (CV 14) is needled obliquely downward 0.5 - 1 cun. Tanzhong (CV 17) is needled 1 cun obliquely toward the left breast root. The needles are retained for 30 minutes and manipulated at intervals. For severe cases, the retention of needles may be prolonged for one or several hours. Back-Shu, Front-Mu acupoints and Qihai (CV 6), Guanyuan (CV 4), Shenque (CV 8) and Zusanli (ST 36) can be moxibusted after needling.

操作:巨阙向下斜刺0.5~1寸。膻中向左乳根方向斜刺1寸左右。留针30分钟,间歇行针。病情严重者适当延长留针时间达1至数小时。俞、募穴及气海、关元、神阙、足三里等穴针灸并用。

2. Ear acupuncture

Prescription: Heart (CO_{15}), Kidney (CO_{10}), Spleen (CO_{13}), Sympathetic (AH_{6a}), Endocrine (CO_{18}), Subcortical (AT_4) and Ear Shenmen (TF_4).

Performance: Each time 3 - 5 acupoints are selected. In the stage of attack, filiform needles are used with strong stimulation and retained for 30 - 60 minutes. The needles are manipulated once every 5 - 10 minutes. In the remission stage, filiform needles are used with mild stimulation, retained for 30 minutes and manipulated once every 10 minutes. Or Wangbuliuxingzi (Semen Vaccariae) is used for ear pressure.

2. 耳针

处方:心,肾,脾,交感,内分泌,皮质下,神门。

操作:每次选用3~5穴,发作期毫针用强刺激,留针30~60分钟,每隔5~10分钟行针1次;缓解期毫针用弱刺激,留针30分钟,每隔10分钟行针1次。或用王不留行籽压耳法。

5.3.3 Hypertension

[Introduction]

Hypertension is a series of clinical symptoms marked by increase of blood pressure in the arteries of body circulation. According to the criteria suggested by WHO in

三、高血压病

【概述】

高血压病是以体循环动脉压增高为主的临床症候群。根据1996年世界卫生组织

1996, adults with systolic pressure ≥ 140 mmHg (18.72 kPa) and/or diastolic pressure ≥ 90 mmHg (12.3 kPa) can be diagnosed with hypertension (result of three times of test done not continually in one day). Hypertension should be differentiated from secondary hypertension (symptomatic hypertension). This disease is similar to dizziness and headache in TCM. It is usually caused by emotional factors, constitutional defects, diet and overstrain that lead to imbalance of yin and yang in the liver, spleen and kidney, eventually resulting in hyperactivity of liver fire, or phlegm disturbing the upper, or frequent asthenia of kidney yin and failing of yin to control yang. It may be caused by consumption of yin involving yang and asthenia of both yin and yang in prolonged disease.

(WHO)建议的血压判别标准，成年人血压收缩压≥140 mmHg(18.72 kPa)和/或舒张压≥90 mmHg (12.3 kPa)，就可诊断为高血压(非同一日连续测量 3 次以上结果)。本病须与继发性高血压(症状性高血压)相区别。本病相当于中医的“眩晕”、“头痛”等病症。主要由情志、禀赋、饮食、劳倦等多种因素，导致肝、脾、肾三脏阴阳失衡，致使肝火亢盛，或痰浊上扰，或肾阴素亏，阴不制阳而引起；病久阴损及阳，可致阴阳两虚之候。

[**Syndrome differentiation**]

【辨证】

1. Hyperactivity of liver fire

Headache and dizziness, susceptibility to restlessness and rage, flushed cheeks and redness of eyes, bitter taste in the mouth and dry throat, constipation and brown urine, red tongue and yellow fur, taut and rapid pulse.

1. 肝火亢盛

头痛眩晕，急躁易怒，面红目赤，口苦咽干，便秘尿赤，舌红苔黄，脉弦数。

2. Phlegm disturbing the upper

Headache and dizziness, distension and heaviness of head, fullness and oppression in the chest and epigastrium, anorexia and lassitude, white and greasy tongue fur, taut and slippery pulse.

2. 痰浊上扰

头痛眩晕，头胀重，胸脘痞闷，纳呆疲乏，舌苔白腻，脉弦滑。

3. Yin asthenia and yang hyperactivity

Dizziness, headache, tinnitus, top-heaviness, dysphoria and insomnia, aching and weakness of loins and knees, numbness of limbs or tremor of hands and feet, red tongue with scanty fur and thin and taut pulse.

3. 阴虚阳亢

头晕目眩，头痛，耳鸣，头重脚轻，心烦失眠，腰膝酸软，肢麻或手足颤抖，舌质偏红，苔少，脉细弦。

4. Asthenia of yin and yang

Dizziness, pale complexion, cold limbs and aching of

4. 阴阳两虚

头目昏花，面色皖白，肢

loins, frequent urination in the night, or vexation, thirst, flushed cheeks, mirror-like tongue with light-red color, deep and thin pulse.

冷腰酸,夜尿频数,或虚烦、口渴、颧红,舌质光而淡红,脉沉细。

[**Treatment**]

【治疗】

1. Body acupuncture

1. 体针疗法

Prescription: Fengchi (GB 20), Quchi (LI 11), Hegu (LI 4), Xuehai (SP 10), Fenglong (ST 40) and Taichong (LR 3).

处方:风池,曲池,合谷,血海,丰隆,太冲。

Modification: For hyperactivity of liver yang, Xingjian (LR 2) and Baihui (GV 20) are added; for phlegm-fire disturbing the upper; Fenglong (ST 40) and Yinlingquan (SP 9) are added; for yin asthenia and yang hyperactivity, Ganshu (BL 18), Shenshu (BL 23), Sanyinjiao (SP 6) and Taixi (KI 3) are added; for asthenia of both yin and yang, Shenshu (BL 23), Guanyuan (CV 4), Zusanli (ST 36) and Sanyinjiao (SP 6) are added; for insomnia and dysphoria, Shenmen (HT 7) is added; for constipation, Zhigou (TE 6) is added; for oppression and fullness in the chest and epigastrium, Neiguan (PC 6) and Zusanli (ST 36) are added; for numbness of limbs, Yanglingquan (GB 34) is added.

随证配穴:肝阳上亢,加行间、百会;痰火上扰,加丰隆、阴陵泉;阴虚阳亢,加肝俞、肾俞、三阴交、太溪;阴阳两虚,加肾俞、关元、足三里、三阴交;失眠烦躁者,加神门;便秘者,加支沟;胸脘痞闷者,加内关、足三里;肢麻者可配阳陵泉。

Performance: The needling techniques are selected according to the manifestations of syndromes. For asthenia of both yin and yang, moxibustion can be used or electropuncture may be resorted to for supplementary purpose.

操作:根据证候虚实施行补泻手法。阴阳两虚者,可适当加灸。并可配合使用电针。

2. Ear acupuncture

2. 耳针疗法

Prescription: Ear Shenmen (TF_4), Upper Fossa (TF_1), Liver (CO_{12}), Kidney (CO_{10}), Tubercule (HX_8), Adrenal Gland (TG_{2p}), Sympathetic (AH_{6a}) and Subcortical (AT_4).

处方:神门,角窝上,肝,肾,结节,肾上腺,交感,皮质下。

Performance: Each time 3 - 5 acupoints can be selected and needled with filiform needles with moderate and strong stimulation. The needles are retained for 30 minutes and manipulated once every 5 - 10 minutes, once

操作:每次选用 3~5 穴,毫针用中强刺激,留针 30 分钟,每隔 5~10 分钟行针 1 次,每日或隔日 1 次。或用王不

a day or once every other day. Or Wangbuliuxingzi (Semen Vaccariae) is used for ear pressure. Or three-edged needle is used for bloodletting on the tip of the ear or back of the ear, once every other day.

留行籽压耳法。亦可用三棱针在耳尖、耳背沟点刺放血，隔日1次。

5.4 Diseases of digestive system

第四节 消化系统疾病

5.4.1 Acute gastritis

[**Introduction**]

Acute gastritis is classified into simple, corrosive, infective and suppurative types of gastritis according to the pathogenic factors. Acute corrosive gastritis is caused by intake of corrosive agents and needs emergent treatment. Acute infective gastritis and suppurative gastritis are caused by general infection. The following discussion focuses on acute simple gastritis marked by pain and discomfort in the upper abdomen, reduced appetite or distension and belching as well as nausea and vomiting. This disease pertains to epigastralgia, vomiting and diarrhea in TCM. Acute gastritis is usually caused by exogenous pathogenic factors and improper diet that lead to dysfunction of the spleen and stomach, failure of gastric qi to descend and upward adverse flow of turbid qi.

[**Syndrome differentiation**]

1. Cold-dampness attacking the middle energizer

Sudden onset of stomachache, severe pain, aversion to cold and preference for warmth, alleviation with warmth, nausea and vomiting, or diarrhea with thin fluid, or even watery diarrhea, or accompanied by aversion to cold and fever, light-colored tongue with white fur as well

一、急性胃炎

【概述】

急性胃炎的种类因致病因素的不同，分为单纯性、腐蚀性、感染性和化脓性四种。急性腐蚀性胃炎由于吞食腐蚀剂，病情险恶，必须及时抢救。急性感染性和化脓性胃炎多继发于全身感染。本节叙述的是急性单纯性胃炎，以上腹部疼痛不适、食欲减退或饱胀嗳气、恶心呕吐为主要临床表现。本病分属于中医的“胃脘痛”、“呕吐”、“泄泻”等病证。大多是由于外邪侵袭，饮食不慎等，导致脾胃纳运失常，胃失和降，浊气上逆所致。

【辨证】

1. 寒湿伤中

胃痛暴作，痛势较剧，畏寒喜暖，得热痛减，恶心呕吐，或泻下清稀，甚则水样便，或伴恶寒发热，舌淡苔白，脉弦紧。

as taut and tense pulse.

2. Retention of damp-heat in the middle energizer

Burning sensation, distension and pain in the epigastrium, aggravation after meal, or postcibal vomiting, foul breath, bitter taste and dryness in the mouth, urgent diarrhea or unsmooth diarrhea, burning sensation in the anus, red tongue with yellow and greasy fur as well as slippery and rapid pulse.

3. Retention of food

Distension and fullness in the epigastrium, unpressable pain, acid regurgitation, alleviation of pain after vomiting, unsmooth defecation with putrefaction and foul odor, thick and greasy tongue fur as well as taut and slippery pulse.

[**Treatment**]

1. Body acupuncture

Prescription: Zhongwan (CV 12), Neiguan (PC 6), Tianshu (ST 25) and Zusanli (ST 36).

Modification: For cold-dampness damaging the middle energizer, Hegu (LI 4) and Yinlingquan (SP 9) are added; for retention of damp-heat in the middle energizer, Hegu (LI 4) and Quchi (LI 11) are added; for retention of food, Neiting (ST 44) and Xuanji (CV 21) are added; for acute epigastralgia, Liangqiu (ST 34) is added.

Performance: Reducing needling technique is used. For the treatment of cold syndrome, moxibustion can be used. This treatment is given once or twice a day.

2. Ear acupuncture

Prescription: Stomach (CO_4), Large Intestine (CO_7), Small Intestine (CO_6) and Sympathetic Nerve (AH_{6a}).

Performance: The needles are manipulated at intervals with strong stimulation. Or Wangbuliuxingzi (Semen

2. 湿热中阻

胃脘灼热胀痛，得食加剧，或食入即吐，口气重浊，口苦而干，泻下急迫或泻下不爽，肛门灼热，舌红苔黄腻，脉滑数。

3. 食积停滞

胃脘胀满，疼痛拒按，嗳腐酸臭，吐后痛减，大便不爽、腐败臭秽，苔厚腻，脉弦滑。

【治疗】

1. 体针疗法

处方：中脘，内关，天枢，足三里。

随证配穴：寒湿伤中，加合谷、阴陵泉；湿热中阻，加合谷、曲池；食积停滞，加内庭、璇玑；胃脘急痛加梁丘。

操作：针用泻法。寒证加灸。每日1～2次。

2. 耳针疗法

处方：胃，大肠，小肠，交感。

操作：用捻转强刺激间歇运针，或用王不留行籽压

Vaccariae) is used for ear pressure.

耳法。

5. 4. 2 Chronic gastritis

二、慢性胃炎

［**Introduction**］

Chronic gastritis refers to various chronic inflammation of gastric mucus due to different pathogenic factors. According to the pathological changes, chronic gastritis can be divided into superficial, atrophic and hypertrophic types of gastritis. The clinical manifestations are atypical. The main symptoms are recurrent fullness, oppression and pain in the middle and upper abdomen as well as anorexia, dyspepsia, nausea, vomiting and belching. This disease is similar to epigastralgia and abdominal fullness in TCM. Chronic gastritis is usually caused by emotional upsets, improper diet, overstrain and weakness due to prolonged disease that lead to depression of liver and qi stagnation, asthenia-cold in middle energizer and insufficiency of stomach yin; or by involvement of the collaterals in prolonged disease and stagnation of blood in the collaterals.

【概述】

慢性胃炎是指由于不同病因引起的各种慢性胃粘膜炎性病变，根据其病理改变，分为浅表性、萎缩性和肥厚性三种。临床表现一般不典型，缺乏明显的特点，主要症状有长期反复发作的中上腹部饱闷感、疼痛，食欲不振，消化不良，恶心，呕吐，嗳气等。本病相当于中医的“胃脘痛”、“痞满”等病证，多由情志不畅，饮食失调，劳倦过度，久病体弱，导致肝郁气滞、中焦虚寒、胃阴不足等而发病；病久入络，则呈现血络瘀阻。

［**Syndrome differentiation**］

1. Liver depression and qi stagnation

Epigastralgia involving the rib-sides, migratory pain, frequent belching and sighing, red tongue with thin and yellow fur as well as taut and rapid pulse.

2. Asthenia-cold in the spleen and stomach

Dull stomachache, preference for warmth and pressure, emaciation and spiritual lassitude, lusterless complexion, loose stool, aversion to cold and cold limbs, light-colored and bulgy tongue with thin, white and slippery fur as well as thin and weak pulse.

3. Insufficiency of stomach yin

Irregular pain in the stomach, heartburn like hunger, hunger without appetite, dry mouth with desire to drink,

【辨证】

1. 肝郁气滞

胃脘疼痛连及两胁，痛无定处，嗳气频作，善太息，舌红苔薄黄，脉弦数。

2. 脾胃虚寒

胃痛隐隐，喜暖喜按，形瘦神疲，面色少华，大便稀溏，畏寒肢冷，舌淡形胖，苔薄白而滑，脉细弱无力。

3. 胃阴不足

胃痛无定时，嘈杂如饥，饥不欲食，口干思饮，舌红少

red tongue with scanty fur, taut and thin or thin and rapid pulse.

苔，脉弦细或细数。

4. Stagnation of blood in the collaterals

4. 血络瘀阻

Stabbing epigastralgia with fixed and unpressable pain, occasional hematemesis or hematochezia, purplish tongue or with ecchymoses and unsmooth pulse.

胃脘刺痛，痛处固定且拒按，时有呕血或便血，质紫暗或见瘀斑，脉涩不利。

[**Treatment**]

【治疗】

1. Body acupuncture

1. 体针疗法

Prescription: Zhongwan (CV 12), Neiguan (PC 6), Gongsun (SP 4), Liangmen (ST 21) and Zusanli (ST 36).

处方：中脘，内关，公孙，梁门，足三里。

Modification: For liver qi invading the stomach, Taichong (LR 3), Qimen (LR 14) and Ganshu (BL 18) are added; for asthenia-cold in the spleen and stomach, Pishu (BL 20) and Weishu (BL 21) are added; for insufficiency of stomach yin, Taixi (KI 3) and Sanyinjiao (SP 6) are added; for stagnation of blood in the collaterals, Xuehai (SP 10) and Geshu (BL 17) are added; for stomach heat, Neiting (ST 44) is added; for fullness and distension in the epigastrium and abdomen, Zhangmen (LR 13), Burong (ST 19) and Pishu (BL 20) are added.

随证配穴：肝气犯胃，加太冲、期门、肝俞；脾胃虚寒，加脾俞、胃俞；胃阴不足，加太溪、三阴交；血络瘀阻，加血海、膈俞；胃热者，加内庭；脘腹胀满者，加章门、不容、脾俞。

Performance: For liver qi invading the stomach and stagnation of blood in the collaterals, mild reducing and reinforcing needling techniques or reducing needling technique can be used; for asthenia-cold in the spleen and stomach and insufficiency of stomach yin, reinforcing needling technique can be used. For the treatment of asthenia-cold syndrome, moxibustion can be used in addition.

操作：肝气犯胃和血络瘀阻证可用平补平泻或泻法；脾胃虚寒和胃阴不足证可用补法，虚寒证加灸。

2. Ear acupuncture

2. 耳针疗法

Prescription: Stomach (CO_4), Spleen (CO_{13}), Liver (CO_{12}), Triple Energizer (CO_{17}), Sympathetic (AH_{6a}), Ear Shenmen (TF_4) and Subcortical (AT_4).

处方：胃，脾，肝，三焦，交感，神门，皮质下。

Performance: Each time 2 - 3 acupoints are selected.

操作：每次选2～3穴，留

The needles are retained for 30 minutes and manipulated at intervals. Or electropuncture may be used. Or Wangbuliuxingzi (Semen Vaccariae) can be used for ear pressure. Two ears are needled in alternation.

针 30 分钟,间歇捻转或用电针;或用王不留行籽压耳法。两耳交替使用。

5.4.3 Gastric and duodenal ulcer

三、胃、十二指肠溃疡

[Introduction]

Gastric and duodenal ulcer is clinically marked by periodic and rhythmic attack and abdominal pain, often accompanied by belching, acid regurgitation, nausea and vomiting. This disease usually occurs among youth and people prime in life, especially among the male. It pertains to the conceptions of epigastralgia, acid regurgitation, heartburn, hematemesis and hematochezia in TCM. It is usually caused by improper diet, emotional changes and overstrain due to dysfunction of the liver in dispersion and conveyance and impairment of the spleen and stomach.

【概述】

胃、十二指肠溃疡是指胃与十二指肠部位的慢性溃疡。临床以周期性发作、节律性上腹部疼痛为特征,常伴有嗳气泛酸,恶心呕吐等症。以青壮年和男性居多。根据其临床症状分属于中医学的"胃脘痛"、"吞酸"、"嘈杂"、"呕血"、"便血"等范畴。主要由饮食、情志、劳倦所伤,导致肝失疏泄、脾胃损伤而发病。

[Syndrome differentiation]

【辨证】

1. Disharmony between the liver and stomach

Epigastralgia involving the rib-sides, belching and acid regurgitation, even nausea and vomiting, aggravation after emotional changes, yellow and thin tongue fur and taut pulse.

1. 肝胃不和

胃脘胀痛连及两胁,嗳气吐酸,甚至恶心呕吐,每因情绪波动而加重,苔薄黄,脉弦。

2. Retention of heat in the stomach and intestines

Burning sensation in the stomach, dryness and bitter taste in the mouth, foul breath, yellow urine and retention of dry feces, red tongue with yellow fur and rapid pulse.

2. 胃肠积热

胃中灼热,口干而苦,口臭,尿黄便结,舌红苔黄,脉数。

3. Qi stagnation and blood stasis

Stabbing and unpressable epigastralgia, aggravation after meal, or hematemesis, hematochezia, purplish tongue with ecchymoses and unsmooth pulse.

3. 气滞血瘀

胃脘刺痛,拒按,食则痛剧,或见呕血,便血,舌紫暗有瘀点,脉涩。

4. Asthenia-cold in the spleen and stomach

Dull epigastralgia, preference for warmth and pressure, regurgitation of clear fluid, spiritual lassitude, lusterless complexion, loose stool, light-colored tongue with white fur and thin and weak pulse.

[Treatment]

1. Body acupuncture

Prescription: Pishu (BL 20), Weishu (BL 21), Zhongwan (CV 12), Neiguan (PC 6) and Zusanli (ST 36).

Modification: For liver qi invading the stomach, Taichong (LR 3) and Qimen (LR 14) are added; for retention of heat in the stomach and intestines, Neiting (ST 44) and Qiangu (SI 2) are added; for qi stagnation and blood stasis, Hegu (LI 4) and Geshu (BL 17) are added; for asthenia-cold in the spleen and stomach, Zhangmen (LR 13) and Qihai (CV 6) are added; for severe stomachache, Liangqiu (ST 34) is added; for constipation and loose stool, Tianshu (ST 25) and Xiajuxu (ST 39) are added; for hematemesis or hematochezia, Zhongwan (CV 12) is deleted while Xuehai (SP 10) and Geshu (BL 17) are added.

Performance: The acupoints on the abdomen should not be vertically needled too deeply. Qimen (LR 14) should be needled obliquely medial or lateral along the costal space with moderate stimulation. Liangqiu (ST 34) is needled with strong stimulation and reducing needling technique. For asthenia-cold in the spleen and stomach, Back-Shu acupoints and Front-Mu acupoints as well as Qihai (CV 6) and Zusanli (ST 36) are needled with the addition of moxibustion and cupping.

2. Ear acupuncture

Prescription: Stomach (CO_4), Duodenum (CO_5), Spleen (CO_{13}), Liver (CO_{12}), Triple Energizer (CO_{17}), Sympathetic Nerve (AH_{6a}), Ear Shenmen (TF_4) and

4. 脾胃虚寒

胃脘隐痛,喜温喜按,泛吐清水,神疲乏力,面色无华,大便溏薄,舌淡苔白,脉细无力。

【治疗】

1. 体针疗法

处方:脾俞,胃俞,中脘,内关,足三里。

随证配穴:肝气犯胃,加太冲、期门;胃肠积热,加内庭、前谷;气滞血瘀,加合谷、膈俞;脾胃虚寒,加章门、气海;胃疼剧烈者,加梁丘;便秘或便溏者,加天枢、下巨虚;呕血或便血者,去中脘,加血海、膈俞。

操作:腹部腧穴应注意掌握针刺的深度,不宜直刺过深,期门宜沿肋间隙向内、外侧斜刺,刺激也不宜过强;梁丘应施强刺激泻法;脾胃虚寒者,俞、募穴和气海、足三里可加用灸法和拔罐。

2. 耳针疗法

处方:胃,十二指肠,脾,肝,三焦,交感,神门,皮质下。

Subcortex (AT_4).

Performance: Each time 3 - 5 acupoints are selected and needled with routine techniques or embedded with needles. Wangbuliuxingzi (Semen Vaccariae) is used for ear pressure. The two ears are treated in alternation.

操作：每次选3～5穴，常规针刺或施行埋针、王不留行籽压耳法。两耳交替。

5.4.4 Gastroptosis

［Introduction］

Gastroptosis refers to the condition that the lesser curvature notch of the stomach is lower than the iliac crest level in standing position due to looseness of the ligament supporting the stomach and decline of the gastrotonia. The clinical manifestations are dragging distension in the abdomen and stomachache which are immediately alleviated when the patient lies flat. This problem is usually seen among women with emaciation, narrow thorax and looseness of abdominal muscles. This disease is usually caused by improper diet, overstrain and lack of caring after illness that lead to hypofunction of the spleen and stomach as well as sinking of gastrosplenic qi. Gastroptosis is usually complicated by retention of dampness and phlegm due to abnormal activities of the spleen and stomach in transformation and transportation, leading to the syndrome of mixture of asthenia and sthenia as well as the syndrome of root asthenia and branch sthenia.

四、胃下垂

【概述】

胃下垂是指胃支持韧带松弛和胃张力减退，以致站立时胃小弯切迹低于髂嵴水平线以下的一种疾病。临床以食后腹部坠胀、胃痛，平卧后症状旋即减轻为主要特征。多见于形体瘦弱、胸廓狭长、腹肌松弛的女性。胃下垂相当于中医的“胃下”、“胃缓”等病证。本病多因饮食、劳倦、病后失调，以致中焦脾胃虚弱、中虚气陷所致。由于脾胃运化失常，留湿停饮，往往兼挟水湿、痰饮，成为虚实夹杂、本虚标实之证。

［Syndrome differentiation］

1. Disharmony between liver and stomach

Distending pain in the epigastrium involving the ribsides, aggravation after meal, frequent belching, vomiting of acid fluid, dysphoria and susceptibility to rage, red tongue with thin and yellow fur, taut and rapid pulse.

2. Spleen asthenia and qi sinking

Fullness and mass in the epigastrium and abdomen, dragging and distending sensation in the abdomen,

【辨证】

1. 肝胃不和

胃脘胀痛，连及两胁，食后尤甚，嗳气频作，呕吐酸水，心烦易怒，舌红苔薄黄，脉弦数。

2. 脾虚气陷

脘腹痞满，坠胀不适，食后尤甚，平卧减轻，或泛吐清

aggravation after meal, alleviation in flat supination, or regurgitation of clear fluid, phlegm and saliva, dizziness and lassitude, loose stool, light-colored tongue with white fur, soft and slow pulse.

水痰涎,头晕乏力,大便溏薄,舌淡苔白,脉濡缓。

3. Asthenia of both qi and yin

Dragging and distending sensation in the epigastrium and abdomen, aggravation after meal, bitter taste and dryness in the mouth, or dry vomiting and hiccup, hunger without appetite, red tongue with scanty fur and thin and rapid pulse.

3. 气阴两虚

脘腹坠胀,食后为甚,口苦口干,或干呕呃逆,形瘦神疲,饥不欲食,舌红少苔,脉细数无力。

[Treatment]

1. Body acupuncture

Prescription: (1) Qihai (CV 6), Baihui (GV 20), Pishu (BL 20), Weishu (BL 21), Zhongwan (CV 12) and Zusanli (ST 36).

(2) Tiwei located 4 cun lateral to Zhongwan (CV 12) or Weishang located 4 cun below Zhongwan (CV 12) penetrating Tianshu (ST 25).

These two groups of acupoints are used in alternation.

Modification: For disharmony between the liver and stomach, Qimen (LR 14), Taichong (LR 3) and Ganshu (BL 18) are added; for asthenia of both qi and yin, Sanyinjiao (SP 6) and Neiguan (PC 6) are added; for fluid gurgling in the stomach, Shuifen (CV 9) and Yinlingquan (SP 9) are added; for stomachache, Liangmen (ST 21) is added; for abdominal distension and diarrhea, Tianshu (ST 25) and Xiajuxu (ST 39) are added; for constipation, Zhigou (TE 6) and Daheng (SP 15) are added.

Performance: The first group of acupoints can be needled and moxibusted. When needling Tiwei and Weishang for the penetration of Tianshu (ST 25), reinforcing needling technique by twirling and rotating the needle is used. When needling sensation is felt, the needle is

【治疗】

1. 体针疗法

处方:(1) 气海,百会,脾俞,胃俞,中脘,足三里。

(2) 提胃(中脘旁开 4 寸)或胃上(下脘旁开 4 寸)透天枢。

两组腧穴交替使用。

随证配穴:肝胃不和,加期门、太冲、肝俞;气阴两虚,加三阴交、内关;胃中有振水声者,加水分、阴陵泉;胃痛加梁门;腹胀、腹泻加天枢、下巨虚;便秘加支沟、大横。

操作:第一组腧穴可针灸并用。提胃、胃上二穴透刺天枢穴时,行捻转补法,得气后,将针向单一方向捻搓,待针下有紧涩感为止,以胃部有升提

rotated uni-directionally till tense and astringent sensation being felt beneath the needle and stomach-lifting sensation being felt. Cautions must be taken not to puncture into the abdominal cavity lest the viscera be impaired.

感为佳。注意不可刺入腹内，以防刺穿脏器。

2. Electro-acupuncture

Prescription: The same as that for needling.

Performance: Electro-acupuncture is used with routine operation and intermittent or sparse and dense wave for 20 minutes of strong stimulation till appearance of tic in the abdominal muscles. This treatment is given once a day and 15－20 times make up one course of treatment.

2. 电针疗法

处方：同针刺处方、配穴。

操作：常规操作，用断续波或疏密波中强刺激 20 分钟，以腹肌出现抽动为佳。每日 1 次，15 ～ 20 次为 1 个疗程。

5.4.5 Acute and chronic enteritis

五、急、慢性肠炎

[**Introduction**]

Acute and chronic enteritis refers to acute or chronic inflammation of intestinal wall mucus due to various factors. The usual manifestations are abdominal pain, frequent defecation, loose stool or watery stool. This disease is similar to the conception of diarrhea in TCM.

Acute enteritis is usually caused by bacteria, virus, fungus and chemical toxin in improper foods or intestinal parasites. The most commonly seen are viral enteritis and bacterial food poisoning. The clinical symptoms are acute diarrhea, abdominal pain and vomiting, accompanied by aversion to cold and fever, etc. The major causes of acute enteritis are exogenous pathogenic factors and improper foods that lead to dysfunction of the spleen in transformation and transportation due to encumbrance by dampness.

Chronic enteritis refers to a series of symptoms of intestinal chronic inflammation due to various factors, pertaining to chronic inflammation of intestinal mucus and

【概述】

急、慢性肠炎是指各种原因引起的急性或慢性肠壁粘膜的炎症性改变。以腹痛、大便次数增多、粪质稀薄甚至成水样便为主要特征。相当于中医的“泄泻”病症。

急性肠炎多是由不洁净食物中的细菌、病毒、霉菌、化学毒素或肠道寄生虫引起的急性肠道感染性炎症，其中以病毒性肠炎和细菌性食物中毒最为常见。临床以急性腹泻、腹痛、呕吐，多伴有恶寒发热等全身症状。外感时邪和饮食不慎是引起本病的两大原因，致使脾为湿困，运化失健而发生泄泻。

慢性肠炎是一个多因素的肠道慢性炎性症候群，属于非特异性细菌感染引起的肠

disturbance of intestinal absorption due to non-specific bacterial infection. The clinical symptoms are abdominal pain, diarrhea, abdominal distension, borborygmus, loose stool or stool with mucus and pus-blood, or alternation of diarrhea and constipation, slow progression of pathological conditions, recurrence and difficulty to heal. Chronic enteritis is usually caused by lingering diarrhea due to exogenous factors, improper diet and overstrain that lead to hypofunction of the spleen and stomach; or by mental upsets, failure of the liver to disperse and convey as well as invasion of liver qi into the spleen. Prolonged diarrhea will lead to involvement of the kidney in spleen disease and insufficiency of kidney yang, consequently resulting in failure in transportation and transformation.

壁粘膜慢性炎性改变和肠道吸收功能紊乱。临床表现为腹痛腹泻,腹胀肠鸣,大便稀薄或间夹粘液和脓血,或腹泻与便秘相交替,病变过程缓慢,反复发作,缠绵难愈。多因外感泄泻迁延日久、饮食劳倦内伤,致使脾胃虚弱;或情志不调,肝失疏泄,横逆犯脾。久泄不已,脾病及肾,肾阳不足,更致运化失司。

[**Syndrome differentiation**]

【辨证】

1. Acute enteritis

1. 急性肠炎

Cold-dampness type: Abdominal pain, borborygmus, watery stool without odor, heaviness of head and body, or accompanied by aversion to cold, fever, white and greasy tongue fur as well as soft and slow pulse.

(1) 寒湿型:腹痛肠鸣,便如水样,无臭味,头重身重,或伴恶寒发热,苔白腻,脉濡缓。

Damp-heat type: Abdominal pain, diarrhea, urgent diarrhea with brown color or with pus-blood and foul odor, burning sensation in the anus, fever, thirst, scanty and brown urine, or accompanied by vomiting and nausea, red tongue with yellow and greasy fur as well as slippery and rapid pulse.

(2) 湿热型:腹痛腹泻,泻下急迫,便色黄褐,或间夹脓血,气味秽臭,肛门灼热,烦热口渴,小便短赤,或兼呕恶,舌红苔黄腻,脉滑数。

Dyspepsia type: Diarrhea with the odor of putrid egg, alleviation of abdominal pain after diarrhea, undigested food in diarrhea, fullness and oppression in the chest and epigastrium, beltching and acid regurgitation, greasy tongue fur and slippery pulse.

(3) 伤食型:泻下粪便臭如败卵,泻后痛减,便中多夹不消化食物,脘腹痞闷,嗳腐酸臭,苔腻,脉滑。

2. Chronic enteritis

2. 慢性肠炎

Liver depression subjugating the spleen: Occurrence of diarrhea with abdominal pain following psychological

(1) 肝郁乘脾:每于精神刺激、情绪紧张时发生,腹痛

stimulation or nervousness, alleviation of pain after diarrhea, frequent flatus, accompanied by distension and oppression in the chest and rib-side, belching and poor appetite, light-red tongue with white fur and taut pulse.

即泻,泻后痛缓,矢气频作,伴胸胁胀闷,嗳气食少,舌淡红苔白,脉弦。

Hypofunction of the spleen and stomach: Loose stool, or occasional loose stool and diarrhea with undigested food, frequent defecation after slight intake of greasy food, no appetite, spiritual lassitude, light-colored tongue with white fur, soft, slow and weak pulse.

(2) 脾胃虚弱:大便溏薄,或时溏时泻,内夹不消化食物,稍进生冷油腻,便次即增,食欲不振,神疲,舌淡苔白,脉濡缓而弱。

Decline of kidney yang: Morning diarrhea, dull abdominal pain, diarrhea right after borborygmus, relief of pain after diarrhea, cold body and limbs, aching and weakness of loins and knees, light-colored tongue with white fur, deep, thin and weak pulse.

(3) 肾阳虚弱:每于黎明泄泻,腹痛隐隐,肠鸣即泄,泄后即安,形寒肢冷,腰膝酸软,舌淡苔白,脉沉细无力。

[**Treatment**]

【治疗】

1. Body acupuncture

1. 体针疗法

Prescription:

处方:

Acute enteritis: Shangjuxu (ST 37), Xiajuxu (ST 39), Liangmen (ST 21), Tianshu (ST 25) and Yinlingquan (SP 9).

(1) 急性肠炎:上巨虚,下巨虚,梁门,天枢,阴陵泉。

Chronic enteritis: Zhongwan (CV 12), Guanyuan (CV 4), Tianshu (ST 25) and Zusanli (ST 36).

(2) 慢性肠炎:中脘,关元,天枢,足三里。

Modification: In acute enteritis, for cold-dampness type, Shenque (CV 8) and Sanyinjiao (SP 6) are added; for damp-heat type, Quchi (LI 11), Dazhui (GV 14) and Neiting (ST 44) are added; for fever, Hegu (LI 4) and Quchi (LI 11) are added; for dyspepsia, Zhongwan (CV 12) and Gongsun (SP 4) are added. In chronic enteritis, for liver depression subjugating the spleen, Zhangmen (LR 13) and Taichong (LR 3) are added; for hypofunction of the spleen and stomach, Pishu (BL 20) and Weishu (BL 21) are added; for decline of fire in mingmen (gate of life), Mingmen (GV 4) and Shenshu (BL 23) are added; for prolonged diarrhea and prolapse of rectum, Baihui

随证配穴:急性肠炎之寒湿型,加神阙、三阴交;湿热型,加曲池、大椎、内庭;发热者,加合谷、曲池;伤食型,加中脘、公孙。慢性肠炎之肝郁乘脾,加章门、太冲;脾胃虚弱,加脾俞、胃俞;命门火衰加命门、肾俞;久泄脱肛加百会。

(GV 20) is added.

Performance: For acute diarrhea, filiform needles and reducing techniques are used. For chronic diarrhea, Zhangmen (LR 13) and Taichong (LR 3) are needled with mild reducing and reinforcing techniques or reducing technique, the rest acupoints are needled with reinforcing techniques. For predominance of cold and asthenia of qi and yang, the needling is followed by moxibustion and cupping.

操作：急性腹泻，用毫针泻法。慢性腹泻，除章门、太冲用平补平泻或泻法外，余均宜用补法。寒盛和气虚、阳虚者加灸和拔罐。

2. Ear acupnucture

Prescription: Large Intestine (CO_7), Small Intestine (CO_6), Spleen (CO_{13}), Stomach (CO_4), Liver (CO_{12}), Abdomen (AH_8), Sympathetic Nerve (AH_{6a}), Triple Energizer (CO_{17}) and Ear Shenmen (TF_4).

Performance: Each time 3 - 5 acupoints are selected and needled with routine procedure. For acute enteritis, strong stimulation in needling is required, once or twice a day; for chronic enteritis, moderate stimulation in needling is required, once a day or once every other day; or Wangbuliuxingzi (Semen Vaccariae) is used for ear pressure.

2. 耳针

处方：大肠，小肠，脾，胃，肝，腹，交感，三焦，神门。

操作：每次选 3～5 穴，常规操作。急性肠炎用强刺激，每日 1～2 次；慢性肠炎用中等刺激，每日或隔日 1 次；或用王不留行籽压耳法。

5.4.6 Biliary tract infection and cholelithiasis

［**Introduction**］

Biliary tract infection includes acute and chronic cholecystitis and cholangitis; cholelithiasis includes cholelithiasis, choledocholithiasis and calculus of intrahepatic duct. Biliary tract infection and cholelithiasis often exist simultaneously and are responsible for each other. Chronic cholecystitis usually occurs after cholelithiasis and is often the sequela of acute cholecystitis, clinically marked by pain in the upper or right upper abdomen. According to the clinical symptoms, biliary tract infection and cholelithiasis pertain to the conceptions of hypochondriac pain, jaundice

六、胆管系统感染和胆石症

【概述】

胆管系统感染包括急、慢性胆囊炎、胆管炎等；胆石症包括胆囊内、胆总管、肝内胆管结石等。两者常同时存在，互为因果，临床症状也相互联系。慢性胆囊炎多发生在胆石症的基础上，且常是急性胆囊炎的后遗症，临床上都有上腹及右上腹疼痛的症状表现。根据其临床症状分属于中医

in TCM. This problem is usually caused by exogenous pathogenic factors, emotional changes and improper diet that lead to interior accumulation of damp-heat and failure of the liver and gallbladder to disperse; or by prolonged accumulation of damp-heat that condenses bile into stone. The clinical manifestations are either of sthenia syndrome or of heat syndrome.

的"胁痛"、"黄疸"等病证。因外邪、情志、饮食所伤，致湿热内蕴，肝胆失疏；湿热日久不化，煎炼胆汁成石。临床多表现为实证、热证。

[**Syndrome differentiation**]

【辨证】

1. Stagnation of liver and gallbladder qi

Oppression and distension in the right upper abdomen, colic at intervals, migratory pain, mental depression, belching and sighing, dysphoria and susceptibility to rage, thin and yellow tongue fur, taut and rapid pulse.

1. 肝胆气滞

右上腹闷胀，间歇性绞痛，痛无定处，精神抑郁，嗳气叹息，心烦易怒，苔薄黄，脉弦数。

2. Damp-heat in the liver and gallbladder

Acute onset, fever, bitter taste in the mouth and dry throat, yellow coloration of eyes and body, yellow urine, constipation, red tongue with yellow and greasy (or dry) fur, taut and rapid pulse.

2. 肝胆湿热

起病急，发热，口苦咽干，目黄，身黄，小便发黄，大便秘结，舌红苔黄腻（或燥），脉弦数。

3. Accumulation of heat-toxin

Chills and fever, flushed cheeks and yellow coloration of body, restlessness, scanty and brown urine, constipation, even delirium and coma, cold limbs, deep-red or purplish tongue with yellow and dry or prickly fur, slippery and rapid or deep and latent pulse.

3. 热毒蕴结

寒战高热，面赤身黄，烦躁不安，小便短赤，大便秘结，甚或神昏谵语，四肢厥冷，舌红绛或紫暗，苔黄燥或生芒刺，脉滑数或沉伏。

[**Treatment**]

【治疗】

1. Body acupuncture

Prescription: Zhongwan (CV 12), Riyue (GB 24), Danshu (BL 19), Taichong (LR 3) and Dannang (EX-LE 6).

1. 体针疗法

处方：中脘，日月，胆俞，太冲，胆囊穴。

Modification: For stagnation of liver and gallbladder qi, Qimen (LR 14) and Yanglingquan (GB 34) are added; for damp-heat in the liver and gallbladder, Yinlingquan (SP 9) and Xiaxi (GB 43) are added; for accumulation of heat-toxin, Quchi (LI 11), Neiting (ST 44) and Xiaxi

随证配穴：肝胆气滞，加期门、阳陵泉；肝胆湿热，加阴陵泉、侠溪；热毒蕴结，加曲池、内庭、侠溪；高热者，加大椎、耳尖；胆绞痛者，加阳陵

(GB 43) are added; for high fever, Dazhui (GV 14) and Erjian (TE 2) are added; for colic of gallbladder, Yanglingquan (GB 34) and Hegu (LI 4) are added; for nausea and vomiting, Neiguan (PC 6) and Zusanli (ST 36) are added; for jaundice, Zhiyang (GV 9) and Zusanli (ST 36) are added; for constipation, Zhigou (TE 6) and Tianshu (ST 25) are added; for coma and prostration, Shuigou (GV 26), Baihui (GV 20), Neiguan (PC 6), Hegu (LI 4) and Zusanli (ST 36) are added.

泉、合谷；恶心呕吐者，加内关、足三里；黄疸者，加至阳、足三里；便秘者，加支沟、天枢；神昏虚脱，加水沟、百会、内关、合谷、足三里。

Performance: Riyue (GB 24) and Qimen (LR 14) are needled obliquely lateral along the costal space, vertical needling should be avoided. Zhongwan (CV 12) is needled obliquely downward to the right hypochondrium to enable the needling sensation radiate to the affected region. Vertical needling should not be too deep. Dazhui (GV 14) and Erjian (LI 2) are pricked for bloodletting. All the acupoints are needled with reducing techniques. At the same time electropuncture can be applied with continuous wave and high frequency for 40 - 60 minutes of strong stimulation.

操作：日月、期门不宜直刺，应沿肋间隙向外侧斜刺；中脘直刺不宜过深，最好向右胁下斜刺，使针感直达病所；大椎、耳尖行点刺出血。均施以泻法。同时亦可加用电针，以连续波、快频率，强刺激40～60分钟。

2. Ear acupuncture

Prescription: Liver (CO_{12}), Gallbladder (CO_{11}), Spleen (CO_{13}), Stomach (CO_4), Triple Energizer (CO_{17}), Duodenum (CO_5), Sympathetic Nerve (AH_{6a}), Ear Shenmen (TF_4), Erjian (LI 2) and Ermigen (R_2).

2. 耳针疗法

处方：肝，胆，脾，胃，三焦，十二指肠，交感，神门，耳尖，耳迷根。

Performance: Each time 3 - 5 acupoints are selected and needled with routine procedure. Strong stimulation is required for acute syndrome (bloodletting from the tip of ear), while moderate stimulation is required for chronic syndrome. Or Wangbuliuxingzi (Semen Vaccariae) is used for ear pressure.

操作：每次选3～5穴，常规操作，急性者宜用强刺激(耳尖点刺出血)，慢性者宜用中强刺激或施行王不留行籽压耳法。

5.4.7 Habitual constipation

七、习惯性便秘

[**Introduction**]

Habitual constipation is marked by unsmooth

【**概述**】

习惯性便秘是指排便艰

defecation, retention of dry feces and an interval of over 48 hours between the two defecations for over 48 hours with discomfort. It is caused either by frequent predominance of yang, partiality to pungent and rich foods and addiction to alcohol and smoking; or by mental upsets; or by interior damage due to overstrain and weakness due to senility; dysfunction of the lung, spleen, stomach and kidney as well as insufficiency of body fluid due to failure of the large intestine to transport after illness or non-restoration of qi and blood after labor.

涩不畅,粪质干燥硬结,排便间隔时间超过 48 小时以上,并有不适感的一种疾病。本病相当于中医的"便秘"、"大便难"、"阳结"、"阴结"、"脾约"等病证。是由于素体阳盛,嗜食辛辣厚味,烟酒过度;或情志不舒;或劳倦内伤,年老体弱,病后或产后气血未复,导致肺、脾胃、肾等脏腑功能失调,津液不足,大肠传导失司所致。

[Syndrome differentiation]

1. Sthenia-constipation

Distension and fullness in the epigastrium and abdomen, unpressable pain, dry feces like goat droppings, fever, flushed cheeks, thirst and foul breath, red tongue with yellow and dry fur, full, large and rapid pulse.

2. Asthenia-constipation

Softness of abdomen, desire to defecate but weakness in trial, lassitude after defecation, dizziness and palpitation, lusterless complexion or flushed cheeks, light-colored tongue with white fur, thin and weak pulse.

3. Cold-constipation

Constipation, cold pain in the abdomen, aversion to cold and preference for warmth, cold limbs, clear and profuse urine, light-colored tongue with white fur, deep and tense pulse.

【辨证】

1. 实秘

脘腹胀满,疼痛拒按,粪便干燥坚硬如羊矢,身热面赤,烦渴口臭,舌红苔黄燥,脉洪大而数。

2. 虚秘

腹软,临厕时虽有便意但常常努责乏力,便后疲乏,头晕心悸,面色无华或两颧泛红,舌淡苔白,脉细无力。

3. 寒秘

大便秘结,腹中冷痛,畏寒喜暖,四肢欠温,小便清长,舌淡苔白,脉沉紧。

[Treatment]

1. Body acupuncture

Prescription: Zhongwan (CV 12), Tianshu (ST 25), Zhigou (TE 6), Shangjuxu (ST 37) and Dachangshu (BL 25).

Modification: For sthenia-heat in the stomach and

【治疗】

1. 体针疗法

处方:中脘,天枢,支沟,上巨虚,大肠俞。

随证配穴:实秘之胃肠实

intestines in sthenia-constipation, Quchi (LI 11) and Neiting (ST 44) are added; for stagnation of the liver and spleen, Hegu (LI 4) and Taichong (LR 3) are added. For asthenia of spleen and lung qi in asthenia-constipation, Pishu (BL 20), Weishu (BL 21), Shenshu (BL 23), Qihai (CV 6) and Zusanli (ST 36) are added; for blood asthenia and yin consumption, Pishu (BL 20), Ganshu (BL 18), Sanyinjiao (SP 6), Taixi (KI 3) and Zhaohai (KI 6) are added; for cold constipation, Dazhong (KI 4) and Guanyuan (CV 4) are added.

热者,加曲池、内庭;肝脾气滞者,加合谷、太冲。虚秘之脾肺气虚者,加脾俞、胃俞、肾俞、气海、足三里;血虚阴亏者,加脾俞、肝俞、三阴交、太溪、照海。寒秘,加大钟、关元。

Performance: Reducing needling technique is used for treating sthenia-constipation, while reinforcing needling technique is used for treating asthenia-constipation. For the treatment of cold-constipation and asthenia-constipation, moxibustion can be used.

操作:实秘用泻法,虚秘用补法,寒秘、虚秘可加用灸法。

2. Ear acupuncture

Prescription: Large Intestine (CO_7), Rectum (HX_2), Lung (CO_{14}), Spleen (CO_{13}), Liver (CO_{12}), Kidney (CO_{10}), Triple Energizer (CO_{17}), Abdomen (AH_8), Sympathetic Nerve (AH_{6a}) and Subcortex (AT_4).

Performance: Each time 3 - 5 acupoints are selected and needled with routine procedure and strong stimulation. The needles are retained for 1 - 2 hours and manipulated twice or 3 times at intervals. Or Wangbuliuxingzi (Semen Vaccariae) is used for ear pressure.

2. 耳针

处方:大肠,直肠,肺,脾,肝,肾,三焦,腹,交感,皮质下。

操作:每次选 3~5 穴,常规操作,强刺激,留针 1~2 小时,间歇捻针 2~3 次;或用王不留行籽压耳法。

5.5 Diseases of blood system

第五节 血液系统疾病

5.5.1 Leukocytopenia

一、白细胞减少症

[**Introduction**]

Leukocytopenia means that the number of white cells in the peripheral blood is kept less than 4×10^9/L and

【概述】

白细胞减少症是指周围血液中白细胞计数持续低于 4

neutrophilic granulocyte percentage is normal or slightly reduced. There are no clinical manifestations or just mild fatigue and infection. This disease pertains to the conception of consumptive disease in TCM due to weakness in constitution, overstrain, lack of proper caring after illness, invasion of virus or improper use of drugs that lead to consumption of healthy qi, asthenia of the spleen and kidney, insufficiency of transformation and decline of nutritive qi, defensive qi, qi and blood.

$\times 10^9$/L,中性粒细胞百分数正常或稍减少。临床可无症状或有轻度乏力和感染等表现。本病属于中医"虚劳"的范畴,多因体质虚弱,劳倦内伤,病后失调,以及病毒侵袭或用药不当,致正气损伤,脾肾亏虚,生化无源,营卫气血衰少而发为本病。

[Syndrome differentiation]

【辨证】

1. Asthenia of the spleen and kidney

1. 脾肾亏虚

No appetite, lassitude, lusterless complexion, palpitation and insomnia, cold body and limbs, loose stool, light-colored tongue with thin fur, weak pulse.

食欲不振,倦怠乏力,面色无华,心悸失眠,形寒肢冷,大便溏薄,舌淡苔薄,脉弱。

2. Insufficiency of the liver and kidney

2. 肝肾不足

Dizziness, insomnia, amnesia, aching and weakness of loins and knees, low fever and night sweating, red tongue with scanty fur, thin and rapid pulse.

头晕目眩,失眠健忘,腰膝酸软,低热盗汗,舌红苔少,脉细数。

[Treatment]

【治疗】

1. Body acupuncture

1. 体针疗法

Prescription: Zusanli (ST 36), Sanyinjiao (SP 6), Xuehai (SP 10), Geshu (BL 17), Shenshu (BL 23) and Guanyuan (CV 4).

处方:足三里,三阴交,血海,膈俞,肾俞,关元。

Modification: For asthenia of the spleen and kidney, Dazhui (GV 14) and Pishu (BL 20) are added; for insufficiency of the liver and kidney, Taichong (LR 3) and Taixi (KI 3) are added; for insomnia, Shenmen (HT 7) is added.

随证配穴:脾肾亏虚,加大椎,脾俞;肝肾不足,加太冲,太溪;失眠者,加神门。

Performance: Reinforcing needling technique is used. Both acupuncture and moxibustion are applied. For evident asthenia of yang, heavy moxibustion is resorted to.

操作:针用补法,针灸并用,阳虚明显者,重用灸法。

2. Ear acupuncture

2. 耳针疗法

Prescription: Spleen (CO_{13}), Kidney (CO_{10}), Liver

处方:脾,肾,肝,内分泌,

(CO_{12}), Endocrine (CO_{18}), Sympathetic Nerve (AH_{6a}) and Ear Shenmen (TF_4).

交感,神门。

Performance: Each time 3 - 4 acupoints are selected and needled with mild stimulation.

操作:每次选3~4穴,弱刺激。

5. 5. 2 Primary thrombocytopenic purpura

二、原发性血小板减少性紫癜

[**Introduction**]

Primary thrombocytopenic purpura, also known as spontaneous immune thrombocytopenic purpura, is a commonly seen disease in hematopathy. The clinical manifestations are spontaneous ecchymoses and hemorrhage from mucus and viscera. It is either acute or chronic. Acute primary thrombocytopenic purpura is usually self-limited and often seen among children. Chronic primary thrombocytopenic purpura is usually seen among young women. This disease is similar to macules and blood syndrome in TCM. Acute primary thrombocytopenic purpura is caused by interior accumulation of heat-toxin that drives blood to flow abnormally; while chronic primary thrombocytopenic purpura is often caused by asthenia-damage of the liver, spleen and kidney, asthenia-fire scorching the collaterals or failure of qi to check blood.

【概述】

原发性血小板减少性紫癜,也称自身免疫性血小板减少性紫癜,是血液病中常见的一种出血性疾病。临床表现为自发性皮肤瘀点或瘀斑,粘膜及内脏出血。分急性和慢性两类,急性者常为自限性,多见于儿童;慢性者以青年女性为常见。本病相当于中医的"斑疹"、"血证"等病症。急性者是因热毒内蕴,迫血妄行;慢性者多为肝、脾、肾等脏器虚损,虚火灼络或气不摄血所致。

[**Syndrome differentiation**]

【辨证】

1. Interior accumulation of heat-toxin

Sudden onset, purplish patches on the skin, often accompanied by hemorrhage, hematuria and hematochezia with fresh red color, or fever, feverish sensation over the palms, soles and chest, yellow and brown urine, deep-red tongue with thin and yellow or yellow and dry fur, slippery and rapid pulse.

1. 热毒内蕴

起病较急,皮肤紫斑,斑色紫赤,量多成片,常伴衄血、尿血、便血,血色鲜红,或有发热,五心烦热,小便黄赤,舌质红绛,苔薄黄或黄燥,脉滑数。

2. Yin asthenia and fire exuberance

Slow onset, purpura with frequent changes of aggravation and alleviation, especially on the lower limbs, or

2. 阴虚火旺

发病较缓,皮肤紫斑时轻时重,斑色紫红,下肢为多,或

epistaxis, dental bleeding, profuse menstruation, often accompanied by tidal fever, flushed cheeks, dysphoria, night sweating, dizziness, amnesia, aching and weakness of loins and knees, red tongue with scanty fur, thin and rapid pulse.

有鼻衄、齿衄,月经过多,常伴潮热颧赤,心烦盗汗,头晕健忘,腰膝酸软,舌红少苔,脉细数。

3. Failure of qi to check blood

3. 气不摄血

Prolonged duration, sparse and light-colored purpura, recurrence, aggravation after overstrain, or accompanied by epistaxis, dental bleeding, hematuria, hematochezia, profuse menstruation, pale complexion, spiritual lassitude, insomnia and anorexia, dizziness, light-colored tongue with white fur, thin and weak pulse.

病情迁延,紫斑稀淡,反复发作,遇劳加重,或兼鼻衄、齿衄、尿血、便血、月经过多,面色无华,神疲倦怠,失眠纳差,头晕目眩,舌淡苔白,脉细弱。

[**Treatment**]

【治疗】

1. Body acupuncture

1. 体针疗法

Prescription: Xuehai (SP 10), Geshu (BL 17) and Sanyinjiao (SP 6).

处方:血海,膈俞,三阴交。

Modification: For interior accumulation of heat-toxin, Quchi (LI 11) and Neiting (ST 44) are added; for yin asthenia and fire exuberance, Taixi (KI 3), Taichong (LR 3), Ganshu (BL 18) and Shenshu (BL 23) are added; for failure of qi to check blood, Pishu (BL 20), Shenshu (BL 23), Qihai (CV 6) and Zusanli (ST 36) are added.

随证配穴:热毒内蕴,加曲池、内庭;阴虚火旺,加太溪、太冲、肝俞、肾俞;气不摄血,加脾俞、肾俞、气海、足三里。

Performance: For interior accumulation of heat-toxin, reducing needling technique is used; for yin asthenia and fire exuberance, reducing needling technique is used first and then reinforcing technique is applied, or mild reinforcing and reducing technique is resorted to; for failure of qi to check blood, reinforcing needling technique is used and moxibustion can also be applied.

操作:热毒内蕴,针用泻法;阴虚火旺,可先泻后补,或用平补平泻法;气不摄血,针用补法,并可加灸。

2. Ear acupuncture

2. 耳针疗法

Prescription: Adrenal Gland (TG_{2p}), Endocrine (CO_{18}), Lung (CO_{14}), Heart (CO_{15}), Spleen (CO_{13}), Liver (CO_{12}) and Middle Ear (HX_1).

处方:肾上腺,内分泌,肺,心,脾,肝,耳中。

Performance: Embedment of needles is used. Or ear pressure with Wangbuliuxingzi (Semen Vaccariae) is applied, pressing three times a day and 3 minutes each time. Two ears are pressed in alternation.

操作：埋针或王不留行籽压耳，每天按压 3 次，每次 3 分钟，两耳交替。

5.6 Diseases of urinary and reproductive systems

第六节 泌尿、生殖系统疾病

5.6.1 Infection of urinary tract

一、泌尿道感染

[**Introduction**]

Infection of urinary tract refers to inflammation of mucus or tissues of the urinary tract due to growth and multiplication of pathogenic bacteria in the urinary tract. The clinical manifestations are frequent urination, urgent urination and painful urination, or accompanied by lumbago and fever. This problem is usually seen among women, similar to stranguria and retention of urine in TCM. This disease originates from the bladder and kidney, but is also related to the spleen. It is caused by accumulation of damp-heat in the lower energizer and dysfunction of the bladder in transforming qi due to exogenous or endogenous factors. It is usually of sthenia syndrome. Prolonged duration may change into asthenia syndrome or syndrome of mixed asthenia and sthenia due to stagnation of heat consuming yin, dampness blocking yang-qi or yin impairing yang.

【**概述**】

泌尿道感染是指病原菌在尿道内生长繁殖，引起泌尿道粘膜或组织的炎症。以尿频、尿急、尿痛等尿路刺激症状为主要临床表现，可伴有腰痛和发热。好发于女性。本病相当于中医的“淋证”、“癃”等病证。病在膀胱和肾，与脾有关。是由外感或内伤等因素引起湿热蕴结下焦，膀胱气化不利所致，多为实证。若迁延不愈，热郁伤阴、湿遏阳气或阴伤及阳，则演变为虚实夹杂或从实转虚。

[**Syndrome differentiation**]

1. Sthenia syndrome

Urgent urination, astringency and burning pain in urination, yellow and turbid urine, distension and pain in lower abdomen, or lumbago, or aversion to cold, fever, red tongue with yellow and greasy fur, slippery and rapid pulse.

【**辨证**】

1. 实证

小便急迫，涩滞热痛，尿黄赤混浊，小腹胀痛，或有腰痛，或有恶寒发热，舌红，苔黄腻，脉滑数。

2. Asthenia syndrome

Unsmooth urination, dripping urination, occasional occurrence or occurrence after overstrain, or tidal fever and night sweating, feverish sensation over palms, soles and chest, red tongue with scanty fur, thin and rapid pulse, or aversion to cold and cold limbs, aching and weakness of loins and knees, edema of lower limbs, light-colored tongue and weak pulse.

2. 虚证

小便不利，淋漓不已，时作时止，遇劳即发，或潮热盗汗，五心烦热，舌红少苔，脉细数；或畏寒肢冷，腰膝酸软，下肢浮肿，舌淡，脉弱。

[Treatment]

1. Body acupuncture

Prescription: Zhongji (CV 3), Yinlingquan (SP 9), Sanyinjiao (SP 6), Shenshu (BL 23) and Pangguangshu (BL 28).

Modification: For severe fever, Hegu (LI 4) and Quchi (LI 11) are added; for asthenia of kidney yin, Taixi (KI 3), Yinxi (HT 6) and Fuliu (KI 7) are added; for asthenia of spleen and kidney yang, Pishu (BL 20) and Zusanli (ST 36) are added; for hematuria, Xuehai (SP 10) and Diji (SP 8) are added; for frequent urination in the night, Qihai (CV 6), Guanyuan (CV 4) and Zusanli (ST 36) are added.

Performance: Zhongji (CV 3) should be needled superficially and obliquely to avoid impairing the bladder. Asthenia syndrome is treated by reinforcing needling technique, while sthenia syndrome is dealt with by reducing needling technique. Yang asthenia syndrome can be treated by moxibustion following acupuncture. Electro-acupuncture can also be applied with continuous or sparse and dense wave and high frequency for stimulation.

【治疗】

1. 体针疗法

处方：中极，阴陵泉，三阴交，肾俞，膀胱俞。

随证配穴：热甚者，加合谷、曲池；肾阴亏虚，加太溪、阴郄、复溜；脾肾阳虚，加脾俞、足三里；血尿者，加血海、地机；夜尿频者，加气海、关元、足三里。

操作：中极应浅刺、斜刺，以免伤及膀胱；虚补实泻，阳虚者可加灸。亦可配合电针疗法，采用连续波或疏密波、快频率刺激。

2. Ear acupuncture

Prescription: Kidney (CO_{10}), Bladder (CO_9), Urethra (HX_3), Ureter ($CO_{9,10i}$), Spleen (CO_{13}), Triple Energizer (CO_{17}), Sympathetic Nerve (AH_{6a}) and Ear Shenmen (TF_4).

2. 耳针疗法

处方：肾，膀胱，尿道，输尿管，脾，三焦，交感，神门。

Performance: Each time 3 - 5 acupoints are selected and needled with routine procedure. The needles are retained for 30 minutes. The needling is done once a day and the two ears are needled in alternation.

操作：每次选 3～5 穴，常规操作，留针 30 分钟。每日 1 次，两耳交替使用。

5.6.2 Urinary tract stones

二、泌尿道结石

[Introduction]

Urinary tract stones refers to formation and retention of crystal clot in the urinary system, including calculus of kidney, ureteral calculus and calculus of urinary tract according to the location of the calculus. The main manifestations are colic in the loins or lower abdomen, astringent pain in urination and hematuria. This disease is similar to stony stranguria, sand stranguria and bloody stranguria in TCM. The location of this disease is in the kidney and bladder, but it is also related to the liver and spleen. It is usually caused by retention of heat in the bladder, asthenia of kidney qi or stagnation of qi and obstruction of the lower energizer. It is of sthenia syndrome in the early stage. However, prolonged duration will change it into asthenia syndrome or syndrome of mixed asthenia and sthenia.

【概述】

泌尿道结石是指泌尿系统中有晶体块形成和停滞。根据结石发生的部位不同，分为肾结石、输尿管结石、膀胱结石和尿道结石。以阵发性腰部或下腹部绞痛、小便涩痛、尿血为主要特征。本病相当于中医“淋证”中“砂淋”、“石淋”、“血淋”的范畴。本病的病位在下焦的肾和膀胱，又与肝、脾有关。多由于热结膀胱、肾气亏虚或气机阻滞，下焦失其通利所致。初起多为实证，病久则每呈虚象或虚实夹杂证。

[Syndrome differentiation]

1. Damp-heat in the lower energizer

Pain in the loins and abdomen like colic, dripping and astringent pain in urination, or sudden anuria, or bloody urine, or fever, bitter taste in the mouth, red tongue with greasy fur, and slippery and rapid pulse.

2. Qi stagnation and blood stasis

Frequent dull pain or vague pain in the loins and abdomen, sudden stoppage of urination, severe pain, even hematuria with deep-red color, grayish complexion, deep-red tongue with purplish appearance, and taut and unsmooth pulse.

【辨证】

1. 下焦湿热

腰腹疼痛如绞，小便淋沥涩痛，或突然尿闭，或尿中带血；或见发热，口苦，舌红苔质腻，脉滑数。

2. 气滞血瘀

平素腰腹隐痛、钝痛，排尿突然中断，疼痛剧烈，甚则尿血，色暗红，面色暗滞，舌质暗红有紫气，脉弦涩。

3. Asthenia of spleen and kidney yang

Occasional dull pain in the loins and abdomen, frequent urination or unsmooth urination, lassitude, cold body and limbs, aching and weakness in the loins and knees, pale complexion, light-colored tongue with white fur, slow and weak pulse.

4. Asthenia of liver and kidney yin

Dripping and burning sensation in urination, dizziness and tinnitus, tidal fever and night sweating, feverish sensation in the palms, soles and chest, insomnia, dreaminess, red tongue with scanty fur, thin and weak pulse.

[**Treatment**]

1. Body acupuncture

Prescription: Zhongji (CV 3), Sanyinjiao (SP 6), Taixi (KI 3), Shenshu (BL 23), Pangguangshu (BL 28) and Jingmen (BL 36).

Modification: For damp-heat in the lower energizer, Shuidao (ST 28), Weiyang (BL 39) and Yinlingquan (SP 9) are added; for qi stagnation and blood stasis, Hegu (LI 4), Taichong (LR 3) and Geshu (BL 17) are added; for asthenia of spleen and kidney yang, Guanyuan (CV 4), Pishu (BL 20), Mingmen (GV 4) and Zusanli (ST 36) are added; for asthenia of liver and kidney yin, Fuliu (KI 7), Ganshu (BL 18), Ququan (LR 8) and Yingu (KI 10) are added; for colic pain, Yanglingquan (GB 34) and tenderness point are added; for hematuria, Xuehai (SP 10) is added; for fever, Hegu (LI 4) and Quchi (LI 11) are added.

Performance: For the treatment of damp-heat in the lower energizer type and qi stagnation and blood stasis type, reducing needling technique is used; for asthenia of spleen and kidney yang type and asthenia of liver and kidney yin, mild reducing needling technique or mild reducing and reinforcing techniques are used. Each time 1 - 2 acupoints are selected and needled with continuous wave,

3. 脾肾阳虚

时有腰腹隐痛,尿频或小便不利,倦怠乏力,形寒肢冷,腰膝酸软,面色皖白,舌淡苔白,脉缓而弱。

4. 肝肾阴虚

小便淋沥灼热,头晕耳鸣,潮热盗汗,五心烦热,失眠多梦,舌红少苔,脉细数无力。

【治疗】

1. 体针疗法

处方:中极,三阴交,太溪,肾俞,膀胱俞,京门。

随证配穴:下焦湿热,加水道、委阳、阴陵泉;气滞血瘀,加合谷、太冲、膈俞;脾肾阳虚,加关元、脾俞、命门、足三里;肝肾阴虚,加复溜、肝俞、曲泉、阴谷;绞痛剧烈,加阳陵泉、压痛点;血尿者加血海;发热者加合谷、曲池。

操作:下焦湿热和气滞血瘀两型用泻法,脾肾阳虚和肝肾阴虚以轻泻法或平补平泻法为主。每次可选用上述诸穴1~2对,以连续波、快频率、强电流连续刺激40~60分钟。脾肾阳虚者,针灸

high frequency and strong electricity for 40 - 60 minutes. For the treatment of asthenia of spleen and kidney yang, acupuncture and moxibustion can be used simultaneously.

并用。

2. Ear acupuncture

Prescription: Kidney (CO_{10}), Ureter ($CO_{9,10i}$), Bladder (CO_9), Urethra (HX_3), Lung (CO_{14}), Spleen (CO_{13}), Triple Energizer (CO_{17}), Sympathetic Nerve (AH_{6a}), Ear Shenmen (TF_4) and Subcortex (AT_4).

Performance: Each time 3 - 5 acupoints are selected and needled with normal procedure, strong stimulation and frequent rotation of the needles. The needles are retained for 30 - 60 minutes. The needling is done once or twice a day. Or Wangbuliuxingzi (Semen Vaccariae) is used for ear pressure.

2. 耳针疗法

处方：肾，输尿管，膀胱，尿道，肺，脾，三焦，交感，神门，皮质下。

操作：每次选 3～5 穴，常规操作，强刺激，多捻针，留针 30～60 分钟。每日 1～2 次。或用王不留行籽压耳法。

5.6.3 Retention of urine

[**Introduction**]

Retention of urine is marked by difficulty in urination or anuria, distension and pain in lower abdomen. It is either acute or chronic according to the pathological conditions. The location of this disease is in the kidney and bladder, but also involves the liver and spleen. It is usually caused by accumulation of damp-heat, obstruction by stagnation, failure of the liver to disperse and convey, asthenia of kidney qi or asthenia of gastrosplenic qi that lead to dysfunction of the bladder in transforming qi due to various factors.

三、尿潴留

【**概述**】

尿潴留是指尿液充胀膀胱而不能排出的病证。以小便困难甚或不通、小腹胀满而痛为主要表现。按病情轻重缓急可分为急性和慢性两类。尿潴留相当于中医的“癃闭”病证，尤其与“闭”证相合。本病的病位在肾与膀胱，涉及肝、脾。若因各种原因，导致湿热蕴结、浊瘀阻塞、肝失疏泄、肾元亏虚或中焦气虚等，使膀胱气化不利，发为癃闭。

[**Syndrome differentiation**]

1. Sthenia syndrome

Obstruction of urine, contraction and pain in lower abdomen, restlessness and hoarse voice, red tongue with yellow and greasy fur, slippery and rapid pulse.

【**辨证**】

1. 实证

小便阻塞不通，努责无效，少腹胀急而痛，烦躁气粗，舌红苔黄腻，脉滑数。

2. Asthenia syndrome

Dripping and weak urination, even discharge several drops of urine or no urine, bulging of lower abdomen, low spirit and deficiency of qi, aching and weakness of loins and knees, dragging sensation in the anus, light-colored tongue with slight greasy fur, thin and weak pulse.

［**Treatment**］

1. Body acupuncture

Prescription: Zhongji (CV 3), Sanyinjiao (SP 6), Weiyang (BL 39) and Pangguangshu (BL 28).

Modification: For accumulation of damp-heat, Quchi (LI 11) and Yinlingquan (SP 9) are added; for liver depression and qi stagnation, Hegu (LI 4), Taichong (LR 3) and Dadun (LR 1) are added; for obstruction of urinary tract, Qugu (CV 2), Jingmen (GB 25), Ciliao (BL 32) and Zhibian (BL 54) are added; for insufficiency of gastrosplenic qi, Qihai (CV 6), Pishu (BL 20) and Zusanli (ST 36) are added; for asthenia of kidney qi, Taixi (KI 3), Fuliu (KI 7) and Shenshu (BL 23) are added; for no desire to urinate or weakness in urination, Qihai (CV 6) and Shenshu (BL 23) are added.

Performance: In needling Zhongji (CV 3), Guanyuan (CV 4) and Qihai (CV 6), percussion is made first to examine the distending degree of the bladder for deciding the direction, angle and depth of needling. Or inter-penetrating technique is used to needle all the acupoints so as to direct the needling sensation to the genitalia to contract the lower abdomen. Zhibian (BL 54) is needled 3 cun obliquely toward the genitalia. The needling technique used is mainly for reducing purpose. For the treatment of asthenia syndrome, mild reducing and reinforcing needling technique can be used with the addition of moxibustion.

2. Ear acupuncture

Prescription: Kidney (CO_{10}), Bladder (CO_9), Lung

2. 虚证

小便淋沥不爽，排出无力，甚则点滴不通，小腹膨隆，面色晄白，神怯气弱，腰膝酸软，时觉肛门下坠，舌淡苔微腻，脉细无力。

【治疗】

1. 体针疗法

处方：中极，三阴交，委阳，膀胱俞。

配穴：湿热蕴结，加曲池、阴陵泉；肝郁气滞，加合谷、太冲、大敦；尿路瘀阻，加曲骨、京门、次髎、秩边；中气不足，加气海、脾俞、足三里；肾元亏虚，加关元、太溪、复溜、肾俞；无尿意或无力排尿者，加气海、肾俞。

操作：针刺中极、关元、气海等下腹部穴位，应首先叩诊，检查膀胱的膨胀程度，以便决定针刺的方向、角度和深浅，或分别采取诸穴互相透刺法，以针感能到达前阴并引起小腹收缩、抽动为好；秩边向前阴方向深刺 3 寸左右。以泻法为主，虚证用平补平泻法，并可加灸。

2. 耳针疗法

处方：肾，膀胱，肺，肝，

(CO_{14}), Liver (CO_{12}), Spleen (CO_{13}), Triple Energizer (CO_{17}), Sympathetic Nerve (AH_{6a}), Ear Shenmen (TF_4), Subcortex (AT_4) and Lumbosacral Vertebrae (AH_9).

脾,三焦,交感,神门,皮质下,腰骶椎。

Performance: Each time 3 - 5 acupoints are selected and needled with routine procedure and medium-strong stimulation. The needles are retained for 30 minutes.

操作：每次选 3～5 穴,常规操作,中强刺激,留针 30 分钟。

5.6.4 Prostatitis

四、前列腺炎

[**Introduction**]

Prostatitis is a commonly encountered disease of urinary system in men. It is either acute or chronic. Acute prostatitis is marked by stimulating symptoms of the urinary tract, bloody urine in the end of urination and perineum pain. Chronic prostatitis is marked by delayed urination, dripping after urination, or discharge of whitish turbid prostate fluid, or seminal emission, premature ejaculation and impotence. It is similar to stranguria, spermatorrhea, gonorrhea and semen in urine in TCM. Prostatitis is usually caused by exogenous damp-toxin, excessive drinking of alcohol, partiality to pungent and greasy foods, or excessive sexual life and endogenous asthenia-heat that lead to accumulation of damp-heat in the lower energizer. The major manifestation is sthenia in branch. Prolonged duration leads to asthenia of liver and kidney yin and asthenia of spleen and kidney yang, further resulting in qi stagnation and blood stasis marked by asthenia of the root or mixture of asthenia and sthenia.

【概述】

前列腺炎是男性泌尿系统的常见疾病,分急性和慢性两大类。急性前列腺炎以尿路刺激症状和终末血尿、会阴部疼痛为主要症状。慢性前列腺炎以排尿延迟、尿后滴尿,或滴出白色前列腺液,或引起遗精、早泄、阳痿等为主要症状。本病相当于中医学“淋证”、“白淫”、“白浊”、“尿精”等病证。主要由外感湿毒,过度饮酒、嗜食辛辣肥甘,或房事过度,虚热内生,以致湿热蕴结下焦,以标实为主;病久则出现肝肾阴虚和脾肾阳虚,进而可致气滞血瘀,以本虚或虚实夹杂为主。

[**Syndrome differentiation**]

1. Downward migration of damp-heat

Burning sensation in the urinary tract, yellow and scanty urine, profuse whitish secreta from the external orifice of urethra, bitter taste and dryness of mouth, thirst and desire to drink water, retention of dry feces, red tongue, yellow and greasy tongue fur, slippery and

【辨证】

1. 湿热下注

尿道灼热,尿黄而少,尿道口白色分泌物偏多,口干苦,口渴而思饮,大便干结,舌红苔黄腻,脉滑数。

rapid pulse.

2. Accumulation of heat-toxin

High fever, aversion to cold, hematuria, pain in defecation, deep-red tongue with yellow and dry fur, taut, rapid and powerful pulse.

3. Stagnation of cold in the liver vessels

Dull pain in the lower abdomen and testis, aggravation with cold and alleviation with warmth, white and slippery tongue fur, deep and taut or slow pulse.

4. Asthenia of liver and kidney yin

Aching in the loins and sacral region, flaccidity of legs, feverish palms, soles and chest, insomnia and dreaminess, seminal emission, dizziness, vague pain in the perineum, burning sensation in the urinary tract, red tongue with scanty fur, deep, thin and rapid pulse.

5. Asthenia of spleen and kidney yang

Dripping urination, profuse urine in the night, pale complexion, cold limbs, flaccidity of limbs, edema, loose stool, spermatorrhea, impotence, light-colored tongue with white fur, thin and weak pulse.

6. Qi stagnation and blood stasis

Prolonged duration, hematuria, bloody semen, fullness and pain in lower abdomen, dripping or silky urination, deep-red tongue or with ecchymoses, taut or unsmooth pulse.

[**Treatment**]

1. Body acupuncture

Prescription: Zhongji (CV 3), Ciliao (BL 32), Sanyinjiao (SP 6) and Yinlingquan (SP 9).

Modification: For downward migration of damp-heat, Qugu (CV 2), Zhibian (BL 54), Pangguangshu (BL 28) and Sanjiaoshu (BL 22) are added; for accumulation of heat-toxin, Quchi (LI 11) and Hegu (LI 4) are added; for stagnation of cold in liver vessels, Dadun (LR 1) and

2. 热毒蕴结

高热,恶寒,血尿,大便疼痛,舌红绛苔黄燥,脉弦数有力。

3. 寒凝肝脉

少腹与睾丸隐隐作痛,遇寒更甚,得热则舒,腹寒阴冷,舌苔白滑,脉沉弦或迟。

4. 肝肾阴虚

腰膂酸楚,腿软乏力,手足心热,失眠多梦,遗精,头目眩晕,会阴部隐痛,时有尿道灼热感,舌红少苔,脉沉细而数。

5. 脾肾阳虚

小便淋沥难尽,夜尿多,面色皖白,肢冷,肢软无力,浮肿,便溏,滑精,阳痿,舌淡苔白,脉细无力。

6. 气滞血瘀

病程久长,血尿,血精,小腹胀满疼痛,尿细如丝或点滴而下,舌暗红或见瘀点,脉弦或涩。

【**治疗**】

1. 体针疗法

处方:中极,次髎,三阴交,阴陵泉。

配穴:湿热下注,加曲骨、秩边、膀胱俞、三焦俞;热毒蕴结,加曲池、合谷;寒凝肝脉,加大敦、太冲;肝肾阴虚,加关元、复溜、太溪、肾俞、肝俞;脾

Taichong (LR 3) are added; for asthenia of liver and kidney yin, Guanyuan (CV 4), Fuliu (KI 7), Taixi (KI 3), Shenshu (BL 23) and Ganshu (BL 18) are added; for asthenia of spleen and kidney yang, Mingmen (GV 4), Pishu (BL 20), Shenshu (BL 23) and Zusanli (ST 36) are added; for qi stagnation and blood stasis, Taichong (LR 3) and Geshu (BL 17) are added; for hematuria, Xuehai (SP 10), Geshu (BL 17) and Zhibian (BL 54) are added; for seminal emission and spermatorrhea, Jinggong (Ext.), Guanyuan (CV 4) and Dahe (KI 12) are added.

肾阳虚,加命门、脾俞、肾俞、足三里;气滞血瘀,加太冲、膈俞;血尿者,加血海、膈俞、秩边;遗精、滑精者,加精宫、关元、大赫。

Performance: Urine is discharged completely, then Zhongji (CV 3), Guanyuan (CV 4) and Qugu (CV 2) are needled vertically for 1.5 - 2 cun to direct the needling sensation to the perineum; Ciliao (BL 32) and Zhibian (BL 54) are needled 1.5 - 3 cun toward the bladder to direct the needling sensation to the lower abdomen and perineum; the other acupoints are needled with routine procedure. The needling technique used is mainly for reducing purpose. For the treatment of asthenia of the spleen and kidney yang, reinforcing needling technique is used together with moxibustion. For the treatment of asthenia of liver and kidney yin, mild reinforcing and reducing needling technique is used.

操作:在排空小便的情况下,中极、关元、曲骨等下腹部穴位直刺 1.5～2 寸,使针感达会阴部;次髎、秩边宜朝膀胱区方向深刺 1.5～3 寸,使针感传到下腹乃至会阴部位;其他腧穴常规针刺。以泻法为主,脾肾阳虚者用补法、加灸,肝肾阴虚者用平补平泻法。

2. Ear acupuncture

2. 耳针疗法

Prescription: Angle of Cymba Concha (CO_8), Kidney (CO_{10}), Bladder (CO_9), Liver (CO_{12}), Triple Energizer (CO_{17}), Ear Shenmen (TF_4), Pelvic Cavity (TF_5), Sympathetic Nerve (AH_{6a}), Endocrine (CO_{18}) and Adrenal Gland (TG_{2p}).

处方:艇角,肾,尿道,膀胱,肝,三焦,神门,盆腔,交感,内分泌,肾上腺。

Performance: Each time 3 - 5 acupoints are selected with normal procedure. For the treatment of acute prostatitis, strong stimulation (with bloodletting from the tip of ear) is used. The needles are retained for a longer (45 - 60 minutes) time and manipulated at intervals. For the

操作:每次选用 3～5 穴,常规操作,急性者用强刺激(并可加耳尖点刺出血),久留针(45～60 分钟),间歇行针;慢性者用中等刺激,留针 20

treatment of chronic prostatitis, moderate stimulation is used. The needles are retained for 20 minutes and the needling is done once a day.

分钟。每日1次。

5.6.5 Seminal emission

［Introduction］

Seminal emission refers to discharge of semen without sexual activity. One or twice seminal emission in a month without evident discomfort in healthy man is regarded as physiological phenomenon. However, several times a week or in a night, accompanied by spiritual lassitude, dizziness and tinnitus, is morbid. Seminal emission in dream is called nocturnal emission, while seminal emission in conscious state is called spermatorrhea. Nocturnal emission is usually caused by over-anxiety, indulgence in sexual life, disharmony between the heart and kidney as well as deficiency of water and exuberance of fire; or by partiality to greasy and pungent foods and accumulation of dampness into heat that disturbs semen. Prolonged duration may exhaust kidney qi and weakens storage of semen, leading to spermatorrhea.

［Syndrome differentiation］

1. Disharmony between the heart and kidney

Dreaminess, priapism, susceptibility to erection, dysphoria and insomnia, dizziness, aching loins and spiritual lassitude, red tongue, thin and rapid pulse.

2. Downward migration of damp-heat

Frequent seminal emission, lassitude and anorexia, dampness or pruritus of pudendum, yellow and brown urine, unsmooth urination or burning sensation in urination, red tongue tip and margins, yellow and greasy fur, slippery or rapid pulse.

3. Asthenia of kidney yang

Seminal emission without dream, even spermatorrhea

五、遗精

【概述】

男子非性生活而精液外泄者称为遗精。一般健康男性,每月遗精1～2次,且无明显不适,属正常生理现象;若一周数次或一夜数次,并伴有神疲困倦,头昏耳鸣等全身症状者,则属于遗精症。有梦而遗者称梦遗;无梦而遗,或清醒时精液自泄者称为滑精。梦遗多由思虑过度,恣情纵欲,心肾不交,水亏火旺;或嗜食肥甘辛辣,蕴湿生热,扰动精室所致。如病延日久,肾元虚惫,精关不固,则成滑精。

【辨证】

1. 心肾不交

梦境纷纭,阳强易举,遗精频繁,心烦少寐,头晕目眩,腰酸神疲,舌质偏红,脉细数。

2. 湿热下注

遗精频作,身倦纳呆,阴部潮湿或痒,尿色黄赤,尿时不爽或有灼热,舌边尖红,苔黄腻,脉滑或数。

3. 肾阳虚衰

无梦而遗,甚至动念则精

with the desire of sex, dizziness and tinnitus, bright-white complexion, aching and weakness of loins and knees, aversion to cold and cold limbs, or accompanied by impotence, spontaneous sweating and shortness of breath, light-colored tongue with white fur, thin and weak pulse.

出,滑泄不禁,头晕耳鸣,面色㿠白,腰膝酸软,畏寒肢冷,或兼阳痿,自汗短气,舌淡苔白,脉细弱。

[**Treatment**]

【治疗】

1. Body acupuncture

1. 体针疗法

Prescription: Shenshu (BL 23), Guanyuan (CV 4) and Sanyinjiao (SP 6).

处方:肾俞,关元,三阴交。

Modification: For disharmony between the heart and kidney, Xinshu (BL 15), Shenmen (HT 7), Neiguan (PC 6) and Taichong (LR 3) are added; for downward migration of damp-heat, Zhongji (CV 3), Yinlingquan (SP 9) and Xingjian (LR 2) are added; for decline of kidney yang, Mingmen (GV 4), Taixi (KI 3) and Zusanli (ST 36) are added.

随证配穴:心肾不交,加心俞、神门、内关、太冲;湿热下注,加中极、阴陵泉、行间;肾阳虚惫,加命门、太溪、足三里。

Performance: For seminal emission, mild reinforcing and reducing or reducing needling techniques are used; for spermatorrhea, reinforcing needling technique is used with the addition of moxibustion.

操作:遗精者针用平补平泻或泻法,不灸;滑精者针用补法,加灸。

2. Ear acupuncture

2. 耳针疗法

Prescription: Internal Genitalia (TF_2), Ear Shenmen (TF_4), Liver (CO_{12}), Kidney (CO_{10}) and Subcortex (AT_4).

处方:内生殖器,神门,肝,肾,皮质下。

Performance: Medium stimulation is required or Wangbuliuxingzi (Semen Vaccariae) is used for ear acupressure.

操作:中等刺激,或用王不留行籽压耳法。

5.6.6 Impotence

六、阳痿

[**Introduction**]

【概述】

Impotence means that the penis in adult cannot erect or erect insufficiently for sexual intercourse. According to TCM, impotence is caused by intemperance of sexual life

阳痿是指成年男子阴茎不能正常勃起,或勃起不坚,以致不能进行性生活的一种

and decline of fire in mingmen (gate of life); or by over-anxiety that impairs the heart and spleen and leads to asthenia of the thoroughfare vessel; or by downward migration of damp-heat in the liver and kidney that leads to flaccidity of the genitalia. Clinically impotence is usually of asthenia syndrome.

疾患。中医认为是恣情纵欲，命门火衰；或思虑忧郁，损伤心脾，冲脉空虚；或肝肾湿热下注，宗筋弛纵，均可导致阳痿。临床以虚证居多。

[**Syndrome differentiation**]

【辨证】

1. Impairment of the heart and spleen

Frigidity in sexual life, or insufficiency of erection, palpitation and susceptibility to fright, insomnia and amnesia, lusterless complexion, spiritual lassitude and fatigue, shortness of breath and spontaneous sweating, light-colored tongue with white fur, thin and weak pulse.

1. 心脾受损

性欲淡漠，或举而不坚，心悸易惊，失眠健忘，面色无华，神疲乏力，气短自汗，舌淡苔白，脉细弱。

2. Decline of fire in mingmen (gate of life)

Impotence, or premature ejaculation, thin and cold semen, blackish eyelids and complexion, dizziness, cold sensation in the body and spiritual lassitude, aching loins and tinnitus, light-colored tongue, deep and thin pulse.

2. 命门火衰

阳事不举，或临房早泄，精稀清冷，面色眼圈黯黑，头晕目眩，形寒神疲，腰酸耳鸣，舌淡，脉沉细。

3. Downward migration of damp-heat

Impotence, insufficiency of erection, eczema of scrotum with foul smell, aching and distension in the lower abdomen, yellow and brown urine, or stabbing pain, itching and burning sensation in urination, yellow tongue fur, soft and rapid pulse.

3. 湿热下注

阴茎萎软，举而不坚，阴囊潮湿、臊臭，睾丸、少腹酸胀不适，小便黄赤，甚者尿时刺痒灼热，苔黄，脉濡数。

[**Treatment**]

【治疗】

1. Body acupuncture

Prescription: Guanyuan (CV 4), Shenshu (BL 23), Sanyinjiao (SP 6) and Taichong (LR 3).

Modification: For impairment of the heart and spleen, Xinshu (BL 15), Pishu (BL 20), Neiguan (PC 6) and Zusanli (ST 36) are added; for decline of fire in mingmen (gate of life), Mingmen (GV 4) and Ciliao (BL 32) are added; for downward migration of damp-heat, Pangguangshu (BL 28), Yinlingquan (SP 9), Ligou (LR

1. 体针疗法

处方：关元，肾俞，三阴交，太冲。

随证配穴：心脾受损，加心俞、脾俞、内关、足三里；命门火衰，加命门、次髎；湿热下注，加膀胱俞、阴陵泉、蠡沟、行间。

5) and Xingjian (LR 2) are added.

Performance: Guanyuan (CV 4) is needled till the needling sensation radiates to the perineum. Sthenia syndrome is treated with reducing needling technique while asthenia syndrome is treated with reinforcing needling technique. For the treatment of decline of fire in mingmen (gate of life), moxibustion is used.

操作：关元针刺时以针感到达前阴为佳，实则泻之，虚则补之，命门火衰者则灸之。

2. Ear acupuncture

Prescription: Internal Genitalia (TF_2), External Genitalia (HX_4), Middle border ($AT_{1,2,4i}$), Liver (CO_{12}), Kidney (CO_{10}), Endocrine (CO_{18}) and Ear Shenmen (TF_4).

2. 耳针疗法

处方：内生殖器，外生殖器，缘中，肝，肾，内分泌，神门。

Performance: Each time 3 - 5 acupoints are selected and needled with filiform needles and medium stimulation. Or embedment of needles or ear pressure with Wangbu liuxingzi (Semen Vaccariae) is used.

操作：每次选3～5穴，用毫针中等刺激，或用揿针埋藏和王不留行籽压耳法。

5.7 Endocrine and metabolism diseases

第七节 内分泌、代谢性疾病

5.7.1 Hyperthyroidism

一、甲状腺功能亢进症

[**Introduction**]

Hyperthyroidism is due to excessive secretion of thyroxin, clinically marked by palpitation, excitation, anxiety, polyphagia, emaciation, aversion to heat and profuse sweating, dry mouth and excessive heat, accompanied by thyroid enlargement and exophthalmia. This disease is usually seen among women, especially among young women. It is similar to goiter and palpitation in TCM. Hyperthyroidism is usually caused by interior damage due to emotional changes; or by improper diet that leads to qi stagnation, blood stasis, fire stagnation and

【概述】

甲状腺功能亢进症是甲状腺病态地分泌过量的甲状腺激素所致。以心悸、情绪亢奋且易于波动、性情急躁、食欲旺盛但消瘦、恶热多汗、口干燥热，以及伴有甲状腺肿大、眼球突出等为主要临床征象。本病多见于女性，中青年发病率较高。本病相当于中医的“瘿气”、“心悸”等病证。

phlegm coagulation, the prolonged duration of which results in exuberant fire and consumes yin. This disease involves the heart, liver, spleen, stomach and kidney.

主要由七情内伤,或饮食失调,形成气滞、血瘀、火郁、痰凝之病理,日久火盛伤阴。病变脏器涉及心、肝、脾胃、肾等。

[Syndrome differentiation]

【辨证】

1. Liver depression and phlegm coagulation

Restlessness and susceptibility to rage, insomnia and dreaminess, dryness and distension of eyes, distension and fullness of chest and hypochondria, exophthalmia, swelling of neck, tremor of hands and tongue, red tongue, yellow and greasy tongue fur, taut and slippery pulse.

1. 肝郁痰凝

烦躁易怒,失眠多梦,眼干目胀,胸胁胀满,眼球突出,颈部肿大,手抖舌颤,舌质红,苔黄腻,脉弦滑。

2. Liver fire and stomach heat

Polyphagia, thirst and polydipsia, emaciation, aversion to heat and profuse sweating, bitter taste in the mouth and dry throat, dizziness, red tongue, yellow tongue fur with scanty fluid, taut and rapid pulse.

2. 肝火胃热

多食善饥,烦渴多饮,形体消瘦,恶热多汗,口苦咽干,头晕目眩,舌质红,苔黄少津,脉弦数。

3. Asthenia of heart and liver yin

Palpitation, feverish palms, soles and chest, insomnia and dreaminess, dry throat and mouth, amnesia and susceptibility to fright, red tongue with scanty fur, thin and rapid pulse or slow pulse with irregular intervals and slow regular intermittent pulse.

3. 心肝阴虚

心悸不安,五心烦热,少寐多梦,咽干口燥,健忘易惊,舌红少苔,脉细数或结代。

[Treatment]

【治疗】

1. Body acupuncture

Prescription: Naohui (TE 13), Renying (ST 9), Neiguan (PC 6), Shenmen (HT 7), Hegu (LI 4), Fenglong (ST 40), Sanyinjiao (SP 6) and Taichong (LR 3).

Modification: For liver stagnation and phlegm coagulation: Futu (ST 32), Tiantu (CV 22), Qimen (LR 14), Taiyuan (LU 9) and Taibai (SP 3) are added; for liver fire and stomach heat syndrome, Zusanli (ST 36), Neiting (ST 44), Yanglingquan (GB 34) and Qiuxu (GB 40) are added; for asthenia syndrome of heart and liver yin,

1. 体针疗法

处方:臑会,人迎,内关,神门,合谷,丰隆,三阴交,太冲。

随证配穴:肝郁痰凝证,加扶突、天突、期门、太渊、太白等;肝火胃热证,加足三里、内庭、阳陵泉、丘墟等;心肝阴虚证,加气舍、心俞、肝俞、巨阙、复溜、照海等。甲状腺肿

Qishe (ST 11), Xinshu (BL 15), Ganshu (BL 18), Juque (CV 14), Fuliu (KI 7) and Zhaohai (KI 6) are added; for goiter, Tianding (LI 17), Tianrong (SI 17), Tianjing (TE 10), Qiying [equivalent to Shuitu (ST 10)] and Pingying [0.5 cun lateral to the median line joining 3 - 5 Jiaji (EX-B2)] are added; for severe goiter, local tumescent mass can be needled; for exophthalmia, Fengchi (GB 20), Shangtianzhu [0.5 cun above Tianzhu (BL 10)], Cuanzhu (BL 2), Yangbai (GB 14) and Sizhukong (TE 23) are added; for dryness and distension of eyes, Jingming (BL 1), Zhaohai (KI 6) and Yanglao (SI 6) are added.

大者,还可选用天鼎、天容、天井、气瘿(相当水突穴,视甲状腺肿大程度,定位稍有出入)、平瘿(颈 3~5 夹脊正中线旁开 0.5 寸)等穴,瘿肿较大者加刺肿块局部;眼球突出加风池、上天柱(天柱穴上 0.5 寸)、攒竹、阳白、丝竹空;眼干目胀加睛明、照海、养老。

Performance: Shallow needling, 0.5 - 0.8 cun, is used to needle acupoints on the neck, such as Futu (ST 32), Tiantu (CV 22), Tianding (LI 17) and Tianrong; for needling Qiying (Goiter Acupoint), the needle is inserted 0.5 cun lateral to the vessel; for needling Pingying [Goiter-Eliminating Acupoint (CO_{13})], the needle is inserted 0.8 - 1 cun and the needling sensation is directed to the region below Adam's apple; for larger enlargement of thyroid, 1 - 2 acupoints on the tumescent mass are selected and the needles are inserted obliquely into the base of the tumescent mass and manipulated with rotating, lifting and thrusting techniques within small range.

操作:颈部诸穴如扶突、天突、天鼎、天容等穴针刺须注意深浅,一般针刺 0.5~0.8 寸为宜,并且注意针刺方向。气瘿穴,避开血管刺入 0.5 寸;平瘿穴,针刺 0.8~1 寸,要求针感达前颈结喉下。瘿肿较大者,再取肿块局部 1~2 个穴位,从外侧斜刺入肿块内至基底部,作小幅度的捻转、提插。以上诸穴按虚实补泻。

2. Ear acupuncture

2. 耳针疗法

Prescription: Ear Shenmen (TF_4), Endocrine (CO_{18}), Liver (CO_{12}), Kidney (CO_{10}), Spleen (CO_{13}), Stomach (CO_4), Subcortex (AT_4) and Sympathetic Nerve (AH_{6a}).

处方:神门,内分泌,肝,肾,脾,胃,皮质下,交感。

Performance: Each time 2 - 3 acupoints are selected and needled once a day. Or 2 - 3 acupoints are selected each time for embedment of needles. Or Wangbuliuxingzi (Semen Vaccariae) is used for ear acupressure. The patient is advised to press the embedment of needles or the

操作:每次取 2~3 穴,每日针 1 次;或每次取 2~3 穴埋针,或用王不留行籽压耳法。嘱病人每天自行按摩埋针或穴贴处数次。

sealed Semen Vaccariae several times a day.

5.7.2　Diabetes

[**Introduction**]

Diabetes refers to disturbance of the metabolism of sugar, fat and protein due to relative or absolute insufficiency of insulin in the body marked by hyperglycemia and glycuresis. The clinical symptoms are polyuria, polydipsia, polyphagia, fatigue and emaciation. In severe cases ketosis and acidosis may be caused. It may also lead to severe complications like coronary heart disease, ischemic cerebrovascular disease, kidney disease, ocular fundus disease, acromelic gangrene and nervous lesion. This disease is similar to "Xiaoke" (diabetes) in TCM. It is usually caused by extreme changes of emotions; or by excessive intake of greasy foods and alcohol; or by intemperance of sexual life leading to consumption of yin due to dryness and heat; or by transformation of dryness from yin asthenia and interior heat that results in lung dryness, stomach heat and kidney asthenia, eventually leading to upper diabetes, middle diabetes and lower diabetes. Prolonged duration will give rise to asthenia of both qi and yin or asthenia of both yin and yang.

[**Syndrome differentiation**]

Upper diabetes: Thirst and polydipsia, dry mouth and tongue, frequent and profuse urination, red tip and margins of the tongue, yellow and thin tongue fur, full and rapid pulse.

Middle diabetes: Polyphagia, heartburn, restlessness and fever, profuse sweating, emaciation, or constipation, profuse cloudy and yellow urine, yellow and dry tongue fur, slippery and rapid pulse.

Lower diabetes: Profuse and frequent urination, turbid urine with sweet taste, thirst and polydipsia, dizzi-

二、糖尿病

【概述】

糖尿病是由于体内胰岛素的相对或绝对不足而引起糖、脂肪和蛋白质代谢的紊乱。其主要特点是表现为高血糖和糖尿。临床上可出现多尿、多饮、多食、疲乏、消瘦等症候群，严重时发生酮症酸中毒。易诱发冠心病、缺血性脑血管病、肾病、眼底病、肢端坏疽以及神经病变等严重并发症。本病相当于中医的"消渴"症。多因为五志过极，或过食肥甘、醇酒厚味，或恣情纵欲，导致燥热伤阴，或阴虚内热化燥，致肺燥、胃热、肾虚而发为上、中、下三消。迁延日久，可见气阴两虚或见阴阳两虚之证。

【辨证】

上消证：烦渴多饮，口干舌燥，尿频量多，舌边尖红，苔薄黄，脉洪数。

中消证：多食善饥，嘈杂，烦热，汗多，形体消瘦，或大便秘结，尿多混黄，苔黄而燥，脉滑数。

下消证：尿频量多，尿液混浊、味甜，渴而多饮，头晕，

ness, blurred vision, red cheeks and vexation, aching of loins and flaccidity of knees, or dry skin, general pruritus, red tongue, thin and rapid pulse.

视物模糊,颧红虚烦,腰酸腿软,或皮肤干燥,全身瘙痒,舌红,脉细数。

Asthenia of yin and yang: Frequent urination, turbid urine like paste, blackish complexion, dryness of earlobe, aversion to cold and cold limbs, sexual hypoesthesia, light and dull colored tongue with white fur, deep, thin and weak pulse.

阴阳两虚:小便频数,混浊如膏,面色发黑,耳轮干萎,畏寒肢冷,性欲减退,舌质淡暗,苔白,脉沉细无力。

[**Treatment**]

【治疗】

1. Body acupuncture

1. 体针疗法

Prescription: Weiwanxiashu (EX-B 3), Geshu (BL 17), Feishu (BL 13), Pishu (BL 20), Shenshu (BL 23), Zusanli (ST 36) and Sanyinjiao (SP 6).

处方:胃脘下俞,膈俞,肺俞,脾俞,肾俞,足三里,三阴交。

Modification: For upper diabetes, Xinshu (BL 15), Taiyuan (LU 9) and Shaofu (HT 8) are added; for middle diabetes, Weishu (BL 21) and Nei-ting (ST 44) are added; for lower diabetes, Ganshu (BL 18), Taixi (KI 3) and Taichong (LR 3) are added; for asthenia of both yin and yang, Guanyuan (CV 4) and Mingmen (GV 4) are added; for thirst and dry mouth, Lianquan (CV 23) and Chengjiang (CV 24) are added; for polyphagia, Zhongwan (CV 12) and Fenglong (ST 40) are added; for profuse sweating, Fuliu (KI 7) is added; for blurred vision, Guangming (GB 37), Touwei (ST 8) and Cuanzhu (BL 2) are added; for skin itching, Fengchi (GB 20), Dazhui (GV 14), Quchi (LI 11), Xuehai (SP 10) and Zhaohai (KI 6) are added.

随证配穴:上消证,加心俞、太渊、少府;中消证,加胃俞、内庭;下消配肝俞、太溪、太冲;阴阳两虚,加关元、命门。烦渴口干者,加廉泉、承浆;多食善饥者,加中脘、丰隆;多汗者,加复溜;视物模糊者,加光明、头维、攒竹;皮肤瘙痒加风池、大椎、曲池、血海、照海。

Performance: Weiwanxiashu (EX-B 6), a key effective acupoint for treating diabetes, should be needled 0.5-0.8 cun obliquely toward the spinal column with reinforcing needling technique. The rest acupoints are needled with reinforcing needling technique or mild reinforcing and reducing needling techniques.

操作:胃脘下俞为治疗糖尿病的有效奇穴,宜斜向脊柱针刺0.5～0.8寸,针用补法;余穴均宜用补法或平补平泻法。

2. Ear acupuncture

Prescription: Pancreas and gallbladder (CO_{11}), Endocrine (CO_{18}), Lung (CO_{14}), Stomach (CO_4), Kidney (CO_{10}), Bladder (CO_9), Thirst point (midpoint on the line joining External Nose and Ear Apex) and Hunger Point (External Nose).

Performance: Each time 3 - 4 acupoints are selected and needled with filiform needles and mild stimulation. Or Wangbuliuxingzi (Semen Vaccariae) is used for ear acupressure. The two ears are pressed in alternation.

2. 耳针疗法

处方：胰胆，内分泌，肺，胃，肾，膀胱，渴点（外鼻与屏尖连线中点），饥点（外鼻）。

操作：每次取 3～4 穴，用毫针轻刺激；或用王不留行籽压耳法，两耳交替使用。

5.7.3 Simple obesity

[**Introduction**]

Obesity refers to accumulation of fat in the body due to changes of the biochemical and physiological functions. Clinically body weight increase by 20% more than the standard level is regarded as obesity, usually accompanied by abnormal changes of appetite and sleep, sweating, dry mouth and disorder of stool. TCM believes that obesity is mainly due to disorder of the spleen and stomach as well as dyfunction of defensive qi. The pathological changes are blood sthenia and qi asthenia, exuberance of yin and deficiency of yang as well as disorder of qi and blood. Insufficiency of primordial qi in the triple energizer affects metabolism of water and transformation of qi, consequently leading to obesity.

[**Syndrome differentiation**]

1. Heat in the stomach and intestines

Hyperorexia, polyphagia, dry mouth and preference for drinking water, aversion to heat and profuse sweating, irritability and susceptibility to rage, constipation, yellow and scanty urine, red tongue with yellow and greasy fur, slippery and powerful pulse or slippery and rapid pulse.

三、单纯性肥胖

【概述】

肥胖系机体生化或生理功能改变，致使体内积聚过多脂肪引起的病证。临床上一般以体重超过标准体重 20%，且往往伴有食欲异常、睡眠异常、出汗、口干、大便异常等症状者为肥胖症。中医认为，脾胃失调，卫气失常是导致本症的重要因素，病理变化为血实气虚，阴偏盛阳偏亏，气血阴阳失调；而三焦元气之不足影响人体的水液代谢和气化功能，也可发生肥胖。

【辨证】

1. 胃肠腑热

食欲旺盛，消谷善饥，口干喜饮，恶热多汗，多急躁易怒，大便秘结，小便黄短，舌质红，苔黄腻，脉滑有力或滑带数。

2. Asthenia of spleen and stomach qi

Pale complexion and lips, poor appetite, abdominal distension after meal, spiritual lassitude and fatigue, palpitation and shortness of breath, somnolence and no desire to talk, loose stool or scanty urine and dropsy, light-colored tongue with tooth prints on the margins, thin and white tongue fur, thin, slow and weak pulse or deep and slow pulse.

2. 脾胃气虚

面唇少华,纳食不多,食后腹胀,神疲乏力,心悸气短,嗜睡懒言,大便稀溏,或尿少浮肿,舌淡边有齿印,苔薄白,脉细缓无力或沉迟。

3. Insufficiency of renal primordial qi

Bright-white complexion, preference for quietness and aversion to activity, normal appetite or reduced appetite, shortness of breath and asthma, sweating in movement, dizziness and aching loins, or afternoon fever, thirst without much drinking, or aversion to cold and edema of limbs, often accompanied by irregular menstruation in women and impotence in men, light-colored tongue with tender texture and tooth prints on the margins, scanty tongue fur, deep, thin and weak pulse.

3. 真元不足

面色皖白,喜静恶动,胃纳正常或偏少,气短而喘,动则汗出,头晕腰酸,或午后烘热,口渴饮少,或畏冷肢肿。女性多伴月经不调,男子或见阳痿。舌质淡嫩,边有齿印,苔少,脉沉细无力。

[**Treatment**]

1. Body acupuncture

Prescription: Quchi (LI 11), Shangjuxu (ST 37), Neiting (ST 44), Yinlingquan (SP 9) and Sanyinjiao (SP 6).

Modification: For heat in the stomach and intestines: Hegu (LI 4), Zusanli (ST 36) and Fenglong (ST 40) are added; for asthenia of stomach and spleen qi, Pishu (BL 20), Weishu (BL 21), Zusanli (ST 36) and Taibai (SP 3) are added; for insufficiency of renal primordial qi, Zhongwan (CV 12), Guanyuan (CV 4) and Sanjiaoshu (BL 22) are added; for constipation, Tianshu (ST 25), Zhigou (TE 6) and Yanglingquan (GB 34) are added; for profuse sweating, Zhongwan (CV 12), Shangwan (CV 13) and Zusanli (ST 36) are added; for somnolence, Zhaohai (KI 6), Shenmai (BL 62) and Tianshu (ST 25) are

【治疗】

1. 体针疗法

处方:曲池,上巨虚,内庭,阴陵泉,三阴交。

随证配穴:胃肠腑热,加合谷、足三里、丰隆;脾胃气虚,加脾俞、胃俞、足三里、太白;真元不足,加中脘、关元、肾俞、三焦俞。便秘加天枢、支沟、阳陵泉;汗出量多加中脘、上脘、足三里;嗜睡加照海、申脉、天枢;腹胀加小肠俞、下巨虚、腕骨;心悸气短加神门、内关、巨阙;口渴多饮加足三里、承浆、太溪;下肢水肿

added; for abdominal distension, Xiaochangshu (BL 27), Xiajuxu (ST 39) and Wangu (SI 4) are added; for palpitation and shortness of breath, Shenmen (HT 7), Neiguan (PC 6) and Jugue (CV 14) are added. For thirst with polydipsia, Zusanli (ST 36), Chengjiang (CV 24) and Taixi (KI 3) are added; for edema of lower limbs, Shangqiu (SP 5), Shuifen (CV 9) and Sanjiaoshu (BL 22) are added; for irregular menstruation, Xuehai (SP 10), Diji (SP 8) and Ququan (LR 8) are added; for impotence, Shenshu (BL 23), Mingmen (GV 4) and Guanyuan (CV 4) are added.

加商丘、水分、三焦俞;月经不调加血海、地机、曲泉;阳痿加肾俞、命门、关元等穴。

Performance: Heat in the stomach and intestines is treated with reducing needling technique; asthenia of spleen and stomach qi or insufficiency of renal primordial qi is treated with reinforcing or mild reinforcing and reducing needling techniques. In the early stage 4 - 5 acupoints are selected each time. Eventually ten or more acupoints are selected for each treatment. Deep needling is required for all acupoints except the ones on the limbs.

操作:胃肠腑热型用泻法,脾胃气虚或真元不足型用补法或平补平泻法。开始针刺时以每次取 4～5 穴为宜,以后可逐渐增加至每次 10 余穴。四肢除末端腧穴外,均要求深刺。

2. Ear acupoints

2. 耳针疗法

Prescription: Hunger Point (External Nose) ($TG_{1,2i}$), Mouth (CO_1), Esophagus (CO_2), Lung (CO_{14}), Stomach (CO_4), Endocrine (CO_{18}) and Pancreas and gallbladder (CO_{11}).

处方:饥点(外鼻),口,食道,肺,胃,内分泌,胰胆。

Performance: All the acupoints mentioned above are needled with filiform needles once every other day; for embedment of needles and ear pressure with Wangbuliuxingzi (Semen Vaccariae), patients are advised to press themselves three times a day (in hunger, before meal and sleep), each acupoint for 2 - 3 minutes. The two ears are pressed in alternation.

操作:以上诸穴可用毫针刺法,隔日 1 次;耳穴埋针和王不留行籽压耳法,均要求每天在饥时、食前、卧前自行按压 3 次,每穴每次按压 2～3 分钟,两耳交替。

5.8 Neural and mental diseases

第八节 神经、精神系统疾病

5.8.1 Prosopalgia

一、三叉神经痛

[Introduction]

Prosopalgia refers to recurrent, short, paroxysmal, lightning-like, stabbing or burning pain in the trigeminal region. Clinically the second and third branches of trigeminal nerve on one side are often involved. Prosopalgia often occurs among people over 40, especially women. It is either primary or secondary. Clinically primary prosopalgia is usually encountered. The following discussion mainly focuses on primary prosopalgia. This disease pertains to the conception of "facial pain" in TCM. It is usually caused by wind attacking the meridians, or upward adverse flow of liver and stomach fire, or consumption of qi and blood as well as stagnation of the vessels and meridians.

【概述】

本病是在面部三叉神经分布区域内反复发作的、短暂的、阵发性剧痛，呈闪电般的刀割样或烧灼样疼痛。临床以一侧的第二支、第三支发病较多。多发生于 40 岁以上，女性居多。有原发性与继发性之分，临床以原发性多见。本节仅介绍原发性三叉神经痛。本病属中医"面痛"范畴；多因风袭经络，或肝胃之火上逆，或气血亏损、脉络瘀滞而作痛。

[Syndrome differentiation]

1. Wind attacking meridians

Constant severe facial pain like stabbing and burning, accompanied by aversion to wind or sweating, nasal obstruction and running nose, thin and white tongue fur, taut and tense or taut and slippery pulse.

2. Upward adverse flow of liver and stomach fire

Facial pain accompanied by dysphoria and susceptibility to rage, flushed cheeks and excessive eye secretion, dryness and bitter taste in the mouth; yellow urine and constipation, red tongue with yellow fur, taut, rapid and slippery pulse.

【辨证】

1. 风袭经络

面痛阵作，如刺如灼，痛势剧烈，伴见恶风或出汗，鼻塞流涕，舌苔薄白，脉弦紧或弦滑。

2. 肝胃之火上逆

面痛兼见心烦易怒，面赤多眵，口干而苦，尿黄便结，舌红苔黄，脉弦数滑。

3. Consumption of qi and blood as well as stagnation in the vessels and meridians

Lingering illness, moderate pain, spiritual lassitude and fatigue, lusterless complexion, light-colored tongue or with purplish appearance and ecchymoses, thin and weak pulse.

［Treatment］

1. Body acupuncture

Prescription: Hegu (LI 4); Taiyang (EX-HN 5), Cuanzhu (BL 2) and Yangbai (GB 14) for pain of the first branch; Sibai (ST 2), Yingxiang (LI 20) and Quanliao (SI 18) for pain of the second branch; Xiaguan (ST 7), Daying (ST 5) and Jiachengjiang (Ext.) for pain of the third branch.

Modification: For wind attacking the meridians, Waiguan (TE 15) and Fengchi (GB 20) are added; for upward adverse flow of liver and stomach fire, Taichong (LR 3) and Neiting (ST 44) are added; for consumption of qi and blood as well as stagnation in the vessels and meridians, Sanyinjiao (SP 6), Zusanli (ST 36) and Geshu (BL 17) are added.

Performance: Local selection of acupoints is made according to the pathological conditions. Twirling and rotating or mild reinforcing and reducing needling techniques are used. Hegu (LI 4) is needled with reducing needling technique; Sanyinjiao (SP 6) and Zusanli (ST 36) are needled with reinforcing needling technique with the addition of moxibustion; Geshu (BL 17) is needled with mild reinforcing and reducing needling techniques. The manipulative techniques for the local acupoints should be mild, while the manipulative techniques for the distal acupoints should be drastic. The needles are retained for 30 minutes or for 1 hour for severe cases and manipulated several times at intervals according to the pathological

3. 气血亏损、脉络瘀滞

病久不愈，痛势较缓，神疲乏力，面色无华，舌淡，或有紫气、瘀点，脉细弱。

【治疗】

1. 体针疗法

处方：主穴：合谷。第一支痛，太阳，攒竹，阳白；第二支痛，四白，迎香，颧髎；第三支痛，下关，大迎，夹承浆。

随证配穴：风袭经络证，加外关、风池。肝胃之火上逆证，加太冲、内庭。气血亏损、脉络瘀滞证，加三阴交、足三里、膈俞。

操作：局部用穴，可据病情适当精简，用捻转泻法或平补平泻法。合谷用泻法；三阴交、足三里用补法，可加灸；膈俞用平补平泻法。局部诸穴手法宜轻，远端穴位手法可重。留针 30 分钟，痛势剧烈者可延长到 1 小时；留针期间可依病情间歇行针数次。每日治疗 1 次；病久体虚者，隔日治疗 1 次。

conditions. The needling is done once a day or once every other day for patients with chronic disease or weak constitution.

2. Ear acupuncture

Prescription: Forehead (AT_1), Mandible (LO_3), Ear Shenmen (TF_4), Cheeks ($LO_{5,\ 6i}$) and Sympathetic (AH_{6a}).

Performance: Each time 2 - 3 acupoints are selected and needled with strong stimulation. The needles are retained for 30 minutes. Or Wangbuliuxingzi (Semen Vaccariae) is used for ear pressure on both ears in alternation. The patients are advised to press themselves 3 - 4 times a day and 2 - 3 minutes each time.

2. 耳针疗法

处方：额，颌，神门，面颊，交感。

操作：每次取 2～3 穴，强刺激，留针 30 分钟。或用王不留行籽压耳，左右耳交替使用，嘱病人每日自行按压 3～4 次，每次 2～3 分钟。

5. 8. 2 Peripheral facial paralysis

[**Introduction**]

Peripheral facial paralysis is due to acute and non-suppurating inflammation in stylomastoid foramen, marked by sudden onset in the morning with the manifestations of stiffness, numbness and looseness of the face, enlargement of palpebral fissure, deviation of the mouth to the healthy side, disappearance of wrinkles on the forehead, flattening of the nasolabial groove and inability to draw eyebrows, frown, close eyes, show teeth, bulge cheeks and pout lips. In some patients pain appears behind the ear and in the face in the early stage. It is similar to distortion of face in TCM. It is mainly caused by wind attacking the meridians in the face, leading to obstruction of meridian qi, malnutrition of tendons and flaccidity of muscles.

[**Syndrome differentiation**]

1. Wind attacking superficies

Sudden distortion of face, numbness of face, or pain behind the ear, aversion to cold and fever, thin and white

二、周围性面瘫

【**概述**】

本病为茎乳突孔内急性非化脓性炎症所致的周围性面神经麻痹。临床表现为起病突然，多在晨起时发现病侧面部板滞、麻木、松弛，眼裂增大，口角歪向健侧，额纹消失，鼻唇沟平坦，不能蹙额、皱眉、闭目、露齿、鼓腮、撅嘴等。部分病人初起时有耳后、面部疼痛等症。中医称为“口僻”、“口眼㖞斜”。主要由于风邪乘虚侵袭面部经络，经气阻滞，经筋失养、肌肉不收而致。

【**辨证**】

1. 风邪外袭

突然口眼㖞斜，面部板滞麻木，或见耳后疼痛，恶寒发

tongue fur, floating and tense or floating and rapid pulse.

2. Insufficiency of qi and blood as well as obstruction of pathogenic factors in the vessels and meridians

Prolonged duration of illness, distortion of face, stiffness of face, even spasm of face, or difficulty in opening eyes, light-colored tongue and thin pulse.

[**Treatment**]

1. Body acupuncture

Prescription: Fengchi (GB 20), Jiache (ST 6), Dicang (ST 4), Hegu (LI 4) and Taichong (LR 3).

Modification: For pain behind ear: Yifeng (TE 17) is added; for inability to close eyes, Yangbai (GB 14) and Cuanzhu (BL 2) are added; for flattening of nasolabial groove, Yingxiang (LI 20) is added; for deviation of nasolabial groove, Shuigou (GV 26) is added; for deviation of mentolabial groove, Chengjiang (CV 24) is added; for prolonged duration of illness, Zusanli (ST 36) is added.

Performance: Jiache (ST 6) and Dicang (ST 4) are needled horizontally toward each other; Yangbai (GB 14) is needled horizontally downward. The acupoints on the face are needled with mild reinforcing and reducing needling techniques; Fengchi (GB 20) is needled with rotating and twirling techniques; Hegu (LI 4) and Taichong (LR 3) are needled with reducing techniques; Zusanli (ST 36) is needled with reinforcing technique with the addition of moxibustion. The needling technique in the early stage should be mild.

2. Electro-acupuncture

Prescription: Jiache (ST 6), Dicang (ST 4), Yangbai (GB 14) and Sibai (ST 2).

Performance: Electricity is attached to the needles for 10 minutes when the acupoints mentioned above are needled till needling sensation is felt. The frequency of

热,苔薄白,脉浮紧或浮数。

2. 气血不足,邪阻脉络

病延日久,口眼㖞斜,面部板滞,甚或面肌抽搐,或闭目难睁,舌淡,脉细。

【治疗】

1. 体针疗法

处方:风池,颊车,地仓,合谷,太冲。

随证配穴:耳后疼痛者,加翳风;目不能合,加阳白、攒竹;鼻唇沟平坦,加迎香;人中沟歪斜,加水沟;颏唇沟歪斜,加承浆。病久者,加足三里。

操作:颊车、地仓两穴相互向对方平刺;阳白向下平刺。面部诸穴用平补平泻法;风池用捻转泻法;合谷、太冲用泻法。足三里用补法,加灸。病初起针刺手法宜轻。

2. 电针疗法

处方:颊车,地仓,阳白,四白。

操作:上述诸穴针刺得气后,通以脉冲电流约10分钟,以面部肌肉微见跳动为宜。

stimulation is monitored to mild jerk of the facial muscles. The needling is done once a day or once every other day.

每日或隔日1次。

5.8.3 Sciatica

三、坐骨神经痛

[**Introduction**]

Sciatica is marked by pain radiating to the foot from lumbar region, buttocks, posterior side of the thigh and lateral side of the shank. The pain is usually unilateral and will be aggravated when the waist is bent or the lower limbs are moved. The causes of sciatica are various. Clinically it is divided into primary and secondary types. The secondary type is further classified into root and trunk types. Sciatica pertains to the conceptions of obstructive syndrome, lumbago and pain of loins and legs in TCM. It is mainly caused by exogenous pathogenic wind, cold and dampness that obstruct meridians; or by asthenia of kidney qi and malnutrition of meridians; or by trauma, sprain, contusion and stagnation of qi and blood in meridians.

【**概述**】

是指在坐骨神经通路及其分布区内的疼痛。临床表现为疼痛由腰部经臀部、大腿后侧、小腿后外侧向足部放散,多为一侧的疼痛,弯腰或活动下肢时加重。可由多种原因所致。临床分为原发性和继发性两类,后者按受损部位又可分为根性和干性两种。本症属中医的"痹证"、"腰痛"、"腰腿痛"等范畴。主要由感受风寒湿邪,经络闭阻;或肾气虚损,经络失养;或外伤闪挫,经络气血瘀滞,而致腰腿疼痛。

[**Syndrome differentiation**]

【**辨证**】

1. Obstruction by cold-dampness

1. 寒湿痹阻

Frequent attack after invasion of cold-dampness, pain and heaviness of loins and legs, inflexibility, subjective cold sensation in the affected region, aggravation in rainy and cold weather, white or white and greasy tongue fur, deep pulse.

多发于感受寒湿之后,腰腿疼痛重着,屈伸不便,自觉患部寒凉,每遇阴雨寒冷病势加重。苔白或白腻,脉沉。

2. Asthenia of kidney qi

2. 肾气虚损

Slow onset, lingering duration, recurrence, aching pain in the loins, aggravation after work, weakness of waist and legs, pale complexion, light-colored tongue, deep and thin pulse.

起病缓慢,日久不愈,反复发作,腰部酸痛,遇劳则重,腰腿乏力,面色不华。舌淡,脉沉细。

3. Stagnation of qi and blood

3. 气血瘀滞

Traumatic injury history of waist, stabbing pain in the

多有腰部外伤史,腰腿疼

waist and legs, aggravation in movement, purplish tongue, taut or unsmooth pulse.

痛如刺,活动则痛甚,舌质紫暗,脉弦或涩。

[**Treatment**]

【治疗】

1. Body acupuncture

1. 体针疗法

Prescription: 3 - 5 lumbar Jiaji (EX-B 2), Ashi point, Huantiao (GB 30) and Yanglingquan (GB 34).

处方:腰3～5夹脊,阿是穴,环跳,阳陵泉。

Modification: For obstruction by cold-dampness, Yaoyangguan (GV 3), Dachangshu (BL 25), Zhibian (BL 54), Chengfu (BL 36), Chengshan (BL 57), Feiyang (BL 58) and Kunlun (BL 60) are added; for asthenia of kidney qi, Shenshu (BL 23), Zusanli (ST 36) and Dazhong (KI 4) are added; for stagnation of qi and blood, Shuigou (GV 26), Weizhong (BL 40) and Geshu (BL 17) are added.

随证配穴:寒湿痹阻,加腰阳关、大肠俞、秩边、承扶、承山、飞扬、昆仑。肾气虚损,加肾俞、足三里、大钟。气血瘀滞,加水沟、委中、膈俞。

Performance: Each time 4 - 9 acupoints are selected according to the pathological conditions. For the treatment of cold-dampness, reducing needling technique, warmed needling or moxibustion with moxa roll are used with the addition of cupping; for the treatment of kidney asthenia, reinforcing needling technique, warmed needling or moxibustion with moxa cone are used; for the treatment of stagnation, bloodletting is done on Weizhong (BL 40) or on the collaterals around.

操作:根据病情,每次选用4～9穴。寒湿者,针用泻法,温针灸或艾条灸,并可加拔火罐;肾虚者,针用补法,温针灸或艾炷灸;有瘀滞者,用泻法,在委中穴及其附近的瘀阻络脉点刺出血。

2. Electro-acupuncture

2. 电针疗法

Prescription: Lumbar Jiaji (EX-B 2), Yanglingquan (GB 34) and Weizhong (BL 40).

处方:腰部夹脊穴,阳陵泉,委中。

Performance: After needling sensation is felt, impulse current is attached to the needles for 10 - 15 minutes, once a day.

操作:针刺得气后,通以脉冲电流10～15分钟,每日1次。

5.8.4 Intercostal neuralgia

四、肋间神经痛

[**Introduction**]

【概述】

Intercostal neuralgia is marked by puncturing or lightning pain in the region with the distribution of

肋间神经痛是指一个或几个肋间部的疼痛。其表现

intercostal nerves. It may be worsened by laughing, sneezing or deep breath. In severe cases, pain may radiate to the shoulder and back. Intercostal neuralgia is usually secondary, primary case is rare. This syndrome pertains to pain in rib-side in TCM. It is usually caused by stagnation of liver qi, damp-heat in the liver and gallbladder, obstruction of blood stasis and insufficiency of blood in the liver and kidney that lead to obstruction or malnutrition of the liver and gallbladder meridians.

为沿病变的肋间神经分布区出现针刺样或闪电样疼痛，可因嬉笑、喷嚏、深呼吸而加重，痛甚者可向同侧肩背部放射。原发性者较少，继发性者多见。本症属中医“胁痛”范围，多由肝气郁结、肝胆湿热、瘀血阻滞、肝肾阴血不足等，致肝胆经络受阻或失养而发为胁痛。

[Syndrome differentiation]

【辨证】

1. Liver depression and qi stagnation

Distending pain in the rib-side and hypochondria, oppression and discomfort in the chest, anorexia, bitter taste in the mouth, aggravation with depression and rage, thin and white or yellow tongue fur, taut pulse.

1. 肝郁气滞

胁肋胀痛，胸闷不舒，食欲不振，口苦，郁怒则症状加重，苔薄白或黄，脉弦。

2. Obstruction of collaterals by blood stasis

Fixed stabbing pain in the rib-side, or caused by sprain, contusion and falling with purplish tongue and unsmooth pulse.

2. 瘀血阻络

胁痛如刺，痛处不移，或由闪挫跌扑而起，舌质紫暗，脉涩。

3. Insufficiency of blood

Vague hypochondriac pain, dry mouth and dysphoria, dizziness, red tongue with scanty fur, thin and rapid pulse.

3. 阴血不足

胁痛隐隐，口干心烦，头昏目眩，舌红少苔，脉细数。

[Treatment]

【治疗】

1. Body acupuncture

Prescription: Zhigou (TE 6) and Yanglingquan (GB 34).

Modification: For liver depression and qi stagnation, Qimen (LR 14) and Taichong (LR 3) are added; for obstruction of the collaterals by blood stasis, Geshu (BL 17), Ganshu (BL 18) and Taichong (LR 3) are added; for insufficiency of blood, Ganshu (BL 18), Shenshu (BL 23), Sanyinjiao (SP 6), Zusanli (ST 36) and Xingjian

1. 体针疗法

处方：支沟，阳陵泉。

随证配穴：肝郁气滞，加期门、太冲。瘀血阻络，加膈俞、肝俞、太冲。阴血不足，加肝俞、肾俞、三阴交、足三里、行间。

(LR 2) are added.

Performance: Liver depression and qi stagnation as well as obstruction of the collaterals by blood stasis are sthenia syndromes and should be treated with reducing needling technique; Qimen (LR 14) and Back-Shu acupoints should be needled obliquely with rotating reducing technique or mild reinforcing and reducing techniques; insufficiency of blood pertains to asthenia syndrome and should be treated with reinforcing needling technique; Xingjian (LR 2) and Taichong (LR 3) should be needled with rotating manipulation.

操作：肝郁气滞、瘀血阻络两证为实，针用泻法；期门、背俞要斜刺，用捻转泻法或平补平泻法。阴血不足属虚证，针用补法。行间、太冲宜用捻转法。

2. Ear acupuncture

2. 耳针疗法

Prescription: Chest (AH_{10}), Ear Shenmen (TF_4), Liver (CO_{12}) and Gallbladder (CO_{11}).

处方：胸，神门，肝，胆。

Performance: Moderate and strong stimulation, retention of needles for 15 - 30 minutes.

操作：中、强刺激，留针15～30分钟。

5.8.5 Angioneurotic headache

五、血管神经性头痛

[**Introduction**]

Angioneurotic headache is usually believed to be caused by disturbance of cerebral vessels and nerves and to be related to various active agents in blood. Clinically angioneurotic headache is unilateral and recurrent, often accompanied by nausea, vomiting and premonitory signs. It is usually of family history and frequently seen among women. It is similar to headache and migraine in TCM. The causes are either attack by exogenous pathogenic wind or dysfunction of the liver, spleen and kidney that lead to retention of pathogenic factors in the meridians, or hyperactivity of liver yang, or obstruction by phlegm and stagnation, or failure of qi and blood to nourish the head.

【概述】

血管神经性头痛又称血管性头痛，一般认为是由于脑血管神经功能紊乱所致，与血液中多种血管活性物质有关。临床多表现为偏于一侧的头痛，呈反复发作性，常伴有恶心、呕吐，发作前可有先兆。常有家族史，多见于女性。本病相当于中医的“头痛”、“厥头痛”、“头风”、“偏头痛”等病证。病因有感受外风和肝、脾、肾功能失调两类，致邪客经络，或肝阳上亢，或痰瘀阻滞，或气血不能上荣，发为头痛。

[Syndrome differentiaton]

1. Wind attacking meridians

Frequent severe headache, onset with the attack of cold and wind, pain involving the neck and back, thin and white tongue fur, taut and tense pulse.

2. Hyperactivity of liver yang

Headache, dizziness, occurrence with mental upsets or nervousness, dysphoria and susceptibility to rage, insomnia, flushed cheeks and bitter taste in the mouth, red tongue with yellow fur and taut pulse.

3. Asthenia of both qi and blood

Continuous headache, dizziness, relapse with overstrain, spiritual lassitude and fatigue, pale complexion, light-colored tongue, thin and weak pulse.

4. Interior obstruction of phlegm and turbid substance

Headache, chest oppression, nausea, vomiting of phlegm and drool, white and greasy tongue fur, slippery pulse.

5. Qi stagnation and blood stasis

Prolonged duration, fixed location of pain, prickly pain, or history of traumatic injury of the head, purplish tongue or with ecchymoses, thin and unsmooth pulse.

[Treatment]

1. Body acupuncture

Prescription: Baihui (GV 20) and Taiyang (EX-HN 5).

Modification: For wind attacking meridians, acupoints should be selected according to the location of headache. Yintang (EX-HN 3), Shangxing (GV 23) and Hegu (LI 4) are added for pain in the forehead; Touwei (ST 8), Fengchi (GB 20), Waiguan (TE 15) and Xiaxi (GB 43) are added for pain in the side of the head; Fengchi (GB 20) and Kunlun (BL 60) are added for pain in the

【辨证】

1. 风袭经络

头痛时作,痛势较剧,遇风受寒则发,或痛连项背,苔薄白,脉弦紧。

2. 肝阳上亢

头痛目眩,每因情志不舒或精神紧张而发,心烦易怒,失眠,面赤口苦,舌红苔黄,脉弦。

3. 气血两虚

头痛绵绵,头晕目眩,遇劳则发,神疲乏力,面色无华,舌淡,脉细弱。

4. 痰浊内阻

头痛昏重,胸闷,恶心、呕吐痰涎,苔白腻,脉滑。

5. 气滞血瘀

病延日久,痛有定处,痛如针刺,或有头部外伤史,舌质紫暗,或有瘀点,脉细涩。

【治疗】

1. 体针疗法

处方:百会,太阳。

随证配穴:风袭经络证,按头痛部位配穴,前额痛,加印堂、上星、合谷;侧头痛,加头维、风池、外关、侠溪;后头痛,加风池、昆仑;头顶痛,加风池、太冲。肝阳上亢,加风池、行间。气血两虚,加气海、

back of the head; Fengchi (GB 20) and Taichong (LR 3) are added for pain in the vertex of the head; for hyperactivity of liver yang, Fengchi (GB 20) and Xingjian (LR 2) are added; for asthenia of both qi and blood, Qihai (CV 6), Zusanli (ST 36), Pishu (BL 20) and Shenshu (BL 23) are added; for interior obstruction of phlegm and turbid substance, Fenglong (ST 40) and Neiguan (PC 6) are added; for qi stagnation and blood stasis, Fengchi (GB 20), Hegu (LI 4), Taichong (LR 3), Sanyinjiao (SP 6) and Geshu (BL 17) are added.

足三里、脾俞、肾俞。痰浊内阻,加丰隆、内关。气滞血瘀,加风池、合谷、太冲、三阴交、膈俞。

Performance: Each time 4 - 6 acupoints are selected according to the pathological conditions. For the treatment of asthenia of both qi and blood, reinforcing needling technique and moxibustion are used. The rest syndromes are needled with reducing or mild reinforcing and reducing needling techniques. For the treatment of blood stasis, Taiyang (EX - HN 5) is pricked for bloodletting.

操作:随证每次选用4~6穴。气血两虚证予补法并灸,其余诸证用泻法或平补平泻法,瘀血者可点刺太阳出血。

2. Ear acupuncture

2. 耳针疗法

Prescription: Subcortical (AT_4), Occipital (AT_3), Forehead (AT_1), Temple (AT_2), Liver (CO_{12}) and Gallbladder (CO_{11}).

处方:皮质下,枕,神门,额,颞,肝,胆。

Performance: Each time 3 - 4 acupoints are selected and the needles are retained for 30 minutes. Or Wangbu liuxingzi (Semen Vaccariae) is used for ear pressure.

操作:每次选3~4穴,留针30分钟。或用王不留行籽压耳法。

5.8.6 Sequela of apoplexy

六、中风后遗症

[**Introduction**]

【概述】

Sequela of apoplexy refers to paralysis of limbs, distortion of face and difficulty in speaking after the attack of acute cerebrovascular disease, similar to wind stroke and paralysis in TCM. It is caused by non-restoration of the visceral functions, retention of phlegm and blood stasis in the meridians as well as abnormal flow of meridian qi.

中风后遗症是指由急性脑血管疾患后遗的肢体瘫痪,口眼歪斜,言语不利等症。属中医的"中风"、"偏枯"、"半身不遂"等范畴。是由脏腑功能尚未复常,痰浊、瘀血阻滞经络,经气运行失常所致。

[Syndrome differentiation]

Paralysis of limbs on one side, accompanied by numbness or pain or susceptibility to sweating, distortion of face, stiffness of tongue and difficulty in speaking and swallowing.

【辨证】

多为一侧肢体瘫痪，伴有麻木或疼痛或易出汗，口眼歪斜，舌强语謇，吞咽困难等。

[Treatment]

1. Body acupuncture

Prescription: Baihui (GV 20), Hegu (LI 4) and Taichong (LR 3).

Modification: For paralysis of upper limbs, Jianyu (LI 15), Quchi (LI 11), Shousanli (LI 10) and Waiguan (TE 15) are added; for paralysis of lower limbs, Huantiao (GB 30), Zusanli (ST 36), Yanglingquan (GB 34), Fenglong (ST 40), Xuanzhong (GB 39) and Kunlun (BL 60) are added; for distortion of face, Jiache (ST 6), Dicang (ST 4), Yangbai (GB 14), Cuanzhu (BL 2) are added; for stiffness of tongue, Lianquan (CV 23) and Tongli (HT 5) are added; for difficulty in swallowing, Lianquan (CV 23) and Fengchi (GB 20) are added.

Performance: The acupoints are selected and needled according to the pathological conditions. Usually mild reinforcing and reducing needling techniques are used. The acupoints on the four limbs are needled with the addition of moxibustion. Jiache (ST 6) and Dicang (ST 4) are needled with the needles pointing to each other. Lianquan (CV 23) is needled with the needle pointing to the root of the tongue. Fengchi (GB 20) is needled with rotating and twirling manipulations.

【治疗】

1. 体针疗法

处方：百会，合谷，太冲。

随证配穴：上肢瘫痪，加肩髃、曲池、手三里、外关。下肢瘫痪，加环跳、足三里、阳陵泉、丰隆、悬钟、昆仑。口眼歪斜，加颊车、地仓、阳白、攒竹。舌强，加廉泉、通里。吞咽困难，加廉泉、风池。

操作：视病情所需，选穴针刺，宜用平补平泻法。四肢腧穴可加灸法。颊车、地仓相互对刺。廉泉向舌根刺。风池行捻转法。

2. Scalp acupuncture

Prescription: Motor zone, sensory zone, zone of pedal movement and sensation and lingual zone on the opposite side.

Performance: The needles are inserted 0.5 - 1 cun with intermittent manipulation. The needles are retained

2. 头针疗法

处方：对侧的运动区，感觉区，足运感区，语言区。

操作：平刺 0.5～1 寸，间歇捻针，留针 30 分钟。也可

for 30 minutes. Impulse current can be attached to the needles with moderate and strong stimulation for 30 minutes.

通以脉冲电流,中、强刺激,留针30分钟。

5.8.7 Insomnia

[Introduction]

Insomnia refers to inability to have normal sleep, marked by difficulty to sleep, or easiness to wake up, or inability to sleep after waking up, or shallow sleep, keeping awake all night. Insomnia often occurs together with headache, dizziness, palpitation and amnesia. It is usually caused by anxiety, overstrain, emotional upsets, weakness and prolonged duration of illness as well as improper diet that lead to dysfunction of the heart, liver, spleen and kidney as well as insufficiency of blood. Insomnia is mainly seen in neurosis in modern medicine.

[Syndrome differentiation]

1. Exuberance of fire in the heart and liver

Dreaminess and easiness to wake up, dysphoria and susceptibility to rage, dizziness, distension or pain in the head, distending pain in the chest, bitter taste in the mouth, thirst, yellow urine and dry feces, red tongue with yellow fur, taut and rapid pulse.

2. Phlegm-heat disturbing heart

Dysphoria and insomnia, dizziness and heaviness of the head, fullness, oppression or pain in the chest and epigastrium, or vomiting of thick phlegm, bitter taste and sticky sensation in the mouth, red tongue with yellow and greasy fur, slippery and rapid pulse.

3. Qi stagnation and blood stasis

Prolonged insomnia, mental depression, oppression and pain in the chest, belching, grayish complexion,

七、失眠

【概述】

失眠又称不寐,是指经常不能获得正常睡眠为特征的一种病证。临床表现为难以入眠,或易醒,或醒后不能再寐,或时寐时醒,甚或整夜不能入眠。常与头痛、眩晕、心悸、健忘等证同时出现。多由思虑劳倦、情志不调、体虚久病、饮食不节等原因,使心、肝、脾、肾功能失调,阴血不足,影响心神而致病。本证主要见于现代医学的"神经官能症"。

【辨证】

1. 心肝火旺

多梦易醒,心烦易怒,头目昏胀或痛,胸胁胀痛,口苦口渴,尿黄便结,舌红苔黄,脉弦而数。

2. 痰热扰心

心烦不寐,头昏而重,胸脘痞闷或疼痛,或咳吐稠痰,口苦而粘,舌红,苔黄腻,脉滑数。

3. 气滞血瘀

失眠日久不愈,精神抑郁,心胸闷痛,嗳气,面色发

purplish tongue and unsmooth pulse.

暗，唇舌紫暗，脉涩。

4. Asthenia of both heart and spleen

4. 心脾两虚

Difficulty to sleep, dreaminess and easiness to wake up, palpitation and amnesia, spiritual lassitude and fatigue, anorexia, pale complexion, light-colored tongue with thin fur, thin and weak pulse.

难以入眠，多梦易醒，心悸健忘，神疲乏力，食欲不振，面色不华，舌淡苔薄，脉细弱。

5. Disharmony between heart and kidney

5. 心肾不交

Dyphoria and insomnia, dizziness and tinnitus, feverish sensation in the palms, soles and chest, dry mouth with scanty fluid, aching and weakness of loins and knees, or palpitation, amnesia, seminal emission, red tongue, thin and rapid pulse.

心烦不寐，头晕耳鸣，五心烦热，口干津少，腰膝酸软，或有心悸，健忘，遗精，舌红，脉细数。

[**Treatment**]

【治疗】

1. Body acupuncture

1. 体针疗法

Prescription: Shenmen (HT 7) and Sanyinjiao (SP 6).

处方：神门，三阴交。

Modification: For exuberance of heart and liver fire: Fengchi (GB 20), Jianshi (PC 5), Laogong (PC 8) and Xingjian (LR 2) are added; for phlegm-fire disturbing the heart, Fengchi (GB 20), Neiguan (PC 6), Zusanli (ST 36), Fenglong (ST 40) and Lidui (ST 45) are added; for qi stagnation and blood stasis, Geshu (BL 17), Jueyinshu (BL 14), Neiguan (PC 6) and Taichong (LR 3) are added; for asthenia of both the heart and spleen, Baihui (GV 20), Xinshu (BL 15), Pishu (BL 20) and Zusanli (ST 36) are added; for disharmony between the heart and kidney, Xinshu (BL 15), Shenshu (BL 23) and Taixi (KI 3) are added.

随证配穴：心肝火旺，加风池、间使、劳宫、行间。痰热扰心，加风池、内关、足三里、丰隆、厉兑。气滞血瘀，加膈俞、厥阴俞、内关、太冲。心脾两虚，加百会、心俞、脾俞、足三里。心肾不交，加心俞、肾俞、太溪。

Performance: Each time 3～5 acupoints are selected. For exuberant liver-fire and heart-fire, phlegm-heat attacking the heart, qi stagnation and blood stasis, reducing techniques are used; for asthenia of both the heart and the spleen, reinforcing techniques should be used with moxibustion applied to Back-Shu acupoints; for disharmony be-

操作：每次随证选用 3～5 穴。心肝火旺，痰热扰心、气滞血瘀等实证，针用泻法；心脾两虚，针用补法，背俞加灸。心肾不交证，神门用捻转泻法，余穴用补法。

tween the heart and the kidney, twirling-rotating techniques for reducing purpose are used for needling Shenmen (HT 7), reinforcing techniques are used for needling other acupoints.

2. Ear acupuncture

Prescription: Ear Shenmen (TF_4), Heart (CO_{15}), Kidney (CO_{10}), Spleen (CO_{13}) and Subcortex (AT_4).

Performance: Each time 2 - 3 points are selected and needled with moderate stimulation and retained for 20 minutes. On Wangbuliuxingzi (Semen Vaccariae) is used for ear-point pressing and pressed 2 - 3 minutes before sleep.

2. 耳针疗法

处方：神门，心，肾，脾，皮质下。

操作：每次取2～3穴，中等刺激，留针20分钟。或用王不留行籽压耳法，于睡前按压2～3分钟。

5.8.8 Globus hystericus

[Introduction]

Globus hystericus refers to abnormal sensation in the throat as if a plum pit or sputum stuck in the throat. However, examination of the throat finds no abnormal changes. It is similar to pharyngeal neurosis or globus hystericus in modern medicine. This problem is usually caused by mental depression, failure of the liver qi to disperse and convey, unsmooth flow of qi and abnormal distribution of body fluid turning into phlegm that stucks in the throat.

[Syndrome differentiation]

It is marked by obstructive sensation in the throat, difficulty to spit and swallow, no pain, normal intake of food, aggravation or alleviation with the changes of emotions, accompanied by mental depression, excessive anxiety, suspicion, migratory pain in the chest, frequent belching, or anorexia, unsmooth defecation, bulgy tongue, thin, white and greasy tongue fur, taut and slippery pulse.

[Treatment]

1. Body acupuncture

Prescription: Neiguan (PC 6), Tanzhong (CV 17),

八、梅核气

【概述】

梅核气是一种咽喉中感觉异常，如有梅核或痰涎塞于咽喉，咽部检查无明显异常的一种病证。相当于现代医学的咽部神经官能症或癔症等病。本病的发生多因情志抑郁，肝失疏泄，气机运行不畅，津液输布失常，聚而成痰，痰气互结于咽喉所致。

【辨证】

咽中如有物阻，吐之不出，咽之不下，无疼痛感，不妨碍进食，常随情绪波动加重或减轻，并伴精神抑郁，过虑多疑，胸胁窜痛，嗳气频作，或食欲不振，大便不畅，舌偏胖，苔薄白腻，脉弦滑。

【治疗】

1. 体针疗法

处方：内关，膻中，丰隆，

Fenglong (ST 40) and Sanyinjiao (SP 6).

三阴交。

Performance: For evident abnormal sensation in the throat, Tiantu (CV 22) is added; for mental depression and migratory pain in the chest and rib-side, Shenmen (HT 7) and Taichong (LR 3) are added; for anorexia and unsmooth defecation, Zusanli (ST 36) is added.

随证配穴：咽部异常感明显，加天突。精神抑郁，胸胁窜痛者，加神门、太冲。食欲不振，大便不畅，加足三里。

Performance: Mild reinforcing and reducing needling techniques are used. Tiantu (CV 22) is needled 0.2 cun vertically first, then the point of the needle is turned downward and slowly inserted 0.5 - 1 cun along the posterior border of the sternum. Tanzhong (CV 17) is needled horizontally 0.5 cun downward.

操作：针刺用平补平泻法。刺天突穴时先直刺约0.2寸，再将针尖转向下方，紧靠胸骨柄后缘慢慢刺入0.5～1寸。膻中向下平刺0.5寸。

2. Ear acupuncture

2. 耳针疗法

Prescription: Ear Shenmen (TF_4), Subcortex (AT_4), Heart (CO_{15}).

处方：神门，皮质下，心。

Performance: Wangbuliuxingzi (Semen Vaccariae) is used for ear pressure. The acupoints are pressed twice or 3 times a day.

操作：以王不留行籽压耳，每日按压2～3次。

5.8.9 Schizophrenia

九、精神分裂症

[**Introduction**]

【概述】

Schizophrenia is clinically marked by incoordination in thinking, perception, sentiment, consciousness and behavior as well as adaptation to environment. The main manifestations are hallucination, illusion, incoherency in thinking, indifference or hyperaffectivity, excitation or stupor and lack of self-awareness. Schizophrenia is similar to mania in TCM. It is usually caused by long-term mental depression, rage and fright that lead to stagnation of liver qi and transformation of fire from qi stagnation; or by production of phlegm from qi stagnation and obstruction by interaction of phlegm and qi; or by prolonged qi stagnation and blood stasis in the vessels; or by impairment of both the heart and spleen and insufficiency of qi and blood that

精神分裂症是一种常见的精神病。临床以思维、知觉、情感、意识、行为及与环境相互之间不协调为主要特征。表现为幻觉、错觉，妄想，思维过程缺乏连贯性、逻辑性，情感淡漠或过度高涨，兴奋躁动或木僵，缺乏自知力等。相当于中医的“癫狂”证。主要因为长期精神抑郁、恼怒、惊恐，致使肝气郁结，气郁化火；或气郁生痰，痰气交阻；或气郁日久，血脉瘀阻；或心脾两伤，

affect cardiac spirit.

气血不足,影响心神而致病。

［Syndrome differentiation］

【辨证】

1. Exuberance of heart and liver fire

Excitation, mania, keeping awake all night, flushed cheeks, glowering eyes, polylogia, coprolalia, abnormal increase of strength, dry feces, yellow and brown urine, tongue with red tip and margins, thin, yellow and dry tongue fur, taut and rapid pulse.

1. 心肝火旺

兴奋躁动,狂乱无知,彻夜不眠,面红目赤,两目怒视,多言叫骂,力大倍常,大便干结,小便黄赤,舌边尖红赤,苔薄黄而干,脉弦数。

2. Stagnation of phlegm and qi

Mental depression, indifference, dementia, dull eyes, grayish and yellowish or dropsy complexion, divagation, anorexia, bulgy tongue, white and greasy tongue fur, taut and slippery pulse.

2. 痰气郁结

精神抑郁,淡漠,神志痴呆,目光呆滞,面色灰黄或虚浮,语无伦次,不思饮食,舌胖大,苔白腻,脉弦滑。

3. Qi stagnation and blood stasis

Long-term mania, mental instability, susceptibility to emotional changes, delusion and insomnia, dull complexion, dry skin, dry feces, purplish tongue, deep and unsmooth pulse.

3. 气滞血瘀

癫狂日久,情绪不稳,哭笑无常,妄想失眠,面色晦滞,皮肤干燥,大便干结,舌紫黯,脉沉涩。

4. Asthenia of both the heart and spleen

Trance, depression, palpitation and susceptibility to fright, susceptibility to sorrow, preference for quietness and inactivity, indifference and silence, lusterless complexion, reduced appetite, light-colored tongue with thin fur, thin, soft and weak pulse.

4. 心脾两虚

精神恍惚,抑郁,心悸易惊,善悲欲哭,喜静懒动,淡漠不语,面色无华,饮食减少,舌淡,苔薄,脉细软无力。

［Treatment］

【治疗】

1. Body acupuncture

Prescription: Baihui (GV 20), Daling (PC 7) and Fenglong (ST 40).

1. 体针疗法

处方:百会,大陵,丰隆。

Modification: For exuberance of heart and liver fire, Shuigou (GV 26), Shaoshang (LU 11), Laogong (PC 8), Dazhui (GV 14) and Yinbai (SP 1) are added; for stagnation of phlegm and qi, Shenmen (HT 7), Jianshi (PC 5) and Tanzhong (CV 17) are added; for stagnation of qi and stasis of blood, Hegu (LI 4), Quchi (LI 11) and Taichong

随证配穴:心肝火旺,加水沟、少商、劳宫、大椎、隐白。痰气郁结,加神门、间使、膻中。气滞血瘀,加合谷、曲池、太冲。心脾两虚,加心俞、脾俞、足三里、三阴交。

(LR 3) are added; for asthenia of both the heart and spleen, Xinshu (BL 15), Pishu (BL 20), Zusanli (ST 36) and Sanyinjiao (SP 6) are added.

Performance: Asthenia of both the heart and spleen can be treated with reinforcing needling technique. Back-Shu acupoints can be moxibusted after needling. The rest of the acupoints can be needled with reducing or mild reinforcing and reducing needling techniques. Shaoshang (LU 11) and Yinbai (SP 1) can be punctured to let out blood. The needles are retained for about 30 - 40 minutes and manipulated at intervals. Cares should be taken to avoid bending and breaking the needles.

操作：心脾两虚证施以补法，背俞可加用灸法。其余诸证采用泻法或平补平泻法。少商、隐白可刺出血。留针时间适当延长，约 30～40 分钟，间歇行针。治疗时注意防止弯针、断针等意外事故的发生。

2. Electro-acupuncture

2. 电针疗法

Prescription: Each time 1 - 2 pairs of acupoints mentioned are selected.

处方：每次在以上腧穴中选用 1～2 对。

Performance: After the needling sensation is felt, impulse current is attached to the needles. The needles are retained for 20 minutes. Such a treatment is given once a day.

操作：针刺得气后，通以脉冲电流，留针 20 分钟，每日 1 次。

5.9 Diseases of locomotor system

第九节 运动系统疾病

5.9.1 Cervical spondylopathy

一、颈椎病

[**Introduction**]

Cervical spondylopathy, also known as cervical vertebral syndrome, is a syndrome due to long-term sprain, osseous hyperplasia, protrusion of intervetebral disc and thickening of ligament that compress the cervical spinal cord, nerve roots and blood circulation. The clinical manifestations are pain in the head, neck, shoulder, arm and chest. This disease pertains to obstructive syndrome in TCM. It is usually caused by invasion of pathogenic wind,

【概述】

颈椎病又称为颈椎综合征，是因颈椎长期劳损、骨质增生、椎间盘突出、韧带增厚，压迫颈脊髓、神经根和血液循环功能障碍所致的综合征。临床主要表现为头颈、肩臂、手及胸部的疼痛。本病主要属中医的"痹证"范畴，由于风

cold and dampness into the meridians, blocking the flow of qi and blood; or by asthenia of the liver and kidney as well as insufficiency of qi and blood in the aged, leading to malnutrition of the tendons; or by impairment of the tendons and vessels due to long-term strain.

寒湿邪侵入经络，闭阻气血；或年老肝肾亏虚，气血不足，筋骨脉络失养；或久劳筋脉受损等，引发本病。

[**Syndrome differentiation**]

【辨证】

1. Exogenous wind-cold attack

1. 外感风寒

Stiffness and pain in the neck or involving the arm and shoulder, cold limbs and numbness of hands, or heaviness sensation, aggravation with wind and cold, accompanied by general aching, thin and white tongue fur, floating and tense pulse.

颈项强痛，或痛连肩臂，肢冷手麻，或觉沉重，受风遇寒加重，伴周身酸痛，苔薄白，脉浮紧。

2. Stagnation of qi and blood

2. 气血瘀滞

Aching, distending pain or prickly pain in the neck, shoulder and arm, or swelling and distension, or pain radiating to the arm, accompanied by dizziness and headache, mental depression, aggravation with nervousness, oppression and pain in the chest, dull tongue, thin and white tongue fur, taut and unsmooth pulse, or deep, thin and unsmooth pulse.

颈项肩臂酸胀疼痛或刺痛，或肿胀，或向手臂放射，伴头昏头痛，精神抑郁紧张时加重，胸闷胸痛，舌暗，苔薄白，脉弦而涩，或沉细涩。

3. Insufficiency of the liver and kidney

3. 肝肾不足

Slow onset, numbness and vague pain in the neck, shoulder and back, prolonged duration, aggravation with overstrain, accompanied by dizziness, blurred vision, tinnitus, deafness, aching and weakness of loins and knees, weakness of lower limbs, tender tongue with thin fur, deep, thin and weak pulse.

起病缓慢，颈项肩背麻木隐痛，日久不愈，劳累后加重，伴眩晕，视力模糊，耳鸣耳聋，腰膝酸软，下肢无力，舌嫩，苔薄，脉沉细无力。

[**Treatment**]

【治疗】

1. Body acupuncture

1. 体针疗法

Prescription: Cervical Jiaji (EX-B 2), Fengchi (GB 20), Dazhui (BL 11) and Ashi acupoints.

处方：颈夹脊，风池，大椎，阿是穴。

Modification: For exogenous wind-cold attack: Hegu (LI 4), Waiguan (TE 15), Fengmen (BL 12) and Jianjing (GB 21) are added; for stagnation of qi and blood,

随证配穴：外感风寒证，配以合谷、外关、风门、肩井。气血瘀滞证，配以合谷、曲池、

Hegu (LI 4), Quchi (LI 11), Jianyu (LI 15), Geshu (BL 17) and Yanglingquan (GB 34) are added; for insufficiency of liver and kidney, Ganshu (BL 18), Shenshu (BL 23), Zusanli (ST 36), Xuanzhong (GB 39) and Taichong (LR 3) are added.

肩髃、膈俞、阳陵泉。肝肾不足证，配以肝俞、肾俞、足三里、悬钟、太冲。

Performance: Reinforcing needling technique is used for the treatment of insufficiency of both the liver and kidney. The rest two syndromes are treated with the reducing needling technique. The acupoints on the neck and back are needled with rotating and twirling manipulations. Moxibustion can be used with the addition of cupping.

操作：肝肾不足证用补法，其他两证用泻法。颈项背部诸穴施以捻转手法。可加用灸法，配合拔火罐。

2. Ear acupuncture

2. 耳针疗法

Prescription: Neck (AH_{12}), Cervical Vertebra (AH_{13}), Shoulder ($SF_{4,5}$), Kidney (CO_{10}) and Ear Shenmen (TF_4).

处方：颈，颈椎，肩，肾，神门。

Performance: Each time 2－3 acupoints are selected and needled with filiform needles and moderate and strong stimulation. The needles are retained for 20－30 minutes. The treatment is given once a day or once every other day. Or Wangbuliuxingzi (Semen Vaccariae) is used for ear point pressing.

操作：每次选用2～3穴，中强刺激，留针20～30分钟，每日或隔日1次。或以王不留行籽压耳。

5. 9. 2 Dysfunction of temporomandibular joint

二、颞颌关节功能紊乱

[Introduction]

Dysfunction of temporomandibular joint is marked by unilateral or bilateral manibular joint pain, aggravation in chewing, joint snap or with frictional noise, limited movement of the mandibular articulation, non-swelling of local skin, chronic duration and recurrence, lingering for several months or several years. This problem is often seen among youngsters and people in the prime of life. It pertains to the conception of cheek pain and lockjaw in TCM. It is usually caused by exogenous wind-cold attack

【概述】

颞颌关节功能紊乱是一种常见的颞颌关节病变。临床主要表现为一侧或双侧颞颌关节处疼痛，咀嚼时加重，关节弹响或有磨擦音，下颌运动受限，局部皮肤不红不肿，并且有慢性和反复发作的特点，常可迁延数月甚至数年。多发于青壮年。属中医“颌

and blockage of the meridians; or by stagnation of qi and blood in the meridians.

痛"、"颊痛"、"口噤不开"等范畴。多为感受风寒，经络闭阻；或气血瘀滞经络所致。

[**Syndrome differentiation**]

Pain, snap or with frictional sound and masticatory dysfunction of unilateral mandible or bilateral mandible joint in closing or opening mouth, accompanied by dizziness, tinnitus and local tenderness.

【辨证】

患者在张口或闭口时，一侧或两侧下颌关节处疼痛、弹响或有摩擦音，咀嚼功能障碍，可伴有头昏耳鸣，局部压痛。

[**Treatment**]

Prescription: Xiaguan (ST 7), Tinggong (SI 19) and Hegu (LI 4).

Modification: For buccal pain, Jiache (ST 6) is added; for pain in auricular region, Yifeng (TE 17) is added; for headache, Taiyang (EX-HN 5) and Fengchi (GB 20) are added.

Performance: Reducing needling technique is used. The acupoints on the head are needled with twirling and rotating techniques. Xiaguan (ST 7) can be moxibusted. Tinggong (SI 19) is located and needled when the mouth is open.

【治疗】

处方：下关，听宫，合谷。

随证配穴：颊部痛，加颊车；耳部痛，加翳风；头痛加太阳、风池。

操作：针用泻法，头面部穴用捻转法。下关穴可予艾条灸。听宫张口取穴进针。

5.9.3 Stiff neck

[**Introduction**]

Stiffness of neck is a commonly encountered damage of cervical soft tissues due to high or low pillow or invasion of wind-cold into the back that prevents the smooth circulation of qi and blood in the meridians. The clinical manifestations are unilateral or bilateral stiffness and pain in the neck as well as restricted movement of the neck due to worsened pain.

[**Syndrome differentiation**]

Stiffness and pain in the neck, aggravation in movement, restricted movement, deviation of the head to the affected side, pain involving the shoulder, back or head,

三、落枕

【概述】

落枕又称颈部伤筋，是临床常见的颈软组织损伤之一。是因睡眠时头部位置过高或过低位，或风寒侵袭项背，使经络气血不畅所致。临床表现为颈部一侧或双侧强痛，转颈活动因痛势加剧而受限。

【辨证】

颈项强痛，动则加剧，活动受限，头部常倾向患侧，痛连肩背或头部。局部有明显

and evident local tenderness.

压痛。

[**Treatment**]

【治疗】

1. Body acupuncture

1. 体针疗法

Prescription: Ashi, Fengchi (GB 20) and Houxi (SI 3).

处方：阿是穴，风池，后溪。

Performance: Reducing needling technique is used and local acupoints also can be moxibusted. When the needle is inserted into Houxi (SI 3), the patient is asked to move the neck. After withdrawal of the needle, cupping is applied to local acupoints.

操作：针用泻法，局部穴可加灸。后溪穴进针后，让病人活动颈部。出针后，可在局部拔火罐。

2. Ear acupuncture

2. 耳针疗法

Prescription: Neck (AH_{12}), Cervical Vertebra (AH_{13}) and Tenderness points.

处方：颈，颈椎，压痛点。

Performance: Strong stimulation is used and the patient is asked to move the neck during the treatment. The needles are retained for 15 - 20 minutes.

操作：强刺激，同时让病人活动颈部，留针 15～20 分钟。

5.9.4 Scapulohumeral periarthritis

四、肩关节周围炎

[**Introduction**]

【概述】

Scapulohumeral periarthritis refers to a kind of soft tissue disorder of the shoulder due to retrograde disease aggravated by long-term sprain and attack of cold or traumatic injury that lead to chronic inflammation of the joint capsule and the soft tissues around the joint, extensive adhesion of the peripheral tissues and restriction of the movement of shoulder joint. It is usually seen among people over 50. Clinical manifestations are aching, heaviness and pain in the shoulder as well as dysfunction of the shoulder in movement. This disease pertains to the conception of obstructive syndrome in TCM. It is caused either by invasion of pathogenic wind, cold and dampness due to asthenia; or by weakness in the aged and malnutrition of tendons and vessels; or by stagnation of qi and blood as well as retention of dampness and phlegm that

肩关节周围炎是一种肩部软组织疾病。由于肩关节退行性病变，加之长期劳损、受寒，或有外伤等原因，使关节囊和关节周围软组织发生慢性炎症反应，周围组织广泛粘连，限制肩关节活动所致。以五十岁左右者多见。临床表现为肩部酸重疼痛和不同程度的肩关节活动障碍。本病属中医的“痹证”范畴，称“肩背痛”、“肩凝”、“漏肩风”、“五十肩”等。多由风寒湿邪乘虚而入；或年老体弱，筋脉失养；或气血凝滞，痰湿留着，

block the meridians, prevent the flow of qi and blood and lead to dysfunction of the tendons and vessels.

皆使经络闭阻,气血不行,经筋失用,发生本病。

[**Syndrome differentiation**]

【辨证】

1. Wind-cold attacking the exterior

1. 风寒外袭

Short duration, pain, aching and heaviness in the shoulder, or pain involving the back and arm, aggravation in the night, restricted movement, alleviation with warmth and aggravation after the attack by wind and cold.

病程较短,肩部疼痛酸重,或痛连背、臂部,入夜为重,活动不利,得温则舒,受风遇寒加重。

2. Retention of pathogenic factors due to asthenia of healthy qi

2. 正虚邪阻

Lingering duration, evident restriction in lifting, abduction and intorsion, or atrophy of local muscles and cold sensation in the arm.

病延日久,上举、外展、内旋活动明显受限,或局部肌肉萎缩,手臂不温。

[**Treatment**]

【治疗】

1. Body acupuncture

1. 体针疗法

Prescription: Jianyu (LI 15), Jianliao (TE 14), Jianqian (Ext.), Quchi (LI 11) and Ashi acupoints.

处方:肩髃,肩髎,肩前,曲池,阿是穴。

Modification: For syndrome of wind-cold attacking the exterior, Jianzhen (SI 9), Jianjing (GB 21), Fengchi (GB 20), Waiguan (TE 15) and Hegu (LI 4) are added; for pain involving the back, Quyuan (SI 13) and Tianzong (SI 11) are added; for pain involving the upper arm, Binao (LI 14) is added; for retention of pathogenic factors due to asthenia, Binao (LI 14), Shousanli (LI 10), Zusanli (ST 36), Yanglingquan (GB 34) and Tiaokou (ST 38) are added.

随证配穴:风寒外袭证,加肩贞、肩井、风池、外关、合谷;痛连背部,加曲垣、天宗;痛连上臂,加臂臑。正虚邪阻证,加臂臑、手三里、足三里、阳陵泉、条口。

Performance: Several acupoints are selected each time according to the pathological conditions. Reducing needling technique is used in treating the syndrome of wind-cold attacking the exterior; retention of pathogenic factors due to asthenia is a syndrome marked by mixture of asthenia and sthenia and should be treated with mild reinforcing and reducing techniques. Zusanli (ST 36) is needled with reinforcing needling technique. Tiaokou (ST

操作:每次依病情选用数穴。风寒外袭证用泻法;正虚邪阻属虚实夹杂证,用平补平泻法。足三里用补法。取患侧条口穴,向承山穴方向刺入,在施手法的同时让病人活动肩关节。加用灸法,可配合拔火罐。

38) located on the affected side is needled with the point of the needle pointing to the direction of Chengshan (BL 57). The patient is asked to move the shoulder joint during the manipulation of the needle. Moxibustion can be used in addition and cupping may be applied for reinforcement of the curative effect.

2. Electro-acupuncture

Prescription: Jianyu (LI 15), Jianliao (TE 14), Jianqian (Ext.), Quchi (LI 11) and Ashi acupoints.

Performance: Each time 1 - 2 acupoints are selected. When needling sensation is felt, impulse current is attached to the needles for 10 minutes. This treatment is given once a day.

3. Ear acupuncture

Prescription: Shoulder ($SF_{4,5}$), Clavicle (SF_6) and Ear Shenmen (TF_4).

Performance: Medium and strong stimulation, retention of the needles for 20 - 30 minutes, once a day.

2. 电针疗法

处方：肩髃，肩髎，肩前，曲池，阿是穴。

操作：每次选用1～2对穴位，针刺得气后，通以脉冲电流10分钟。每日1次。

3. 耳针疗法

处方：肩，锁骨，神门。

操作：中、强刺激，留针20～30分钟。每日1次。

5. 9. 5 External humeral epicondylitis

[**Introduction**]

External humeral epicondylitis is a commonly encountered chronic injury of the elbow due to long-term repeated traction injury of the attaching area of the external humeral epicondyle extensor. The clinical manifestations are pain in the external humeral epicondyle, aggravation in forceful stretching of the wrist to the dorsal side and local tenderness. This problem pertains to the conceptions of elbow sprain and obstructive syndrome in TCM due to strain and invasion of pathogenic wind, cold and dampness that lead to unsmooth circulation of qi and blood in the local meridians.

[**Syndrome differentiation**]

Slow onset, aching pain in the lateral side of the

五、肱骨外上髁炎

【概述】

肱骨外上髁炎，俗称“网球肘”，是常见的肘部慢性损伤。为肱骨外上髁伸肌附着处受到长期反复的牵拉伤所致。临床表现为肱骨外上髁部疼痛，用力向背侧伸腕时疼痛加剧，局部压痛。属中医的“肘劳”、“痹证”范畴。由于劳损、风寒湿邪侵袭等，致局部经络气血不畅而发病。

【辨证】

起病缓慢，肘部外侧酸

elbow radiating to the forearm or shoulder and back, weakness in grasping, aggravation in performing the activities like twisting towel and local tenderness.

痛，可向前臂或肩背放散，握物无力，作拧毛巾等动作时疼痛加剧，局部压痛。

[Treatment]

Prescription: Ashi, Quchi (LI 11), Shousanli (LI 10) and Hegu (LI 4).

Performance: Each time 1 - 2 acupoints on the yangming meridian of the hand are selected and needled with reducing needling technique. Moxibustion can be applied to the local area. The needles are retained for 20 - 30 minutes.

【治疗】

处方：阿是穴，曲池，手三里，合谷。

操作：每次选阿是穴及1～2个手阳明经穴，针用泻法，局部并用灸法，留针20～30分钟。

5.9.6 Thecal cyst

[Introduction]

Thecal cyst usually appears around the joint, especially on the dorsal side of the wrist joint. The main manifestations are painless, hard and small semispheroid lumps. The external membrane of the cyst is fibrous tissue and the internal membrane is white and slippery. The cyst is full of whitish colloidal liquid. Thecal cyst is similar to wrist tendon tumor in TCM due to stagnation of qi, accumulation of fluid into phlegm and coagulation in the meridians.

[Syndrome differentiation]

Local pathological change is semispheroid lumps that are smooth in surface and bear no adhesion with the skin. The smaller ones are the size of soy beans and are hard in texture. The larger ones are the size of dove egges, appears mobile under pressure. There is no pain, only occasional sense of aching, distension and weakness in excessive movement.

[Treatment]

Prescription: Local cyst.

六、腱鞘囊肿

【概述】

腱鞘囊肿为肌腱腱鞘胶样变性的一种疾病。好发于关节周围，以腕关节背侧最为多见。主要表现为无痛性的硬韧的局限性的半球形小肿块。囊肿的外膜为纤维组织，内膜白而光滑，囊内充满白色胶状液体。本病相当于中医的"腕筋瘤"。为气机郁滞，津聚成痰，痰凝经络而成。

【辨证】

病变局部呈一半球形的小肿块，表面光滑，与皮肤无粘连，小者如黄豆大，质地硬韧，大者如鸽蛋大小，按之有囊性波动感，无疼痛，活动过度时或有酸胀无力感。

【治疗】

处方：囊肿局部。

Performance: The thick needle of No. 28 is used to puncture 1 cun vertically from the top of the lump and then puncture obliquely the four sides of the lump with rotating technique. The needle is retained for 15 minutes. When the needle is withdrawn, the needling hole is enlarged by swaying the needle. The needling hole is squeezed to press out colloidal liquid. After needling, the affected part is bandaged with pressure for 3 - 5 days.

操作：用28号粗针，在囊肿顶部直刺入1针，刺破囊壁，并在囊肿周围斜刺4针，行捻转法，留针15分钟，出针时摇大针孔，并加挤压，可见有胶状液体流出。施术后加压包扎3～5日。

5.9.7 Gonitis

[Introduction]

Gonitis is a kind of retrograde disease, usually seen among middle-aged and old people. The clinical manifestations are pain and swelling of the knee joint, aggravation in walking, relief after rest, appearance of frictional sound in movement, stiffness of the joint after long-term sleeping or sitting or standing (which can be relieved gradually after relaxation), mild exudates from the joint cavity in severe cases or even evident swelling due to hemorrhage from the joint cavity. The symptoms in the late stage are restricted movement of the knee joint, disuse atrophy, or even inversion or eversion of the knee. Gonarthritis pertains to the conception of obstructive syndrome in TCM due to insufficiency of liver and kidney, malnutrition of tendons and bones and obstruction of the meridians by pathogenic wind, cold, dampness and heat in the aged; or due to production of phlegm resulting from spleen asthenia and migration of phlegm and dampness in the meridians; or due to long-term stagnation of blood vessels and retention of blood stasis in the joints.

[Syndrome differentiation]

Pain, swelling, aching weakness, unsmoothness of the knees that become aggravated with cold and relieved with warmth; stiffness of the knees after long-term

七、膝骨关节炎

【概述】

膝骨关节炎是膝关节的一种退行性病变。为中老年人的常见多发病。临床主要表现为：膝关节疼痛肿胀，行走时加重，休息后缓解，活动关节时有摩擦音，久卧久坐久站后觉关节僵硬，活动后可逐渐缓解，严重时关节腔中可有少量渗液，甚至关节腔因出血而肿大明显。后期膝关节活动受限，引起废用性肌萎缩，甚至发生膝外翻或内翻畸形。本病属中医的“痹证”、“鹤膝风”范畴。多因中老年后肝肾不足，筋骨失养，风寒湿热等邪痹阻经络；或脾虚生痰，痰湿流注经络关节；或日久血脉瘀滞，瘀血痹阻关节而成。

【辨证】

膝关节疼痛，肿胀，酸软无力，活动不利，遇寒加重，得温则舒，日久关节僵硬，肌肉

duration; muscular atrophy; or accompanied by aching or pain of the waist, vertigo, tinnitus and fatigue.

[Treatment]

1. Body acupuncture

Prescription: Xiyan (EX-LE 5), Heding (EX-LE 2), Xiyangguan (GB 33), Yanglingquan (GB 34) and Ashi acupoints.

Modification: For evident swelling and pain, Liangqiu (ST 34), Xuehai (SP 10) and Yinlingquan (SP 9) are added; for aching and weakness of the waist as well as dizziness and tinnitus, Ganshu (BL 18), Shenshu (BL 23), Zusanli (ST 36) and Sanyinjiao (SP 6) are added.

Performance: The proximal acupoints are needled with reducing needling technique. Ganshu (BL 18), Shenshu (BL 23) and Zusanli (ST 36) are needled with reinforcing needling technique. Moxibustion can be used and cupping is applied for reinforcement of the curative effect.

2. Ear acupuncture

Prescription: Knee (AH_4), Kidney (CO_{10}) and Ear Shenmen (TF_4).

Performance: Medium and strong stimulation, retention of the needles for 20 - 30 minutes. Or Wangbuliuxingzi (Semen Vaccariae) is used for ear acupressure.

5.9.8 Rheumatoid arthritis

[Introduction]

Rheumatoid arthritis is a kind of chronic and general immune disease, clinically marked by pain, swelling, stiffness and deformity of the joints. It usually invades the distal small joints in the early stage and is often migratory. Consequently it involves the wrist, knee, elbow, ankle and shoulder, leading to muscular atrophy around the joints and irregular fever. This disease is seem more

萎缩,或伴见腰酸或痛,头晕耳鸣,乏力。

【治疗】

1. 体针疗法

处方:膝眼,鹤顶,膝阳关,阳陵泉,阿是穴。

随证配穴:肿痛明显者,加梁丘、血海、阴陵泉;腰酸乏力,头晕耳鸣者,加肝俞、肾俞、足三里、三阴交。

操作:近部诸穴用泻法;肝俞、肾俞、足三里等穴用补法。可加灸法,配合拔火罐。

2. 耳针疗法

处方:膝,肾,神门。

操作:中、强刺激,留针20~30分钟。或用王不留行籽压耳。

八、类风湿关节炎

【概述】

类风湿关节炎是一种慢性全身性自身免疫性疾病。临床以关节的疼痛、肿胀、僵硬、变形为特征。初起多侵犯四肢远端小关节,往往是游走性的,继则可影响到腕、膝、肘、踝、肩等大关节。并可引

in women than in men. It pertains to the conceptions of severe and migratory arthralgia and gout in TCM. It is usually caused by weak constitution and invasion of pathogenic wind, cold, dampness and heat into the meridians and joints, hindering the flow of qi and blood; or by dysfunction of the liver in dispersion and conveyance, stagnation of qi and unsmooth circulation of blood. Prolongation of the pathological conditions will lead to asthenia of the liver and kidney, failure of the liver to govern the tendons and the kidney to govern bones as well as infusion of phlegm and blood stasis into the joints, resulting in muscular atrophy and deformity of joints.

起关节附近肌肉萎缩,不规则发热等。女性发病多于男性。本病属中医的"历节风"、"白虎风"、"痛风"等病的范畴。多因体质素虚,风寒湿热之邪乘虚入侵经络、关节,阻碍气血之运行;或肝失疏泄,气机郁滞,血行不畅,而留着关节所致。久则肝肾亏虚,肝不主筋,肾不主骨,痰湿瘀血入于关节,以致肌肉萎缩,关节畸形。

[Syndrome differentiation]

【辨证】

1. Cold-dampness type

1. 寒湿型

Severe pain of joints, swelling and heaviness sensation, numbness of skin, aggravation with cold, preference for warmth, or aversion to cold, thin, white and greasy tongue fur, taut and slippery pulse.

关节疼痛较剧,肿胀沉重,肌肤麻木,遇寒加重,喜得温热,或有恶寒,苔薄白腻,脉弦滑。

2. Damp-heat type

2. 湿热型

Reddish swelling and pain of joints, inflexibility, or fever, thirst, yellow urine, retention of dry feces, yellow and greasy tongue fur, slippery and rapid pulse.

关节红肿热痛,屈伸不利,或有发热,口渴,尿黄,便结,苔黄腻,脉滑数。

[Treatment]

【治疗】

1. Body acupuncture

1. 体针疗法

Prescription: Dazhui (GV 14) and Zusanli (ST 36). Upper limbs: Jianyu (LI 15), Shousanli (LI 10), Quchi (LI 11), Waiguan (TE 15), Hegu (LI 4), Yangxi (LI 5), Yangchi (TE 4), Wangu (SI 4) and Baxie (EX-UE 9). Lower limbs: Huantiao (GB 30), Juliao (GB 29), Liangqiu (ST 34), Xiyan (EX-LE 5), Yanglingquan (GB 34), Ququan (LR 8), Xuanzhong (GB 39), Kunlun (BL 60), Jiexi (ST 41) and Bafeng (EX-LE 10). Neck: Cervical Jiaji (EX-B 2) and Fengchi (GB 20).

处方:大椎,足三里。上肢:肩髃,手三里,曲池,外关,合谷,阳溪,阳池,腕骨,八邪。下肢:环跳,居髎,梁丘,膝眼,阳陵泉,曲泉,悬钟,昆仑,解溪,八风。颈部:颈夹脊,风池。

Modification: For migratory pain, Fengchi (GB 20),

随证配穴:疼痛走窜者,

Xuehai (SP 10) and Geshu (BL 17) are added; for heaviness of limbs, Yinlingquan (SP 9) is added; for fever, Hegu (LI 4) and Quchi (LI 11) are added; for prolonged duration, Guanyuan (CV 4), Shenshu (BL 23), Pishu (BL 20) and Sanyinjiao (SP 6) are added.

加风池、血海、膈俞；肢体重着者，加阴陵泉；发热者，加合谷、曲池；病延日久者，加关元、肾俞、脾俞、三阴交。

Performance: Guanyuan (CV 4), Shenshu (BL 23) and Pishu (BL 20) are needled with reinforcing needling technique and combined with moxibustion. The other acupoints are needled with reducing needling technique. Moxibustion can be applied to the location of pain. Local area with evident swelling can be punctured to let out blood.

操作：关元、肾俞、脾俞用补法并灸，其他腧穴用泻法。疼痛部位可加用灸法；局部红肿明显者，可在其处点刺出血。

2. Ear acupuncture

2. 耳针疗法

Prescription: Areas corresponding to the pathological conditions, Ear Shenmen (TF_4), Liver (CO_{12}), Spleen (CO_{13}) and Kidney (CO_{10}).

处方：相应病变部位，神门，肝，脾，肾。

Performance: Each time 2 - 4 acupoints are selected and needled with medium and strong stimulation. The needles are retained for 20 - 30 minutes. The needling is done once a day.

操作：视病情每次选用2～4穴，中、强刺激，留针20～30分钟，每日1次。

5.9.9 Lumbago

九、腰痛

[**Introduction**]

The causes of lumbago are various. The lumbago discussed in the following is mainly caused by chronic sprain of the lumbar muscles and protrusion of lumbar intervertebral disc. Lumbago can be caused by damage of the lumbar muscles, adhesion of muscles and ligaments or joints; or by retrograde pathological changes of the spinal vertebrae complicated by lumbar impairment, rupture of the fibrous ring of the lumbar vertebrae and protrusion of pulpiform nucleus that press on the nerves, periost and ligaments. TCM holds that lumbago is mainly caused by retention of pathological wind, cold and dampness in the

【概述】

腰痛又称腰脊痛，是临床常见症状之一。引起腰痛的原因甚多，本节主要讨论由慢性腰肌劳损、腰椎间盘突出等腰局部原因所致的腰痛症。腰部肌肉损伤，纤维变性，肌肉、韧带或关节内发生粘连；或在脊椎退行性变的基础上腰部受伤、腰椎纤维环破裂、髓核脱出，压迫神经、骨膜、韧带等，均可引起腰痛。中医认

meridians; or by malnutrition of the meridians and tendons due to kidney asthenia; or by inhibited flow of qi and blood in the meridians due to overstrain and impairment.

为主要由于风寒湿邪痹阻经络；或肾虚经络筋骨失于濡养；或过劳、受伤等，使经络气血运行不利而成腰痛。

［Syndrome differentiation］

【辨证】

1. Obstruction by pathogenic cold and dampness

1. 寒湿痹阻

Cold pain and heaviness sensation in the loins, or pain involving the buttocks and legs, inflexibility, aggravation with cold and rain, thin and white tongue fur and deep or slow pulse.

腰部冷痛而沉重，或痛连臀腿，活动不利，遇寒冷阴雨则加重，苔薄白，脉沉或迟。

2. Stagnation of qi and blood

2. 气血瘀滞

Pricking and fixed pain, stiffness of the waist, inflexibility, purplish tongue or with ecchymoses, taut or unsmooth pulse.

腰痛如刺，痛处不移，腰部板滞，仰俯转侧不便或不能，舌紫暗或有瘀点，脉弦或涩。

3. Deficiency of kidney essence

3. 肾虚精亏

Slow onset, vague aching and lingering pain in the loins, aggravation with overstrain, weakness of loins and knees; pale complexion, dizziness, tinnitus, spiritual lassitude, cold limbs, frequent and clear urine, pale tongue, deep and thin pulse in the case of yang asthenia; flushed cheeks, dysphoria, insomnia, dry mouth and throat, feverish sensation over palms and soles, yellow urine and dry feces, red tongue, thin and rapid pulse in the case of yin asthenia.

起病缓慢，腰痛隐隐，酸楚空软，绵绵不已，遇劳为甚，腰膝无力；偏阳虚者，面色皖白，头昏耳鸣，神疲肢冷，尿频而清，舌淡，脉沉细；偏阴虚者，面色潮红，心烦失眠，口燥咽干，手足心热，尿黄便干，舌红，脉细数。

［Treatment］

【治疗】

1. Body acupuncture

1. 体针疗法

Prescription: Shenshu (BL 23), Dachangshu (BL 25) and Ashi acupoints.

处方：肾俞，大肠俞，阿是穴。

Modification: For the syndrome of obstruction due to cold-dampness, Yaoyangguan (GV 3), Huantiao (GB 30), Chengfu (BL 36), Weizhong (BL 40) and Kunlun (BL 60) are added; for the syndrome of stagnation of qi and

随证配穴：寒湿痹阻证，配腰阳关、环跳、承扶、委中、昆仑。气血瘀滞证，配膈俞、次髎、委中、阳陵泉、飞扬。肾

blood, Geshu (BL 17), Ciliao (BL 32), Weizhong (BL 40), Yanglingquan (GB 34) and Feiyang (BL 58) are added; for the syndrome of kidney asthenia and essence consumption, Mingmen (GV 4), Qihaishu (BL 24), Guanyuanshu (BL 26), Ciliao (BL 32), Zusanli (ST 36) and Dazhong (KI 4) are added.

虚精亏证,配命门、气海俞、关元俞、次髎、足三里、大钟。

Performance: Kidney asthenia syndrome is treated with reinforcing needling technique, other syndromes are treated with reducing needling techniques. All the acupoints on the waist can be moxibusted with the supplementation of cupping. If there is blood stagnation, Weizhong (BL 40) is punctured to let blood.

操作:肾虚证用补法,余证用泻法。腰部诸穴可加用灸法,配合拔火罐。有瘀血者,可于委中穴处点刺出血。

2. Ear acupuncture

2. 耳针疗法

Prescription: Lumbosacral Vertebrae (AH_9), Kidney (CO_{10}), Ear Shenmen (TF_4) and Subcortex (AT_4).

处方:腰骶椎,肾,神门,皮质下。

Performance: Each time 2 – 3 acupoints are selected and needled with medium and strong stimulation. The needles are retained for 20 – 30 minutes. Or Wangbuliuxingzi (Semen Vaccariae) is used for ear pressure.

操作:每次选 2～3 穴,中、强刺激,留针 20～30 分钟。或用王不留行籽压耳。

5.9.10 Acute lumbar sprain

十、急性腰扭伤

[Introduction]

【概述】

Acute lumbar sprain is usually caused by improper posture, or excessive exertion or falling and contusion that impair the lumbar muscles, fascia and ligaments. The clinical manifestations are sudden lumbago and limited movement of the waist. TCM holds that lumbago is caused by improper exertion or falling and contusion that lead to impairment of the lumbar tendons and meridians as well as stagnation of qi and blood.

急性腰扭伤是常见的腰部软组织损伤,多因用力姿势不当,或过度负重,或跌扑闪挫等,使腰部肌肉、筋膜、韧带等软组织损伤。临床表现为猝然腰痛,活动受限。属中医"腰痛"范畴。由于用力不当,或跌扑闪挫等原因,导致腰部筋脉受损,气血阻滞,发生腰痛。

[Syndrome differentiation]

【辨证】

Sudden onset of lumbago, aggravation in movement,

腰痛猝发,疼痛剧烈,活

limited movement of the waist, inability of the waist to straighten, difficulty in pronation and turning of the body or even standing, frequent supporting of the waist with the hands; or spasm of the local muscles on the lower limbs, obvious tenderness and evident sprain history.

动受限,腰不能挺直,难以俯仰、转侧,甚或不能站立,动则痛甚,患者常以手按腰;或下肢局部肌肉痉挛,压痛明显。有明显扭伤史。

[**Treatment**]

【治疗】

1. Body acupuncture

1. 体针疗法

Prescription: Shuigou (GV 26), Houxi (SI 3), Weizhong (BL 40), Yaoyangguan (GV 3), Dachangshu (BL 25) and Ashi Acupoints.

处方:水沟,后溪,委中,腰阳关,大肠俞,阿是穴。

Performance: Each time 2 - 4 acupoints are selected and needled with reducing needling technique. Shuigou (GV 26) or Houxi (SI 3) is needled first. Shuigou (GV 26) is needled obliquely upward with rotating manipulation of the needle. The patient is asked to move the waist during the retention of the needle. Weizhong (BL 40) is punctured to let blood with a three-edged needle. The acupoints on the waist can also be moxibusted or treated with cupping. The needles are retained for 20 - 30 minutes and manipulated at intervals.

操作:每次选用2～4穴,针用泻法。先刺水沟或后溪,水沟穴向上斜刺,行捻转法,留针时让患者活动腰部。委中穴可用三棱针点刺出血。腰部穴可并用灸法,也可拔火罐。留针20～30分钟,间歇行针。

2. Ear acupuncture

2. 耳针疗法

Prescription: Lumbosacral Vertebrae (AH_9), reaction points, Ear Shenmen (TF_4) and Subcortical (AT_4).

处方:腰骶椎,反应点,神门,皮质下。

Performance: Strong stimulation, 30 - 60 minutes of needle retention and manipulation of needles at intervals. Or Wangbuliuxingzi (Semen Vaccariae) is used for ear acupressure.

操作:强刺激,留针30～60分钟,间歇行针。或用王不留行籽压耳法。

5.9.11 Sprain of soft tissues of the limbs

十一、四肢软组织扭伤

[**Introduction**]

【概述】

Sprain of the soft tissues of the limbs refers to the sprain of the muscles, tendons and ligaments around the shoulders, elbows, hip joints, knees and ankles due to

四肢软组织扭伤,指肩、肘、腕、髋、膝、踝关节周围的肌肉、筋膜、韧带等软组织,由

twisting or pulling without fracture, dislocation and contusion of the skin. The clinical manifestations are swelling, pain and dysfunction of the joints. This problem pertains to the conception of impairment of tendons in TCM due to improper exertion or falling and contusion that impair the vessels and meridians and result in stagnation of qi and blood.

于过度的扭曲或牵拉等原因引起的损伤,但无骨折、脱臼和皮肤破损。临床主要表现为扭伤部位的肿胀、疼痛、关节活动障碍等。四肢软组织扭伤属中医"伤筋"范畴,因用力不当或闪挫跌扑等,伤及筋肉脉络,气血瘀滞而成。

[**Syndrome differentiation**]

The main manifestations are swelling, pain, dysfunction of the joints and cyanotic color of local skin. If there are signs of protrusive swelling and unsmooth movement of the joints, the sprain is severe.

【辨证】

主要表现为扭伤部位的肿胀、疼痛、关节活动障碍,局部肌肤可见青紫。若红肿高耸,关节屈伸不利,则伤势较重。

[**Treatment**]

1. Body acupuncture

Prescription: Local Ashi acupoints.

Modification: For the treatment of the shoulders, Jianyu (LI 15), Jianliao (TE 14), Jianzhen (SI 9) and Jianjing (GB 21) are added; for the treatment of the elbows, Quchi (LI 11), Xiaohai (SI 8) and Tianjing (TE 10) are added; for the treatment of the wrist, Yangchi (TE 4), Yangxi (LI 5), Yanggu (SI 5) and Waiguan (TE 15) are added; for the treatment of hip joints, Huantiao (GB 30), Zhibian (BL 54) and Chengfu (BL 36) are added; for the treatment of the knees, Xiyan (EX-LE 5), Liangqiu (ST 34), Xiyangguan (GB 33) and Yanglingquan (GB 34) are added; for the treatment of the ankles, Jiexi (ST 41), Kunlun (BL 60) and Qiuxu (GB 40) are added.

Performance: Reducing needling technique is used; local acupoints can be moxibusted or applied with cupping.

2. Ear acupuncture

Prescription: Reaction points and Ear Shenmen (TF_4).

【治疗】

1. 体针疗法

处方:局部阿是穴。

随证配穴:肩部,可加肩髃、肩髎、肩贞、肩井。肘部,可加曲池、小海、天井。腕部,可加阳池、阳溪、阳谷、外关。髋部,可加环跳、秩边、承扶。膝部,可加膝眼、梁丘、膝阳关、阳陵泉。踝部,可加解溪、昆仑、丘墟。

操作:针用泻法;局部穴可加灸,也可加拔火罐。

2. 耳针疗法

处方:反应点,神门。

Performance: Medium and strong stimulation is required, the needles are retained for 20 - 30 minutes and the needling is done once a day. For the treatment of old wound, Wangbuliuxingzi (Semen Vaccariae) can be used for ear acupressure.

操作：中、强刺激，留针20～30分钟，每日1次。陈旧伤可用王不留行籽压耳法。

5.10 Diseases of surgery and dermatology

第十节 外科、皮肤科疾病

5.10.1 Acute mastadenitis

一、急性乳腺炎

[**Introduction**]

Acute mastadenitis refers to infection of the breast due to invasion of bacteria into mammary glands and lactiferous ducts. This problem is frequently encountered among women with breastfeeding, especially primipara. It usually occurs 3 - 4 weeks after labor due to rupture of nipple and invasion of bacteria complicated by unsmooth secretion of milk and stagnation of milk. The clinical manifestations are local swelling, pain, tenderness and hard nodules of the breast, accompanied by aversion to cold, fever and enlargement of lymph nodes over the armpit on the affected side. This disease pertains to breast abscess in TCM due to invasion of pathogenic factors or accumulation of milk; or due to mental upsets and stagnation of liver qi; or due to excessive intake of rich foods and accumulation of heat in the stomach meridian that lead to the obstruction of the vessels and stagnation of qi, blood and milk.

【概述】

急性乳腺炎是因细菌侵入乳腺和乳管组织而引起的乳房感染。病人绝大部分是产后哺乳期的妇女，尤以初产妇为多见，发病多在产后3～4周。多因乳头破损，细菌侵入，兼以排乳不畅，乳汁淤积，致细菌繁殖而发病。临床表现主要为乳房局部的红肿疼痛，触痛、硬块，伴有恶寒发热，患侧腋下淋巴结肿大等。本病属中医“乳痈”范畴，认为是由外邪乘虚而入或乳汁蓄积，而与血气相搏；或情志不舒，肝气郁结；或多食厚味，胃经积热等，致脉络阻塞，气血与积乳蕴结而成痈。

[**Syndrome differentiation**]

Redness, swelling and pain of the breast on the affected side; breast nodules, swelling, pain and difficulty in secreting milk before suppuration; frequently accompanied by headache due to cold and heat, nausea and thirst;

【辨证】

患侧乳房红肿疼痛，初起未成脓时，乳房结块，肿胀疼痛，排乳困难，常兼有寒热头痛，恶心口渴；痈脓形成，则乳

enlargement of the breast lumps, redness and swelling of skin, local continuous throbbing pain and lingering fever.

房肿块增大，皮肤焮红，局部有持续跳痛，发热不退。

［**Treatment**］

【**治疗**】

Prescription: Zusanli (ST 36), Shaoze (SI 1) and Jianjing (GB 21).

处方：足三里，少泽，肩井。

Modification: For headache due to cold and heat, Hegu (LI 4), Quchi (LI 11) and Fengchi (GB 20) are added; for distension and pain of the breast, Qimen (LR 14) and Taichong (LR 3) are added; for chest oppression and hiccup, Neiguan (PC 6) and Tanzhong (CV 17) are added.

随证配穴：寒热头痛，加合谷、曲池、风池；乳房胀痛，加期门、太冲；胸闷呕逆，加内关、膻中。

Performance: Reducing needling technique is used. Fengchi (GB 20) and the acupoints on the chest and back are needled with rotating manipulation. Shaoze (SI 1) is pricked to let blood. Jianjing (GB 21) is needled 0.3-0.5 cun lest the viscera be impaired. Qimen (LR 14) is needled 0.5 cun obliquely toward the breast. Tanzhong (CV 17) is needled horizontally 1 cun toward the affected part. The needles are retained for 30 minutes and manipulated at intervals.

操作：针用泻法，风池及胸背部穴行捻转法。少泽点刺出血。肩井直刺0.3～0.5寸，不可过深，以免伤及内脏。期门向乳房斜刺约0.5寸。膻中向患侧平刺约1寸。留针30分钟，间歇行针。

5.10.2 Hyperplasia of mammary glands

二、乳腺增生病

［**Introduction**］

【**概述**】

Hyperplasia of mammary glands is believed to be caused by disturbance of the ovary, usually seen among young women. The clinical manifestations are multiple different-sized and movable nodules in one or both breasts, distension and pain of the breasts, especially before menstruation. This disease pertains to the conception of mammary stagnation in TCM due to prolonged stagnation of liver qi and coagulation of phlegm; or due to asthenia of the liver and kidney, dysfunction of the thoroughfare vessel and retention of phlegm in the stomach collaterals over the breast since the middle age.

乳腺增生病，又称乳腺囊性增生病。多认为其病变与卵巢功能紊乱有关。常见于青壮年妇女。临床表现主要以一侧或两侧乳房触及多个大小不一、质韧不硬的肿块，可被推动，乳房胀痛，经前期为甚。本病属中医的“乳癖”范畴。多由于长期肝气郁结，气聚痰凝；或因中年后肝肾亏虚，冲任失调，痰气交结于乳房胃络所致。

[**Syndrome differentiation**]

Different-sized, round and hard nodules appear in one or both of the breasts. When the nodules become large, they appear like cysts with unclear margin, no adhesion with the skin and thoracic fascia, local distending pain and aggravation before menstruation. Sometimes the nipple discharges yellowish and greenish, brownish and bloody liquid, accompanied by aching and weakness of loins and fatigue, irregular menstruation, mental depression, dysphoria and insomnia.

【辨证】

单侧或双侧乳房多靠近周边部位触及大小不一、圆形而质地较坚韧的肿块,肿块较大时呈囊性,边界不甚清楚,与皮肤及胸筋膜无粘连,局部胀痛,经前期为甚;有时乳头流出黄绿色、棕色、血性的浆液。可伴见腰酸乏力,月经不调,情志抑郁,心烦失眠等症。

[**Treatment**]

1. Body acupuncture

Prescription: Tanzhong (CV 17), Wuyi (ST 15), Rugen (ST 18), Jianjing (GB 21) and Sanyinjiao (SP 6).

Modification: For irregular menstruation, Qihai (CV 6), Zusanli (ST 36) and Taichong (LR 3) are added; for mental depression, dysphoria and insomnia, Hegu (LI 4), Neiguan (PC 6) and Taichong (LR 3) are added; for aching and weakness of the loins, Shenshu (BL 23) and Taixi (KI 3) are added.

Performance: Tanzhong (CV 17) is needled horizontally toward the breast on the affected side; Wuyi (ST 15) is needled horizontally lateral; Rugen (ST 18) is needled toward the upper direction or horizontally lateral or obliquely. All these three acupoints are needled with rotating and reducing techniques. Shenshu (BL 23) and Taixi (KI 3) are needled with rotating and reinforcing techniques. The needles are retained and manipulated twice or 3 times at intervals.

2. Ear acupuncture

Prescription: Endocrine (CO_{18}), Liver (CO_{12}) and Kidney (CO_{10}).

【治疗】

1. 体针疗法

处方:膻中,屋翳,乳根,肩井,三阴交。

随证配穴:月经不调,加气海、足三里、太冲;情志抑郁,心烦失眠,加合谷、内关、太冲;腰酸乏力,加肾俞、太溪。

操作:膻中向患侧乳房平刺,屋翳向外平刺,乳根向上或向外平刺或斜刺,三穴均用捻转泻法。肾俞、太溪用捻转补法。留针期间间歇行针 2~3 次。

2. 耳针疗法

处方:内分泌,肝,肾。

Performance: Medium and strong stimulation is required, the needles are retained for 30 minutes and the needling is done once a day. Or Wangbuliuxingzi (Semen Vaccariae) is used for ear acupressure.

操作：中、强刺激，留针30分钟。每日1次。或用王不留行籽压耳。

5.10.3 Hemorrhoids

三、痔疮

[**Introduction**]

Hemorrhoids is one of the commonly encountered chronic anal and intestinal diseases and is divided into internal hemorrhoids, external hemorrhoids and complicated hemorrhoids according to the location. TCM holds that hemorrhoids is caused by prolonged sitting, overloading, long distance walking, frequent labor, addiction to pungent and greasy foods, chronic diarrhea and constipation that lead to looseness of tendons and vessels, interior accumulation of damp-heat, stagnatin of qi and blood in the lower part of the body.

【概述】

痔疮是肛肠部的常见慢性疾病，为直肠末端粘膜下和肛管皮下的静脉丛扩大、曲张所形成的静脉团。根据发生部位的不同，分为内痔、外痔和混合痔。中医认为本病的发生主要由于久坐、负重、远行、妊娠多产、嗜食辛辣肥腻、久泄、便秘等多种因素，致筋脉松弛，湿热内蕴，气血瘀滞，结聚于下部而成。

[**Syndrome differentiation**]

1. Sthenia syndrome

Fresh red or blackish red and profuse or scanty blood in stool, protrusion of hemorrhoids nucleus, swelling and pain or severe pain or burning sensation around the anus, retention of dry feces or unsmooth defecation, accompanied by dysphoria, dry mouth, abdominal distension, yellow urine, red tongue, yellowish or yellowish and greasy tongue fur, rapid and sthenic pulse.

2. Asthenia syndrome

Protrusion of hemorrhoids nucleus, prolapsing sensation of the anus; or protrusion of nucleus, light-colored or blackish bleeding, accompanied by palpitation, lusterless complexion, spiritual lassitude and shortness of breath, poor appetite, light-colored tongue and thin pulse.

【辨证】

1. 实证

便时出血色鲜红或暗红，量或多或少，痔核脱出，肛门肿痛或剧痛，或灼热，大便燥结或粘滞不爽，伴心烦，口干，腹胀，尿黄，舌红，苔黄或黄腻，脉数实。

2. 虚证

痔核脱出不能回纳，肛门有下坠感；或痔核脱出，出血色淡，或晦而不鲜，伴头晕心悸，面色少华，神疲气短，食少，舌淡，脉细。

［**Treatment**］

1. Body acupuncture

Prescription：Baihuanshu（BL 30），Changqiang（GV 1），Chengshan（BL 57）and Erbai（EX-UE 2）.

Modification：For sthenia syndrome，Ciliao（BL 32），Huiyang（BL 35）and Sanyinjiao（SP 6）are added；for asthenia syndrome，Baihui（GV 20），Pishu（BL 20）and Zusanli（ST 36）are added.

Performance：Reducing needling technique is used for treating sthenia syndrome while reinforcing needling technique is used for treating asthenia syndrome. Baihuanshu（BL 30）and Changqiang（GV 1）are needled with mild reinforcing and reducing techniques. Changqiang（GV 1）is needled obliquely anterior to the coccyx. Baihui（GV 20）can be moxibusted.

2. Ear acupuncture

Prescription：Rectum（HX_2），Large Intestine（CO_7），Ear Shenmen（TF_4）and Subcortex（AT_4）.

Performance：Each time 2－3 acupoints are selected and needled with medium stimulation. The needles are retained for 20－30 minutes once a day. Or Wangbuliuxingzi（Semen Vaccariae）is used for ear acupressure.

【**治疗**】

1．体针疗法

处方：白环俞，长强，承山，二白。

随证配穴：实证，加次髎、会阳、三阴交。虚证，加百会、脾俞、足三里。

操作：实证用泻法；虚证用补法，白环俞、长强予平补平泻法。长强穴须紧靠尾骨前面斜刺；百会施灸法。

2．耳针疗法

处方：直肠，肛门，大肠，神门，皮质下。

操作：每次选2～3穴，中度刺激，留针20～30分钟，每日1次。或以王不留行籽压耳。

5.10.4 Urticaria

［**Introduction**］

Urticaria is a commonly encountered allergic dermatosis due to eating fish，shrimps and crabs；or due to stinging of flies and injection of animal serum；or due to contact with pollen，nettle and certain chemicals；or due to stimulation of cold or hot air. The clinical manifestations are different-sized red or pale urticaria and abnormal pruritus with sudden onset and sudden disappearance. Acute case may heal in several days，while chronic case may linger for months and years. Urticaria is usually caused by

四、荨麻疹

【**概述**】

荨麻疹是一种常见的过敏性皮肤病。多因食鱼、虾、蟹等；或因蚊虫叮咬，注射动物血清；接触花粉、荨麻及某些化学物质；或冷热空气刺激等而致病。临床表现以皮肤出现鲜红或苍白色风团，大小不等，瘙痒异常，皮疹的发生和消失都很快，此起彼落，消

retention of exogenous pathogenic wind-cold or wind-heat in the skin; or by excessive intake of greasy food leading to retention of endogenous damp-heat in the skin.

退后不留痕迹为特征。急性者数天内痊愈,慢性者可达数月、数年。本病相当于中医"瘾疹"、"风疹块"的范畴。多因外感风寒或风热之邪,客于皮肤;也有因过食油腻荤腥,湿热内生,熏蒸肌肤等引发本病。

[Syndrome differentiation]

【辨证】

1. Exogenous pathogenic wind

1. 外感风邪

Sudden onset, occurrence or aggravation after attack of wind-cold or heat, accompanied by aversion to cold, fever, aching limbs, thin and white tongue fur and floating pulse.

起病急骤,遇风冷或受热后发作或加剧,伴见恶寒发热,肢体酸楚,苔薄白,脉浮。

2. Accumulation of heat in the stomach and intestines

2. 胃肠积热

Urticaria is usually caused by excessive eating of fish and shrimps or drinking of alcohol, accompanied by epigastric and abdominal pain, or nausea and vomiting, diarrhea or constipation, yellow and greasy tongue fur, slippery and rapid pulse.

皮疹多因食鱼虾或饮酒而发,伴有脘腹疼痛,或恶心呕吐,泄泻或便结,苔黄腻,脉滑数。

[Treatment]

【治疗】

1. Body acupuncture

1. 体针疗法

Prescription: Hegu (LI 4), Quchi (LI 11), Xuehai (SP 10), Weizhong (BL 40) and Sanyinjiao (SP 6).

处方:合谷,曲池,血海,委中,三阴交。

Modification: For exogenous pathogenic wind syndrome, Dazhui (GV 14) and Fengchi (GB 20) are added; for accumulation of heat in the stomach and intestines, Zhongwan (CV 12) and Zusanli (ST 36) are added; for nausea and vomiting, Neiguan (PC 6) is added; for abdominal pain, diarrhea or constipation, Tianshu (ST 25) is added.

随证配穴:外感风邪证,配大椎、风池。胃肠积热证,配中脘、足三里。恶心呕吐,加内关;腹痛、泄泻或便结,加天枢。

Performance: Reducing needling technique is used and Weizhong (BL 40) can be pricked for bloodletting.

操作:针用泻法。委中可点刺出血。

2. Ear acupuncture

Prescription: Fengxi (SF_1、Zi), Lung (CO_{14}), Ear Shenmen (TF_4), Spleen (CO_{13}) and Endocrine (CO_{18}).

Performance: Each time 2 - 3 acupoints are selected, medium and strong stimulation is required. The needles are retained for 30 minutes and the needling is done once a day.

2. 耳针疗法

处方：风溪，肺，神门，脾，内分泌。

操作：每次选 2～3 穴，中、强刺激，留针 30 分钟，每日 1 次。

5. 10. 5 Herpes zoster

[**Introduction**]

Herpes zoster is clinically marked by clusters of blisters in the form of a belt in the areas distributing with peripheral nerves or certain part of skin and local burning pain. It usually appears on one side of the chest, face, eye, abdomen and thigh. TCM holds that it is caused by exogenous virulent wind, dampness and heat; or by stagnant liver and gallbladder fire that fumigates meridians and skin with damp-heat in the spleen meridian. Prolonged stagnation of pathogenic factors in the meridians, unsmooth circulation of qi and blood and retention of blood stasis in the meridians may lead to lingering local pain.

[**Syndrome differentiation**]

In the early period there is pricking pain in the affected part and redness of local skin, then followed by clusters of macules, sudden appearance of blisters in the form of belt and severe pain. It may be accompanied by mild fever, general discomfort and anorexia. After 2 - 3 weeks, scab is gradually formed and exfoliates without any scar. In a few cases pain may linger for a longer time.

五、带状疱疹

【概述】

带状疱疹是由水痘-带状疱疹病毒侵犯神经、皮肤而引起的一种病毒性疾病。临床以沿周围神经分布区域皮肤出现数个簇集水疱群，成带状排列，局部有烧灼样疼痛为特征。好发于一侧的胸部、头面部、眼、腹部、股部等处。本病相当于中医的“缠腰火丹”、“蛇丹”等。本病多由外感风湿热毒，或肝胆郁火，挟脾经湿热薰蒸于经络皮肤而致。当邪阻经络日久，气血运行不畅，血瘀阻络，则局部疼痛迁延不愈。

【辨证】

病初起时患部先有刺痛，局部皮肤发红，继而出现集聚的丘疹，并迅速变为水疱，呈带状排列，疼痛较剧。可伴有轻度发热，全身不适，食欲不振等症。约 2～3 周后，疱疹逐渐结痂脱落，一般不留瘢痕。少数患者疼痛仍可持续

[Treatment]

1. Body acupuncture

Prescription: For local area of pathological changes, Hegu (LI 4), Quchi (LI 11), Xuehai (SP 10), Yanglingquan (GB 34), Zusanli (ST 36) and Taichong (LR 3) are selected.

Modification: For fever, Dazhui (GV 14) is added; for herpes zoster on the chest and hypochondria, Zhigou (TE 6), Qimen (LR 14), Geshu (BL 17) and Ganshu (BL 18) are added.

Performance: More needles can be used to perform surrounded needling in the local area of pathological changes. Moxibustion can also be used. Reducing needling technique is required to apply.

2. Ear acupuncture

Prescription: Reaction points, Ear Shenmen (TF_4), Liver (CO_{12}), Lung (CO_{14}) and Subcortex (AT_4).

Performance: Each time 2-4 acupoints are selected, strong stimulation is required and the needles are retained for 20-30 minutes.

较长时间。

【治疗】

1. 体针疗法

处方：病变局部，合谷，曲池，血海，阳陵泉，足三里，太冲。

随证配穴：发热者，加大椎；发于胸胁者，加支沟、期门、膈俞、肝俞。

操作：在病变局部以多针围刺，也可用灸法。针用泻法。

2. 耳针疗法

处方：相应区的反应点，神门，肝，肺，皮质下。

操作：每次取2～4穴，强刺激，留针20～30分钟。

5.10.6 Flat wart

[Introduction]

Flat wart refers to viral small growth in the superficial part of the skin, usually seen among young people on the dorsum of hand or face due to retention of pathogenic wind-heat in the skin or due to liver stagnation and blood asthenia as well as stagnatin of qi and blood.

[Syndrome differentiation]

It usually appears on the face, dorsum of hand and forearm. The flat macules are marked by the size of needle

六、扁平疣

【概述】

扁平疣是发生于皮肤浅表的病毒性小赘生物。为硬性的扁平丘疹，好发于青少年的手背和颜面部。本病中医称为“扁瘊”，多因风热之邪郁于肌表，或肝郁血虚，气血瘀滞而成。

【辨证】

好发于颜面、手背和前臂，为扁平丘疹，如针头、芝麻

point, sesame or soy bean with clear border, slight prominence over the skin, normal or brownish color, scattered or linear distribution and no esthesia.

或黄豆大小,境界清楚,略高于皮面,呈正常肤色或略带褐色,多数散在,或线状分布,一般无感觉。

[**Treatment**]

【治疗】

1. Body acupuncture

1. 体针疗法

Prescription: Fengchi (GB 20), Hegu (LI 4), Quchi (LI 11) and Xuehai (SP 10).

处方:风池,合谷,曲池,血海。

Modification: For wart on the face, Taiyang (EX-HN 5), Yangbai (GB 14), Quanliao (SI 18) and Jiache (ST 6) are added; for wart on the dorsum of hand, Zhongzhu (TE 3) and Waiguan (TE 15) are added; for distension of head and dysphoria, Neiguan (PC 6) and Xingjian (LR 2) are added.

随证配穴:颜面多见者,加太阳、阳白、颧髎、颊车;手背多见者,加中渚、外关;头胀心烦者,配内关、行间。

Performance: Each time several acupoints are selected and needled with reducing needling technique. The needles are retained for 15 - 30 minutes.

操作:每次选数穴,针用泻法。留针15~30分钟。

2. Ear acupuncture

2. 耳针疗法

Prescription: Endocrine (CO_{18}), Cheeks ($LO_{5,6i}$) and Ear Shenmen (TF_4).

处方:内分泌,面颊,神门。

Performance: Medium stimulation is required and the needles are retained for 15 - 30 minutes. The needling is done once a day or Wangbuliuxingzi (Semen Vaccariae) is used for ear acupressure. The patient is advised to press ear acupoints twice or 3 times a day.

操作:中等刺激,留针15~30分钟,每日1次。或以王不留行籽压耳,嘱病人每日按压2~3次。

5.11 Diseases of eyes, ears, nose and throat

第十一节 眼、耳鼻喉科疾病

5.11.1 Acute conjunctivitis

一、急性结膜炎

[**Introduction**]

【概述】

Acute conjunctivitis usually appears in the spring and summer. It is infectious or epidemic. The clinical mani-

急性结膜炎是临床常见的外眼病,由细菌或病毒感染

festations are conjunctival congestion, mucous or suppurating secreta and tendency of fulminant spreading. Acute conjunctivitis is usually caused by retention of exogenous wind-heat and seasonal virulent factors in the meridians and stagnation of fire; or by exuberant liver and lung fire attacking the eyes along the meridians.

而成，多发生于春夏两季，具有传染性或流行性。临床主要表现为显著的结膜充血、有粘液性或脓性分泌物，易造成暴发流行。本病属中医的风热眼范畴，有"暴风客热"、"天行赤眼"、"天行赤眼暴翳"等名称，俗称"红眼"、"火眼"。多因外感风热及时气邪毒，阻滞经脉，火郁不宣；或肝肺火盛，循经上扰，积热交攻于目而致。

[Syndrome differentiation]

1. Pathogenic wind-heat: Redness and swelling of eyes, photophobia and epiphora, sensation of foreign object, excessive secretion of eyes, even swelling and burning pain of the eyelids and hyperemia of bulbar conjunctiva, accompanied by headache, fever, nasal discharge, sore throat, red tongue with yellow fur and rapid pulse.

2. Exuberance of liver and gallbladder fire: Involvement of the pupil, photophobia and epiphora, blurred vision, irritating sensation in the eyes and ciliary hyperemia, accompanied by bitter taste in the mouth, dry throat, uncomfortable fullness in the chest and hypochondria, retention of dry feces, red tongue with yellow fur, taut and rapid pulse.

【辨证】

1. 风热邪毒：目赤肿痛，畏光流泪，有异物感，眵多粘结，甚则胞肿灼痛，白睛溢血；伴头痛发热，流涕咽痛等，舌红苔黄，脉数。

2. 肝胆火盛：病侵黑睛，畏光流泪，视物模糊，涩痛难睁，抱轮红赤，伴口苦咽干，胸胁苦满，大便干结，舌红苔黄，脉弦数。

[Treatment]

1. Body acupuncture

Prescription: Taiyang (EX-HN 5), Jingming (BL 1) and Hegu (LI 4).

Modification: For pathogenic wind-heat, Fengchi (GB 20), Waiguan (TE 15) and Quchi (LI 11) are added; for exuberance of liver and gallbladder fire, Taichong (LR 3), Qimen (LR 14) and Xiaxi (GB 43) are added; for

【治疗】

1. 体针疗法

处方：太阳，睛明，合谷。

随证配穴：风热邪毒，加风池、外关、曲池。肝胆火盛，加太冲、期门、侠溪。头痛者，加上星；咽喉肿痛者，加少商；

headache, Shangxing (GV 23) is added; for sore throat, Shaoshang (LU 11) is added; for hyperemia of bulbar conjunctiva, Geshu (BL 17) is added; for constipation, Zhigou (TE 6) is added.

白睛溢血者,加膈俞;便秘者,加支沟。

Performance: The acupoints are needled with filiform needles and reducing needling technique. Moxibustion is not used. Taiyang is pricked for bloodletting. Before needling Jingming (BL 1), the acupuncturist advises the patient to close the eye and push the eye ball to the lateral side and the right hand inserts the needle 0.5 - 1 cun into the acupoint with mild rotation and without application of lifting-thrusting technique. When the needle is withdrawn, the acupoint is pressed with finger. Fengchi (GB 20) is needled obliquely 0.8 - 1 cun toward the nose tip. Qimen (LR 14) is needled obliquely or horizontally 0.8 - 1 cun.

操作:毫针刺用泻法,不灸。太阳点刺出血。针睛明穴时嘱病人闭眼,医者左手轻推眼球向外侧固定,右手缓慢直刺 0.5～1 寸,少捻转,不提插,出针后按压针孔片刻。风池向鼻尖斜刺 0.8～1 寸。期门斜刺或平刺 0.8～1 寸。

2. Ear acupuncture

Prescription: Eye (LO_5), Liver (CO_{12}), Lung (CO_{14}) and Large Intestine (CO_7).

Performance: Each time 2 - 3 acupoints are selected and needled with medium stimulation. The needles are retained for 30 minutes. The ear tip is pricked for bloodletting. The needling is done once a day. Or Wangbuliuxingzi (Semen Vaccariae) is used for ear acupressure alternatively on the ears. The patient is advised to press the ears 3 - 4 times a day and 2 - 3 minutes each time.

2. 耳针疗法

处方:眼,肝,肺,大肠。

操作:每次取 2～3 穴,中等刺激,留针 30 分钟,耳尖点刺放血,每日 1 次。或用王不留行籽压耳,左右交替使用,并嘱病人每日自行按压 3～4 次,每次 2～3 分钟。

5.11.2 Auditory vertigo

[**Introduction**]

Auditory vertigo, also known as Meniere's disease, is a kind of non-inflammatory disease due to dysfunction of vestibule and retention of fluid in labyrinth. The main clinical manifestations are vertigo, metamorphopsia, inability to stand and sit, nausea, vomiting and sweating,

二、内耳性眩晕

【概述】

内耳性眩晕又称梅尼埃综合征,是由于前庭功能障碍,内耳膜迷路积水所引起的一种非炎症性疾病。临床主要表现为头昏眼花,视物旋转

accompanied by undulatory deafness and tinnitus as well as spontaneous and horizontal nystagmus. This disease pertains to the conception of "dizziness" in TCM usually caused by asthenia of the spleen and stomach, hyperactivity of liver yang, endogenous production of wind and yang as well as wind, fire and phlegm attacking the upper orifices; or by insufficiency of yin essence, qi and blood as well as malnutrition of the lucid orifices.

翻覆,不能坐立,恶心呕吐,出汗,伴有一侧波动性耳聋和耳鸣,并有自发性、水平性的眼球震颤。本病属中医的"眩晕"范畴。多因脾胃虚弱,肝阳上亢,风阳内动,风、火、痰上扰清空或阴精气血不足,清窍失养所致。

[**Syndrome differentiation**]

【辨证】

1. Insufficiency of qi and blood

Vertigo, aggravation in movement, recurrence with overstrain, spiritual lassitude, pale complexion, palpitation, insomnia, light-colored tongue and thin pulse.

1. 气血不足

头晕目眩,动则加剧,劳累即发,神疲乏力,面色苍白,心悸失眠,舌淡,脉细。

2. Hyperactivity of liver yang

Vertigo due to emotional changes, frequent nausea, flushed cheeks, bitter taste in the mouth, dry throat, fullness in the chest and hypochondria, aching and weakness of the loins and knee, reddish tongue with scanty fur, taut, thin and rapid pulse.

2. 肝阳上亢

头晕目眩,多因情志波动而诱发,泛泛欲吐,面红目赤,口苦咽干,胸胁苦满,腰膝酸软,舌红少苔,脉弦细数。

3. Consumption of kidney essence

Frequent vertigo, aggravation in the night, spiritual lassitude, amnesia, aching and weakness of the loins and knees, tinnitus, deafness, hypoacusis, dreaminess and seminal emission, tidal fever and night sweating, reddish tongue with scanty fur and thin and rapid pulse.

3. 肾精亏损

眩晕屡发,入夜尤甚,神疲健忘,腰膝酸软,耳鸣耳聋,听力减退,多梦遗精,潮热盗汗,舌红少苔,脉细数。

4. Retention of dampness and phlegm in the middle energizer

Vertigo, heaviness and wrapped sensation in the head, chest oppression and nausea, even vomiting of phlegm and saliva, somnolence and lassitude, poor appetite, white and greasy tongue fur as well as soft and slippery pulse.

4. 痰湿中阻

眩晕,头重如裹,胸闷泛恶,甚则呕吐痰涎,嗜睡乏力,食欲不振,苔白腻,脉濡滑。

[Treatment]

1. Body acupuncture

Prescription: Baihui (GV 20) and Fengchi (GB 20).

Modification: For insufficiency of qi and blood, Pishu (BL 20), Zusanli (ST 36), Qihai (CV 6) and Guanyuan (CV 4) are added; for hyperactivity of liver yang, Ganshu (BL 18), Shenshu (BL 23), Xingjian (LR 2) and Xiaxi (GB 43) are added; for consumption of kidney essence, Shenshu (BL 23), Taixi (KI 3), Sanyinjiao (SP 6), Guanyuan (CV 4) and Xuanzhong (GB 39) are added; for retention of dampness and phlegm in the middle energizer, Pishu (BL 20), Weishu (BL 21), Fenglong (ST 40), Yinlingquan (SP 9) and Zhongwan (CV 12) are added.

Performance: For asthenia of qi and blood and consumption of kidney essence, mild reinforcing and reducing needling techniques are used to needle Baihui (GV 20) and Fengchi (GB 20), reinforcing needling technique is used to needle the other acupoints or with the combination of moxa-roll moxibusiton. For hyperactivity of liver yang, Fengchi (GB 20) is needled in the direction of the nose tip with rotating and twirling reducing techniques and Baihui (GV 20) is needled horizontally with twirling and rotating reducing technique; Ganshu (BL 18) and Shenshu (BL 23) are needled obliquely toward the spinal column with reinforcing needling technique; Xingjian (LR 2) and Xiaxi (GB 43) are needled with reducing technique. For retention of dampness and phlegm in the middle energizer, Pishu (BL 20) and Weishu (BL 21) are needled with reinforcing needling technique, the rest of the acupoints are needled with reducing technique.

2. Ear acupuncture

Prescription: Kidney (CO_{10}), Ear Shenmen (TF_4), Occiput (AT_3), Internal Ear (LO_6) and Brain ($AT_{3,4i}$).

Performance: Each time 2 - 3 acupoints are selected

【治疗】

1. 体针疗法

处方：百会，风池。

随证配穴：气血不足，加脾俞、足三里、气海、关元；肝阳上亢，加肝俞、肾俞、行间、侠溪；肾精亏损，加肾俞、太溪、三阴交、关元、悬钟；痰湿中阻，加脾俞、胃俞、丰隆、阴陵泉、中脘。

操作：气血虚弱、肾精亏损证，百会、风池针用平补平泻法，余穴针用补法，加温针灸或艾条灸。肝阳上亢证，风池刺向鼻尖，行捻转泻法，百会平刺行捻转泻法；肝俞、肾俞向脊柱斜刺，针用补法，行间、侠溪针用泻法。痰湿中阻证，脾俞、胃俞针用补法，余穴针用泻法。

2. 耳针疗法

选穴：肾，神门，枕，内耳，脑。

操作：每次取穴 2～3 个，

and needled with medium and strong stimulation. The needles are retained for 20 - 30 minutes with manipulation at intervals. Or Wangbuliuxingzi (Semen Vaccariae) is used for ear acupressure alternatively on both ears 3 - 4 times a day.

中强刺激,留针 20～30 分钟,间歇运针。或用王不留行籽压耳,左右交替,每 3～4 日 1 次。

3. Scalp acupuncture

Selection of area: Vertigo-auditory zone on both sides.

Performance: The needling is done once a day with medium and strong stimulation and longer retention of the needles.

3. 头针疗法

选区：双侧晕听区。

操作：每日 1 次,中强刺激,长时间留针。

5.11.3 Nasosinusitis

［**Introduction**］

Nasosinusitis, one of the commonly encountered diseases in the five sensory organs due to inflammation of the nasosinusal mucus, is either acute or chronic. Usually chronic nasosinusitis is more common. The clinical manifestations are profuse nasal thick discharge, nasal obstruction, headache or vertigo, and hyposmia. This disease pertains to the conception of "nasosinusitis" in TCM caused by accumulation of pathogenic factors in the nasal cavity due to failure of pulmonary qi to disperse resulting from exogenous pathogenic cold and heat attack; or by failure of qi and blood to nourish the nose due to asthenia of the spleen and lung.

三、鼻窦炎

【概述】

鼻窦炎是鼻窦粘膜因感染而产生炎症的五官科常见的疾病之一,分急性、慢性两类,以慢性多见。临床主要表现为鼻流浊涕量多、鼻塞、头痛或昏,嗅觉减退。本病属中医"鼻渊"范畴,由外感寒热邪毒袭表犯肺,致肺气失宣,邪气上扰,壅于鼻窍；或脾肺虚弱,气血不能上荣于鼻所致。

［**Syndrome differentiation**］

1. Sthenia syndrome

Nasal discharge of thick snivel with yellow color and foul smell, anosmia, or accompanied by fever, cough, headache and rapid pulse if there is exuberant heat in the lung meridian; or accompanied by headache, bitter taste in the mouth, dry throat, dysphoria, susceptibility to rage, reddish tongue with yellow fur and taut and rapid

【辨证】

1. 实证

鼻流浊涕,色黄腥秽,鼻塞不闻香臭,若肺经热盛可兼有发热咳嗽,头痛脉数；若胆经郁热可兼头痛,口苦咽干,烦躁易怒,舌红苔黄,脉弦数；若脾经湿热可兼头重体倦,脘

pulse if there is stagnant heat in the gallbladder meridian; or accompanied by heaviness of the head and lassitude of the body, distension and oppression in the chest and epigastrium, anorexia, reddish tongue with yellow and greasy fur and soft pulse if there is damp-heat in the spleen meridian.

腹胀闷，纳呆，舌红苔黄腻，脉濡。

2. Asthenia syndrome

Nasal obstruction with whitish and thick nasal discharge, hyposmia, or accompanied by dizziness, cold body and limbs, shortness of breath and weakness, light-colored tongue with thin fur as well as weak and slow pulse if there is asthenia-cold in pulmonary qi; or accompanied by lassitude of the limbs, sallow complexion, reduced appetite and abdominal distension, loose stool and clear urine, light-colored tongue with whitish fur and slow and rapid pulse.

2．虚证

鼻塞流涕，涕白粘稠，嗅觉减退，若肺气虚寒可兼头晕，形寒肢冷，气短乏力，舌淡苔薄，脉缓弱；若脾气虚弱可兼肢困乏力，面色萎黄，食少腹胀，便溏溲清，舌淡苔白，脉缓弱。

[Treatment]

1. Body acupuncture

Prescription: Yingxiang (LI 20), Hegu (LI 4) and Yintang (EX-HN 3).

Modification: For sthenia syndrome, Taiyang (EX-HN 5) is added; if there is heat in the lung meridian, Dazhui (GV 14) and Lieque (LU 7) are added; if there is stagnant heat in the gallbladder meridian, Fengchi (GB 20) and Xingjian (LR 2) are added; if there is stagnant heat in the spleen meridian, Zusanli (ST 36) and Yinlingquan (SP 9) are added. For asthenia syndrome, Zusanli (ST 36) is added; if there is asthenia-cold in pulmonary qi, Feishu (BL 13) and Taiyuan (LU 9) are added; if spleen qi is asthenic, Pishu (BL 20) and Weishu (BL 21) are added.

Performance: For sthenia syndrome, reducing needling technique is used without moxibustion; Yingxiang (LI 20) is needled obliquely toward the inner region;

【治疗】

1．体针疗法

处方：迎香，合谷，印堂。

随证配穴：实证加太阳，若肺经热甚加大椎、列缺；胆经郁热加风池、行间；脾经湿热加足三里、阴陵泉。虚证加足三里，若肺气虚寒加肺俞、太渊；脾气虚弱加脾俞、胃俞。

操作：实证，针用泻法，不灸；迎香针向内斜刺，印堂向下平刺，均用捻转泻法，太阳

Yintang (EX-HN 3) is needled horizontally downward with rotating technique for reducing purpose; Taiyang (EX-HN 5) is pricked for bloodletting. For asthenia syndrome, Yingxiang (LI 20) and Yintang (EX-HN 3) are needled with mild reinforcing and reducing techniques, the rest of the acupoints are needled with reinforcing technique with needle-warming moxibustion or with moxa-roll moxibustion.

点刺出血。虚证,迎香、印堂针用平补平泻法,余穴针用补法,加温针灸或艾条灸。

2. Ear acupuncture

Prescription: Internal Nose (TG_4), Lung (CO_{14}), Forehead (AT_1) and Lower Tragus (TG_2).

Performance: Each time 3 - 4 acupoints are needled with medium stimulation. The needles are retained for 30 minutes. Or 2 - 3 acupoints are selected for embedment of needles. Or Wangbuliuxingzi (Semen Vaccariae) is used for auricular acupressure alternatively on both ears 3 - 4 times a day.

2. 耳针疗法

选穴:内鼻,肺,额,下屏。

操作:每次取3~4穴,中等刺激,留针30分钟,或选单侧2~3穴埋针或埋王不留行籽,左右交替,每3~4日1次。

5.11.4 Rhinallergosis

[**Introduction**]

Rhinallergosis refers to allergic reaction of the nasal mucus due to excessive sensitivity of the certain part of the body to the sensitinogen. It usually occurs all year round or in certain seasons, the former is more frequent and often seen among young people. The clinical manifestations are mainly paroxysmal nasal pruritus, frequent sneezing, nasal obstruction and thin nasal discharge. This problem is caused by insufficiency of yang-qi in the lung, spleen and kidney, weakness of defensive qi and invasion of pathogenic wind and cold into the nose that lead to stagnation of pulmonary qi and obstruction of the nose.

四、过敏性鼻炎

【概述】

过敏性鼻炎又名变态反应性鼻炎,是身体对某些过敏原敏感性增高所致的鼻粘膜的过敏反应。有常年性发作和季节性发作两型,前者居多,多见于青少年。临床主要表现为发作性鼻痒、喷嚏连作、鼻塞、鼻流清涕。本病属中医"鼻鼽"范畴,由于肺、脾、肾三脏阳气不足,卫表不固,风寒之邪侵及鼻窍,邪正相持,肺气不得通调,鼻窍不利而发为本病。

[Syndrome differentiation]

1. Asthenia of the lung

Nasal pruritus, frequent sneezing, thin and profuse nasal discharge, nasal obstruction, sudden onset and disappearance; accompanied by cough, lassitude, no desire to speak, shortness of breath, low voice, spontaneous sweating, light-colored tongue with thin fur and weak pulse.

2. Asthenia of the spleen

Prolonged duration, repeated relapse of nasal pruritus and sneezing, thin and profuse nasal discharge, nasal obstruction, aggravation of the symptoms or occurrence after overstrain; accompanied by anorexia, abdominal distension, heaviness of the limbs, loose stool, light-colored tongue with tooth-prints on the margin, white or whitish greasy tongue fur and soft and weak pulse.

3. Asthenia of the kidney

Prolonged duration, paroxysmal nasal pruritus and sneezing, thin nasal discharge, nasal obstruction, anosmia; accompanied by aversion to cold, cold limbs, aching and weakness of the loins and knees, seminal emission and immature ejaculation, loose stool, light-colored tongue with white fur and deep and thin pulse.

[Treatment]

1. Body acupuncture

Prescription: Yingxiang (LI 20), Hegu (LI 4), Taiyuan (LU 9) and Zusanli (ST 36).

Modification: For asthenia of the lung, Feishu (BL 13) and Fengmen (BL 12) are added; for asthenia of the spleen, Pishu (BL 20) and Weishu (BL 21) are added; for asthenia of the kidney, Shenshu (BL 23) and Mingmen (GV 4) are added; for nasal obstruction, Yintang (EX-HN 3) is added; for profuse sputum, Fenglong (ST 40) is added; for tinnitus, Tinggong (SI 19) is added.

【辨证】

1. 肺虚

鼻痒,喷嚏频作,鼻流清涕量多,鼻塞,发病迅速,消失亦快;兼有咳嗽,倦怠懒言,气短音低,自汗,舌淡苔薄,脉虚弱。

2. 脾虚

发病时间长,反复发作鼻痒、喷嚏,鼻流清涕量多,鼻塞,每在疲劳后发作或症状加重;兼有纳呆腹胀,肢体困重,大便溏薄,舌淡边有齿印,苔白或白腻,脉濡弱。

3. 肾虚

发病时间长,发作鼻痒、喷嚏,鼻流清涕,鼻塞失嗅,伴畏寒肢冷,腰膝酸软,遗精早泄,大便溏薄,舌淡苔白,脉沉细。

【治疗】

1. 体针疗法

处方:迎香,合谷,太渊,足三里。

随证配穴:肺虚加肺俞、风门;脾虚加脾俞、胃俞;肾虚加肾俞、命门。鼻塞甚者加印堂;痰多加丰隆;耳鸣加听宫。

Performance: Yingxiang (LI 20) is needled obliquely toward the inner side with rotating and twirling reducing technique. The other acupoints are needled with needle-warming moxibustion or moxa-roll moxibustion or moxibustion of 3 - 5 moxa cones after needling. Taiyuan (LU 9) is needled 0.3 -0.5 cun with rotating and twirling reinforcing technique, avoiding radial artery.

操作：迎香向内侧斜刺，针用捻转泻法，余穴均用补法，温针灸或艾条灸，或针后加艾炷灸 3～5 壮。太渊避开桡动脉直刺 0.3～0.5 寸，针用捻转补法。

2. Ear acupuncture

2. 耳针疗法

Prescription: Internal Nose (TG_4), Endocrine (CO_{18}), Subcortex (AT_4), Pingchuan (Ext.), Adrenal Gland (TG_{2p}), Lung (CO_{14}) and Kidney (CO_{10}).

处方：内鼻，内分泌，皮质下，平喘，肾上腺，肺，肾。

Performance: Each time 2 - 3 acupoints are needled with medium and strong stimulation. The needles are retained for 20 minutes and manipulated at intervals. Or Wangbuliuxingzi (Semen Vaccariae) is used for auricular acupressure alternatively on both ears, 3 - 4 times a day.

操作：每次取 2～3 穴，中强刺激，间歇捻转，留针 20 分钟；或王不留行籽压耳，左右交替，每 3～4 日 1 次。

3. Acupoint injection

3. 水针疗法

Prescription: Fengchi (GB 20), Yingxiang (LI 20) and Feishu (BL 13) [or Pishu (BL 20) or Shenshu (BL 23)].

处方：风池，迎香，肺俞（或脾俞或肾俞）。

Drugs: Vitamin B_{12}, placental tissue fluid and angelica injection, etc.

药物：维生素 B_{12}，胎盘组织液，当归注射液等。

Performance: 0.5ml is injected into the acupoints each time and once every other day.

操作：每穴注射 0.5 毫升，隔日 1 次。

5.11.5 Acute and chronic laryngopharyngitis

五、急、慢性咽喉炎

[**Introduction**]

【概述】

Laryngopharyngitis refers to acute inflammation of the throat, seen in the premonitory signs of some acute infectious diseases and usually occurring in the winter and spring. The main clinical manifestations are sore throat, burning sensation in the throat, swelling of laryngeal mucus with the sensation of foreign object. Laryngopharyngitis is similar to acute obstructive syndrome of the

急性咽喉炎是咽喉部的急性炎症，见于某些急性传染病的前驱症状，多发于冬春季节，主要临床特点为咽痛、咽部灼热感、咽部粘膜红肿有异物感，相当于中医的“急喉痹”范畴，又称“风热喉痹”，常因

throat or obstructive syndrome of the throat due to wind-heat in TCM, usually caused by sudden change of weather, weakness of defensive qi, invasion of pathogenic wind-heat into the lung meridian and retention of pathogenic wind-heat in the throat.

气候急剧变化，肺卫失固，风热邪毒乘虚侵犯肺经，循经上逆搏结于咽而成。

Chronic laryngopharyngitis refers to chronic inflammation of the laryngeal mucus and lymph tissues, usually caused by repeated relapse of acute laryngopharyngitis and seen among the middle-aged people. The main clinical manifestations are dry throat, burning sensation in the throat and sensation of foreign object in the throat. Chronic laryngopharyngitis pertains to the conception of chronic obstructive syndrome of the throat or obstructive syndrome of the throat due to asthenic fire in TCM, usually caused by remaining of pathogenic factors in prolonged diseases, asthenia of both the lung and kidney, failure of yin fluid to nourish the throat and hyperactivity of asthenic fire.

慢性咽喉炎主要是咽粘膜及淋巴组织的慢性炎症，常由急性咽喉炎反复发作演变而来，多发于中年人，主要临床特点为咽部干燥、灼热、有异物感。本病属中医的“慢喉痹”，又称“虚火喉痹”，多由久病余邪未清，肺肾两虚，阴液不能上润咽喉，虚火上炎而成。

[**Syndrome differentiation**]

【辨证】

1. Sthenia syndrome

1. 实证

Reddish swelling of the throat, burning pain and obstructive sensation in the throat, accompanied by fever, thirst, sweating, headache, cough with sputum, thick and yellow sputum, constipation, brownish urine, reddish tongue with yellow fur and rapid pulse.

咽部红肿，灼热疼痛，咽喉有堵塞感，伴发热口渴，汗出头痛，咳嗽有痰，痰黄粘稠，大便秘结，小便短赤，舌红苔黄，脉数。

2. Asthenia syndrome

2. 虚证

Discomfort in the throat, dryness and mild pain in the throat, preference for little drinking, dry cough without or with scanty and sticky sputum, flushed cheeks in the afternoon, feverish sensation in the palms and soles, aching and weakness of the loins and knees, vexation and insomnia, dizziness, tinnitus, reddish tongue with scanty fur and thin and rapid pulse.

咽中不适，干燥微痛，不喜多饮，干咳无痰或痰少而粘，午后颧红，手足心热，腰膝酸软，虚烦失眠，头晕眼花，耳鸣，舌红少苔，脉细数。

[**Treatment**]

1. Body acupuncture

Prescription: Shaoshang (LU 11), Hegu (LI 4) and Lianquan (CV 23).

Modification: For sthenia syndrome, Fengchi (GB 20), Neiting (ST 44) and Quchi (LI 11) are added; for asthenia syndrome, Taiyuan (LU 9), Yuji (LU 10), Zhaohai (KI 6) and Taixi (KI 3) are added; for severe cough, Chize (LU 5) is added; for profuse sputum, Fenglong (ST 40) is added; for tidal fever and night sweating, Yinxi (HT 6) and Fuliu (KI 7) are added; for aching and weakness of the loins and knees, Zhishi (BL 52) and Weizhong (BL 40) are added.

Performance: For sthenia syndrome, reducing needling technique is used; Shaoshang (LU 11) is pricked with three-edged needle for bloodletting; Fengchi (GB 20) and Hegu (LI 4) are needled with rotating technique for reducing purpose. For asthenia syndrome, the main acupoints are needled with mild reinforcing and reducing techniques while the compatible acupoints are needled with reinforcing technique; no moxibustion is applied.

2. Ear acupuncture

Prescription: Throat (TG_3), Lung (CO_{14}), Kidney (CO_{10}) and Lower Tragus (TG_2).

Performance: Chronic laryngopharyngitis is needled with medium and strong stimulation and chronic laryngopharyngitis is needled with mild stimulation. Each time 2 - 3 acupoints are selected to needle. Or Wangbuliuxingzi (Semen Vaccariae) is used for ear acupressure alternatively on both ears, 3 - 4 times a day.

【治疗】

1. 体针疗法

处方：少商，合谷，廉泉。

随证配穴：实证加风池、曲池、内庭；虚证加太渊、鱼际、照海、太溪。咳嗽甚加尺泽；痰多加丰隆；潮热盗汗加阴郄、复溜；腰膝酸软加志室、委中。

操作：实证，针用泻法，少商用三棱针点刺出血，风池、合谷针用捻转泻法。虚证，主穴用平补平泻法，配穴针用补法，不灸。

2. 耳针疗法

选穴：咽喉，肺，肾，下屏。

操作：急性咽喉炎采用中强刺激，慢性咽喉炎用轻刺激，每次选用 2～3 穴；或王不留行籽压耳，左右交替，每 3～4 日 1 次。

5.12 Gynecological diseases

第十二节 妇科疾病

5.12.1 Dysmenorrhea

［Introduction］

Dysmenorrhea refers to abdominal pain during or before and after menstruation, usually affecting normal work and daily life. It is either primary dysmenorrhea (or functional dysmenorrhea) marked by no evident changes of the genitalia or secondary dysmenorrhea due to organic pathological changes of the genitalia. The clinical manifestations are mainly lower abdominal pain or lumbago before and after or during menstruation, even unbearable pain and regular occurrence with menstrual cycle. This disease pertains to abdominal pain during menstruation in TCM, usually caused by stagnation of liver qi, inhibition of blood flow or attack by cold during menstruation and unsmooth circulation of qi and blood; or by malnutrition of the uterine meridian due to asthenia of qi and blood as well as liver and kidney.

［Syndrome differentiation］

1. Coagulation of cold-dampness

Cold pain in the lower abdomen before or during menstruation, rejection to pressure and preference for warmth, unsmooth and scanty menorrhea with purplish and blackish clot, accompanied by cold body and limbs, aching joints, whitish greasy tongue fur, deep and tense pulse.

2. Qi stagnation and blood stasis

Distending pain in the lower abdomen before or during menstruation, unsmooth and scanty menorrhea with purplish and blackish clot, accompanied by distension in

一、痛经

【概述】

痛经是指妇女在行经前后或经期腹部疼痛，以致影响工作及日常生活者。生殖器官无明显异常者称原发性痛经或功能性痛经，因生殖器官的器质性病变而致者称为继发性痛经。临床主要表现为行经前后或经期小腹及腰部疼痛，甚至剧痛难忍，并随月经周期发作。本病属中医“经行腹痛”范畴，多由肝气郁结，血行受阻或经期受寒，气血运行不畅所致；也可因气血虚弱、肝肾亏损而使胞脉失养引起本病。

【辨证】

1. 寒湿凝滞

经前或经期小腹冷痛，拒按喜热，经行不畅，量少，色紫黑有块，伴形寒肢冷，关节酸痛，苔白腻，脉沉紧。

2. 气滞血瘀

经前或经期小腹胀痛，经行不畅，量少，色紫黑有块，伴胸胁乳房作胀，舌质紫或有瘀

the chest, hypochondria and breast, purplish tongue or with ecchymoses, deep and taut pulse.

点,脉沉弦。

3. Insufficiency of qi and blood

Vague pain in the lower abdomen during or after menstruation, preference for pressure, light-colored and thin menorrhea, accompanied by pale complexion, lassitude, dizziness, light-colored tongue and thin and weak pulse.

3. 气血不足

经期或经后小腹隐隐作痛,喜按,月经色淡质清稀,伴面色少华,倦怠无力,头晕眼花,舌淡,脉细弱。

4. Asthenia of both the liver and kidney

Vague pain in the lower abdomen after menstruation, irregular menstruation, profuse or scanty menorrhea with light-red color and no blood clot, accompanied by aching and weakness of the loins and knees, restless sleep in the night, dizziness and tinnitus, reddish tongue with scanty fur and thin pulse.

4. 肝肾两虚

经后小腹隐隐作痛,月经先后不定期,经量或多或少,色淡红无血块,伴腰膝酸软,夜卧不宁,头晕耳鸣,舌红少苔,脉细。

[**Treatment**]

【治疗】

1. Body acupuncture

Prescription: Zhongji (CV 3), Ciliao (BL 32), Diji (SP 8) and Sanyinjiao (SP 6).

Modification: For coagulation of cold-dampness, Guanyuan (CV 4) and Shuidao (ST 28) are added with heavy and frequent moxibustion; for qi stagnation and blood stasis, Taichong (LR 3) and Xuehai (SP 10) are added; for insufficiency of qi and blood, Pishu (BL 20) and Zusanli (ST 36) are added; for asthenia of both the liver and kidney, Ganshu (BL 18), Shenshu (BL 23) and Taixi (KI 3) are added; for nausea and vomiting, Neiguan (PC 6) and Zhongwan (CV 12) are added.

Performance: The treatment begins 3-5 days before menstruation. Ciliao (BL 32) is needled 1.5 cun into the posterior sacral foramen obliquely toward the spinal column with reducing needling technique and repeated manipulation to enable warm sensation to transmit to the lower abdomen; for severe pain, electropuncture can be

1. 体针疗法

处方:中极,次髎,地机,三阴交。

随证配穴:寒湿凝滞,加关元、水道,宜多灸重灸;气滞血瘀加太冲、血海;气血不足加脾俞、足三里;肝肾两虚加肝俞、肾俞、太溪。恶心呕吐者加内关、中脘。

操作:经前3～5天开始治疗,次髎用泻法,应稍斜向脊柱,沿骶后孔刺入1.5寸,反复行针,使温热感传入小腹,疼痛甚者可加电针;中极穴,先排空小便,向下斜刺,使

used. Zhongji (CV 3) is needled (urination is done first) obliquely downward to enable needling sensation to transmit to the lower region. Diji (SP 8) is needled with reducing needling technique. Sanyinjiao (SP 6) is needled obliquely upward to enable needling sensation to transmit to the upper region. For the treatment of coagulation of cold-dampness, reducing needling technique can be used and local acupoints are dealt with needle-warming moxibustion or moxa-roll moxibustion; for qi stagnation and blood stasis, reducing needling technique is used and no moxibustion is applied; for insufficiency of qi and blood as well as asthenia of the liver and kidney, reinforcing needling technique is used with the addition of moxibustion.

针感向下传导；地机用泻法；三阴交向上斜刺使针感上传。寒湿凝滞证，针用泻法，局部穴温针灸或艾条灸；气滞血瘀证，针用泻法，不灸；气血不足、肝肾两虚均针用补法，加灸。

2. Ear acupuncture

Prescription: Internal Genitalia (TF_2), Subcortex (AT_4), Sympathetic Nerve (AH_{6a}), Endocrine (CO_{18}), Liver (CO_{12}) and Kidney (CO_{10}).

Performance: Each time 2 - 4 acupoints are needled with medium and strong stimulation. Or Wangbuliuxingzi (Semen Vaccariae) is used for ear acupressure alternatively on both ears, 3 - 4 times a day. The treatment begins 3 days before menstruation to prevent relapse.

2. 耳针疗法

选穴：内生殖器，皮质下，交感，内分泌，肝，肾。

操作：每次取 2～4 穴，毫针中强刺激，亦可用王不留行籽压耳，左右交替，每 3～4 日 1 次。为防止复发，每于月经来潮前 3 天开始治疗。

5.12.2 Irregular menstruation

[**Introduction**]

Irregular menstruation refers to abnormal changes of the menstrual cycle, volume and color of menorrhea, often accompanied by other symptoms. It is usually caused by endocrine disorder. Menstrual cycle 7 days earlier than usual or even occurrence of menorrhea twice in a month is called early menstruation; menstrual cycle 7 days later than usual or even occurrence of menorrhea once in 40 - 50 days is called delayed menstruation; menstruation

二、月经不调

【概述】

月经不调是指月经周期、经量、经色等发生异常，并伴有其他症状。多由内分泌功能失调而致。若月经周期提前 7 天以上，甚至一月两至，为月经先期，亦称经早；若月经周期推迟 7 天以上，甚至四五十天一次为月经后期，亦称

either early or delayed without a cycle is called irregular menstruation or disordered menstruation. TCM believes that irregular menstruation is caused by exogenous cold and heat or internal impairment due to emotional disorder, excessive sexual activity and frequent labor that lead to disorder of qi and blood as well as impairment of the thoroughfare and conception vessels.

经迟；若月经不按周期来潮，或先或后，为月经先后不定期，亦称经乱。中医认为本病主要由外感寒热或内伤七情、房劳多产等导致气血失调，冲任损伤而致。

［**Syndrome differentiation**］

【辨证】

1. Early menstruation

1. 经早

The menstruation occurs earlier than usual and even twice in a month. The sthenia-heat syndrome is marked by the symptoms of profuse menorrhea with fresh red color and sticky texture, dysphoria with smothery sensation, dry mouth and thirst, preference for cold drinks, reddish tongue with yellowish fur and rapid pulse; the asthenia-heat syndrome is marked by scanty red and sticky menorrhea, tidal fever and night sweating, feverish sensation over palms and soles, reddish tongue with scanty fur, thin and rapid pulse; qi-asthenia syndrome is marked by profuse light-colored and thin menorrhea, spiritual lassitude, palpitation and shortness of breath, light-colored tongue with thin fur and weak pulse.

月经先期而至，甚至经行一月两次。若月经量多，经色鲜红，质粘稠，烦热，口干渴，喜冷饮，舌红苔黄，脉数者为实热证；若月经量少色红，经质粘稠，潮热盗汗，手足心热，舌红少苔，脉细数者为虚热证；若月经量多色淡，质清稀，精神疲倦，心悸气短，舌淡苔薄，脉弱者为气虚证。

2. Delayed menstruation

2. 经迟

The menstruation is scanty and occurs even once in 40 - 50 days. Blood-asthenia syndrome is marked by light-colored menorrhea, sallow complexion, dizziness, light-colored tongue with scanty fur and thin and weak pulse; cold-sthenia syndrome is marked by blackish-colored menorrhea, cold pain in the lower abdomen, alleviation of pain with warmth, thin and white tongue fur as well as deep and slow pulse; qi stagnation syndrome is marked by blackish-colored menorrhea, oppression in the chest, distension in the hypochondria and breasts, thin and white tongue fur and taut pulse.

月经期推迟，甚至四五十天一次，量少。若经色淡，面色萎黄，头昏眼花，舌淡红少苔，脉虚细者为血虚证；若经色黯，小腹冷痛，得热痛减，苔薄白，脉沉迟者为寒实证；若经色黯，胸痞不舒，胁肋乳房作胀，苔薄白，脉弦者为气滞证。

3. Disordered menstruation

The menstruation is irregular and is either profuse or scanty. Liver depression syndrome is marked by blackish-colored, sticky and unsmooth menorrhea, distending pain in the lower abdomen, thin and white tongue fur and taut pulse; kidney-asthenia syndrome is marked by light-colored and thin menorrhea, dizziness and tinnitus, aching and weakness of the loins and knees, light-colored tongue and deep and weak pulse.

[Treatment]

1. Body acupuncture

Prescription: Qihai (CV 6) and Sanyinjiao (SP 6).

Modification: For sthenia-heat syndrome in early menstruation, Quchi (LI 11) and Xuehai (SP 10) are added; for asthenia-heat syndrome, Taichong (LR 3) and Taixi (KI 3) are added; for qi-asthenia syndrome, Zusanli (ST 36) and Pishu (BL 20) are added; for blood-asthenia syndrome in delayed menstruation, Zusanli (ST 36), Pishu (BL 20) and Weishu (BL 21) are added; for cold-sthenia syndrome, Guanyuan (CV 4) and Mingmen (GV 4) are added; for qi stagnation, Qimen (LR 14) and Taichong (LR 3) are added; for liver depression syndrome in disordered menstruation, Taichong (LR 3) and Ganshu (BL 18) are added; for kidney asthenia, Shenshu (BL 23) and Taixi (KI 3) are added.

Performance: The treatment begins 3 - 5 days before menstruation. The reducing needling technique is used to treat sthenia syndrome while the reinforcing needling technique is used to treat asthenia syndrome. Qihai (CV 6) is needled obliquely downward and Sanyinjiao (SP 6) is needled obliquely upward to enable the needling sensation to transmit to the lower abdomen. Quchi (LI 11), Xuehai (SP 10), Taichong (LR 3) and Qimen (LR 14) are needled with the reducing needling technique, while the

3. 经乱

经期先后不定期，经量或多或少。若经色紫，质粘稠，经行不畅，少腹胀痛，苔薄白，脉弦者为肝郁证；若经色淡，质清稀，头晕耳鸣，腰膝酸软，舌淡，脉沉弱者为肾虚证。

【治疗】

1. 体针疗法

处方：气海，三阴交。

随证配穴：经早之实热证加曲池、血海；虚热证加太冲、太溪；气虚证加足三里、脾俞。经迟之血虚证加足三里、脾俞、胃俞；寒实证加关元、命门；气滞证加期门、太冲。经乱之肝郁证加太冲、肝俞；肾虚证加肾俞、太溪。

操作：于经前3～5天开始治疗。实证用泻法，虚证用补法。气海向下斜刺，三阴交向上斜刺，使针感传至下腹。曲池、血海、太冲、期门针用泻法，余穴针用补法，寒实证、气虚证、血虚证、肾虚证均可加温针灸或艾条灸。

rest acupoints are needled with the reinforcing needling technique. For the treatment of cold-sthenia syndrome, qi-asthenia syndrome, blood-asthenia syndrome and kidney-asthenia syndrome, needling-warming moxibustion or moxa-roll moxibustion can be added.

2. Ear acupuncture

Acupoints: Internal Genitalia (TF_2), Subcortex (AT_4), Kidney (CO_{10}), Liver (CO_{12}) and Endocrine (CO_{18}).

Performance: Each time 2 - 3 acupoints are needled with medium stimulation and the needles are retained for 20 minutes. Or Wangbuliuxingzi (Semen Vaccariae) is used for ear acupressure alternatively on both ears. The patient is advised to press the sealed seeds on the ear several times a day. And the sealed seeds are changed once every 3 - 4 days.

2. 耳针疗法

选穴：内生殖器，皮质下，肾，肝，内分泌。

操作：选 2～3 穴，中等刺激，留针 20 分钟。或以王不留行籽压耳，嘱患者自行按压数次，左右交替；每 3～4 日更换。

5.12.3 Amenorrhea

[**Introduction**]

Amenorrhea refers to no occurrence of menarche over 18 years old or stoppage of menstruation for 3 months. The former is primary amenorrhea and the latter is secondary amenorrhea. This syndrome pertains to the conception of amenorrhea in TCM, also known as unsmooth menorrhea and stoppage of menstruation. Amenorrhea is usually caused by insufficient transformation of blood from the spleen and stomach as well as severe consumption of yin blood and exhaustion of blood source; or by retention of blood coagulation in the meridians and vessels due to retention of pathogenic factors in the uterus resulting from cold attack or cold drinks or due to mental depression.

三、闭经

【概述】

凡女子年龄超过 18 周岁，月经尚未来潮或曾来过月经，但又连续停经 3 个月以上者称为闭经。前者为原发性闭经，后者为继发性闭经。本病属中医“经闭”范畴，又称“经闭不利”、“歇经”等。由脾胃气血生化乏源，阴血亏耗过甚，血源枯竭，无血以下而成血枯经闭；或因受寒饮冷，邪气客于胞宫或情志抑郁气机不畅，瘀血凝结，经脉阻滞成为血滞经闭。

[Syndrome differentiation]

1. Asthenia syndrome

The main symptoms are gradual reduction of menstrual flow, or even amenorrhea. Amenorrhea due to asthenia of qi and blood is usually accompanied by sallow complexion, emaciation, dispiritedness, vertigo, palpitation, light-colored tongue and thin pulse. Amenorrhea due to insufficiency of the liver and kidney is accompanied by vertigo, tinnitus, aching weakness of the loins and knees, feverish sensation in the five centers (palms, soles and chest), tidal fever, night sweating, darkish-colored tongue and taut and thin pulse.

2. Sthenia syndrome

The main symptoms are amenorrhea and stoppage of menstruation for several months. Amenorrhea due to qi stagnation and blood stasis is accompanied by unpressable pain in lower abdomen, restlessness, susceptibility to anger, distending fullness in the chest and hypochondria, blackish-colored tongue or with ecchymoses and deep-taut pulse. Amenorrhea due to cold coagulation and blood stagnation is accompanied by cold body and limbs, cold pain in the lower abdomen, blackish-colored tongue with ecchymoses and deep-tense pulse. Amenorrhea due to phlegmatic dampness obstruction is accompanied by obesity, fullness and oppression in the chest and hypochondria, dispiritedness and lassitude, anorexia and profuse sputum, leukorrhagia, greasy tongue fur and slippery pulse.

[Treatment]

1. Body acupuncture

(1) Asthenia syndrome:

Prescription: Qihai (CV 6), Zusanli (ST 36) and Sanyinjiao (SP 6).

Modification: For asthenia of blood, Pishu (BL 20) and Geshu (BL 17) are added; for insufficiency of the

【辨证】

1. 虚证

经量逐渐减少，以至经闭，若兼面色萎黄，形体消瘦，精神不振，头晕心悸，舌淡脉细者为气血虚弱；若兼头晕耳鸣，腰膝酸软，五心烦热，潮热盗汗，舌暗淡脉弦细者为肝肾不足。

2. 实证

月经闭阻，数月不行，若兼少腹胀痛，拒按，烦躁易怒，胸胁胀满，舌紫黯或有瘀点，脉沉弦者为气滞血瘀；若兼形寒肢冷，小腹冷痛，舌暗有瘀，脉沉紧者为寒凝血滞；若兼形体肥胖，胸胁满闷，神疲倦怠，纳少痰多，白带量多，苔腻脉滑者为痰湿阻滞。

【治疗】

1. 体针疗法

(1) 虚证：

处方：气海，足三里，三阴交。

随证配穴：气血虚弱加脾俞、膈俞；肝肾不足加肝俞、肾

liver and kidney, Ganshu (BL 18), Shenshu (BL 23) and Guanyuan (CV 4) are added; for aching and weakness of the loins and knees, Mingmen (GV 4) and Zhishi (BL 52) are added; for tidal fever and night sweating, Fuliu (KI 7) and Taixi (KI 3) are added; for palpitation, Neiguan (PC 6) and Shenmen (HT 7) are added.

俞、关元。腰膝酸软加命门、志室；潮热盗汗加复溜、太溪；心悸加内关、神门。

Performance: The reinforcing needling technique is used. Qihai (CV 6) is needled obliquely downward with rotating reinforcing technique; Sanyinjiao (SP 6) is needled obliquely upward to enable the needling sensation to transmit to the upper part; for asthenia of qi and blood, moxibustion can be added.

操作：针用补法。气海向下斜刺，施捻转补法；三阴交向上斜刺使针感上传。气血虚弱证可加用灸法。

(2) **Sthenia syndrome**:

(2) 实证：

Prescription: Zhongji (CV 3), Xuehai (SP 10) and Sanyinjiao (SP 6).

处方：中极，血海，三阴交。

Modification: For qi stagnation and blood stasis, Hegu (LI 4), Taichong (LR 3) and Diji (SP 8) are added; for cold coagulation and blood stagnation, Guanyuan (CV 4) is added; for retention of phlegmatic dampness in the middle energizer, Zhongwan (CV 12) and Fenglong (ST 40) are added.

随证配穴：气滞血瘀加合谷、太冲、地机；寒凝血滞加关元；痰湿中阻加中脘、丰隆。

Performance: The filiform needles are used with reducing techniques. In needling Zhongji (CV 3), urination is done first and the needle is inserted obliquely downward with rotating reducing technique; Guanyuan (CV 4) is needled with the addition of moxa-roll moxibustion or moxa-cone moxibustion. The rest acupoints are needled with reducing techniques.

操作：毫针刺用泻法。中极穴，排空小便后向下斜刺行捻转泻法，关元加艾条灸或艾炷灸，余穴均用泻法。

2. Electro-acupuncture

2. 电针疗法

Prescription: Guilai (ST 29) is combined with Sanyinjiao (SP 6), Zhongji (CV 3) is combined with Diji (SP 8), and Qugu (CV 2) is combined with Xuehai (SP 10).

处方：归来配三阴交，中极配地机，曲骨配血海。

Performance: Each time one couple of the acupoints are selected or the couples of acupoints are selected

操作：每次选其中 1 对穴位，或各对穴交替使用，针刺

alternatively. After the needling sensation is felt, the impulse current is attached to the needles for 10 - 15 minutes. Electropuncture is performed once a day or once every other day.

得气后，通以脉冲电流 10～15 分钟，每日或隔日 1 次。

5.12.4 Premenstrual tension syndrome

四、经前期紧张综合征

［Introduction］

Premenstrual tension syndrome refers to emotional changes occurring regularly before menstruation. The clinical manifestations are restlessness, sorrow and sweeping, or mental depression, murmuring and insomnia which disappear when menstruation is over. This syndrome is called "abnormal emotional changes during menstruation" usually caused by stagnant liver qi attacking the spleen and failure of the spleen to produce blood to nourish the cardiac spirit due to asthenia; or by transformation of mental depression into fire that heats fluid into phlegm and disturbs the mind.

【概述】

经前期紧张综合征是指妇女每值行经之前出现的情志异常。临床主要表现为行经之前烦躁不安，悲伤啼哭，或情志抑郁，喃喃自语，彻夜不眠，经净后情志逐渐恢复正常。中医称之为"经行情志异常"，多由肝气郁结，木郁克土，脾虚不能生血，心神失养；或情志郁结化火，炼液成痰，扰乱神明而成。

［Syndrome differentiation］

1. Stagnation of liver qi

Mental depression and irritability, oppression and distension in the chest, no appetite, thin and greasy tongue coating as well as taut and thin pulse.

2. Phlegm-fire attacking the upper

Mania, headache, insomnia, flushed complexion and red eyes, oppression in the chest and dysphoria, reddish or deep red tongue, yellowish thick or greasy tongue coating as well as taut and rapid pulse.

【辨证】

1. 肝气郁结

精神抑郁不乐，情绪不宁，胸闷胁胀，不思饮食，苔薄腻，脉弦细。

2. 痰火上扰

狂躁不安，头痛失眠，面红目赤，心胸烦闷，舌红或绛，苔黄厚或腻，脉弦数。

［Treatment］

Prescription: Shenmen (HT 7), Neiguan (PC 6) and Taichong (LR 3).

Modification: For stagnation of liver qi, Qimen (LR 14), Zhongwan (CV 12) and Zusanli (ST 36) are added;

【治疗】

处方：神门，内关，太冲。

随证配穴：肝气郁结加期门、中脘、足三里；痰火上扰加

for phlegm-fire attacking the upper, Daling (PC 7), Fenglong (ST 40) and Neiting (ST 44) are added.

大陵、丰隆、内庭。

Performance: Filiform needle is used with reducing needling technique. Shenmen (HT 7), Taichong (LR 3), Daling (PC 7) and Neiting (ST 44) are needled vertically 0.3-0.5 cun with rotating manipulation for reducing purpose; Qimen (LR 14) is needled obliquely inward with twirling manipulation for reducing purpose; the rest acupoints are needled with reducing manipulation.

操作：毫针刺用泻法。神门、太冲、大陵、内庭直刺0.3～0.5寸，行捻转泻法；期门向内斜刺，行捻转泻法；余穴均用泻法。

5.12.5 Perimenopausal syndrome

五、围绝经期综合征

[Introduction]

Perimenopausal syndrome refers to a series of symptoms related to the dysfunction of automatic nerve before and after menopause. The clinical manifestations are menstrual disorder, tidal fever, irritability and susceptibility to rage, vertigo and tinnitus, amnesia and suspicion and abnormal sensation due to hypofunction of ovary, hyperthyroidism and hyperadrenalism as well as endocrine disorder. This syndrome is similar to the conceptions of "syndromes before and after menopause" and "visceral irritability" in TCM due to decline of kidney qi, exhaustion of reproductive essence, insufficiency of essence and blood, asthenia of the thoroughfare and conception vessels, imbalance between kidney yin and yang as well as dysfunction of the viscera.

【概述】

围绝经期综合征是妇女在绝经前后出现的以自主神经功能失调为主的症候群，临床主要表现为月经紊乱，潮热，烦躁易怒，头晕耳鸣，健忘多疑，感觉异常等，由卵巢功能减退，甲状腺、肾上腺功能亢进，内分泌失调而致。相当于中医"绝经前后诸证"、"脏躁"等证的范畴，由于肾气日衰，天癸将竭，精血不足，冲任亏虚，肾之阴阳失衡，脏腑功能失常而成。

[Syndrome differentiation]

1. Asthenia of liver and kidney yin

Dizziness and tinnitus, flushed complexion, night sweating and fever, aching pain in loins and knees, irregular menstruation with fresh red color and profuse or scanty menorrhea, reddish tongue with scanty coating, thin and rapid pulse.

【辨证】

1. 肝肾阴虚

头晕耳鸣，面部潮红，盗汗烦热，腰膝酸痛，月经不调，经色鲜红，量或多或少，舌红少苔，脉细数。

2. Asthenia of spleen and kidney yang

Pale complexion, dispiritedness, cold body and limbs, edema of lower limbs, thin and profuse leukorrhea, loose stool and dyspepsia, frequent urination in the night, deep and weak pulse.

2. 脾肾阳虚

面色皖白,精神委靡,形寒肢冷,下肢浮肿,带下清稀量多,纳呆便溏,夜尿频,脉沉弱。

3. Imbalance between the heart and kidney

Palpitation and insomnia, restlessness, dreaminess and susceptibility to fright, bitter taste in the mouth and dry throat, reddish tongue with scanty coating, thin and rapid pulse.

3. 心肾不交

心悸失眠,烦躁不安,多梦易惊,口苦咽干,舌红少苔,脉细数。

4. Stagnation of phlegm and qi

Obesity, chest oppression and profuse phlegm, epigastric and abdominal distension and fullness, belching and acid regurgitation, edema and loose stool, greasy tongue coating and slippery pulse.

4. 痰气郁结

形体肥胖,胸闷痰多,脘腹胀满,嗳气吞酸,浮肿便溏,苔腻,脉滑。

［**Treatment**］

【治疗】

1. Body acupuncture

Prescription: Sanyinjiao (SP 6), Qihai (CV 6), Shenmen (HT 7) and Baihui (GV 20).

Modification: For asthenia of the liver and kidney, Taixi (KI 3), Taichong (LR 3) and Ganshu (BL 18) are added; for asthenia of spleen and kidney yang, Pishu (BL 20), Zusanli (ST 36), Yinlingquan (SP 9) and Zhongwan (CV 12) are added; for imbalance between the heart and the kidney, Tongli (HT 5), Xinshu (BL 15), Shenshu (BL 23) and Zhishi (BL 52) are added; for stagnation of phlegm and qi, Fenglong (ST 40) and Tanzhong (CV 17) are added.

Performance: Each time 5 - 6 acupoints are selected according to the pathological conditions. Sanyinjiao (SP 6), Qihai (CV 6) and Shenmen (HT 7) are needled with reinforcing technique; while Fengchi (GB 20) and Baihui (GV 20) are needled with reducing technique. For the treatment of asthenia of liver and kidney yin, Taixi

1. 体针疗法

处方:三阴交,气海,风池,神门,百会。

随证配穴:肝肾阴虚加太溪、太冲、肝俞;脾肾阳虚加脾俞、足三里、阴陵泉、中脘;心肾不交加通里、心俞、肾俞、志室;痰气郁结加丰隆、膻中。

操作:根据病情每次选用5～6穴。三阴交、气海、神门针用补法,风池、百会针用泻法。肝肾阴虚证,太溪、肝俞针用补法,太冲针用泻法;脾肾阳虚证,针用补法,温针灸

(KI 3) and Ganshu (BL 18) are needled with reinforcing technique, while Taichong (LR 3) is needled with reducing technique; for the treatment of asthenia syndrome of spleen and kidney yang, reinforcing needling technique is used and needle-warming moxiubstion or moxa-roll moxibustion is used; for the treatment of imbalance between the heart and the kidney, Tongli (HT 5) is needled with reducing technique and the rest acupoints are needled with reinforcing technique; for the treatment of stagnation of phlegm and qi, reducing needling technique is used.

或艾条灸；心肾不交证，通里针用泻法，余穴均用补法；痰气郁结证，针用泻法。

2. Ear acupuncture

Prescription: Endocrine (CO_{18}), Internal genitalia (TF_2), Sympathetic Nerve (AH_{6a}), Subcortex (AT_4), Kidney (CO_{10}) and Liver (CO_{12}).

Performance: Each time 2 - 3 acupoints on one side are selected to seal with Wangbuliuxingzi (Semen Vaccariae). The patient is advised to press the sealed seeds on the selected ear acupoints 3 times a day. The sealed seeds are changed once every 3 - 4 days. Five to ten days make up one course of treatment.

2. 耳针疗法

选穴：内分泌，内生殖器，交感，皮质下，肾，肝。

操作：选单侧 2～3 穴用王不留行籽压耳，左右交替，嘱病人每日按压 3 次；每 3～4 日更换，5～10 次为 1 个疗程。

5.12.6 Sterility

[**Introduction**]

Sterility refers to inability to conceive three years after marriage with normal sexual life and without contraception, or inability to conceive for two years after giving birth to a baby or after abortion without contraception. It is usually caused by dysfunction of ovary secretion and ovum formation or deformity of genital organs. TCM believes that sterility is caused by kidney asthenia and dysfunction of the thoroughfare and conception vessels due to asthenia of kidney essence, liver depression and qi stagnation, blockage of the uterus by phlegm and dampness as well as blood stasis and cold coagulation.

六、不孕症

【**概述**】

凡育龄妇女，婚后夫妇同居 3 年以上，配偶生殖功能正常，未避孕而未能怀孕者；或曾生育或流产后，无避孕而又两年以上不再受孕者称为不孕症。主要由卵巢分泌及卵子生成障碍，生殖道畸形等所致。相当于中医“无子”、“绝产”等范畴，因肾精亏损，肝郁气滞，痰湿阻胞，血瘀寒凝等致肾虚不养，冲任失调而致不孕。

[Syndrome differentiation]

1. Kidney asthenia type

Sterility long after marriage, aching and weakness of loins and knees; the symptoms in delayed menstruation are scanty menorrhea with light color, even amenorrhea, profuse clear urine, loose stool, light-colored tongue with whitish color, thin and deep or slow pulse due to asthenia of kidney yang; the symptoms of early menstruation are scanty menorrhea with red color and without blood clot, emaciation, dizziness, palpitation, insomnia, dry mouth, fever, reddish tongue with scanty fur as well as thin and rapid pulse due to asthenia of kidney yin.

2. Liver depression type

The symptoms are sterility for years, irregular menstruation, abdominal pain during menstruation, unsmooth scanty menorrhea with blackish color and clot, distending pain in the breasts before menstruation, mental depression, dysphoria, susceptibility to anger, reddish tongue and taut pulse.

3. Phlegm-dampness type

The symptoms are sterility long after marriage, obesity, delayed menstruation, even amenorrhea, sticky leukorrhea, palpitation, dizziness, chest oppression, nausea, whitish greasy tongue coating and slippery pulse.

4. Blood stasis type

The symptoms are sterility long after marriage, delayed menstruation with scanty menorrhea, purplish menorrhea with clot, dysmenorrhea, unpressable abdominal pain during menstruation, blackish tongue with ecchymoses, taut and unsmooth pulse.

[Treatment]

1. Body acupuncture

Prescription: Zhongji (CV 3), Sanyinjiao (SP 6), Qixue (Ext.) and Zigong (EX-CA 1).

【辨证】

1. 肾虚型

婚久不孕，腰膝酸软，若月经后期，量少色淡，甚则闭经，小便清长，大便不实，舌淡苔白，脉沉细或迟者，为肾阳虚；若月经先期，量少色红，无血块，形体消瘦，头昏眼花，心悸失眠，口干烦热，舌红少苔，脉细数者，为肾阴虚。

2. 肝郁型

多年不孕，经期先后不定，经行腹痛，行而不畅，量少色黯，有块，经前乳房胀痛，精神抑郁，烦躁易怒，舌红，脉弦。

3. 痰湿型

婚后久不受孕，形体肥胖，经行延后，甚则闭经，带下量多粘稠，心悸头晕，胸闷呕恶，苔白腻，脉滑。

4. 血瘀型

婚久不孕，月经后期量少，色紫暗有块，痛经，痛时拒按，舌暗有瘀斑，脉弦涩。

【治疗】

1. 体针疗法

处方：中极，三阴交，气穴，子宫。

Modification: For kidney asthenia, Shenshu (BL 23) and Rangu (KI 2) are added; for asthenia of kidney yang, Mingmen (GV 4) and Guanyuan (CV 4) are added; for asthenia of kidney yin, Taixi (KI 3) is added; for liver depression, Ganshu (BL 18), Taichong (LR 3) and Yanglingquan (GB 34) are added; for phlegm-dampness, Yinlingquan (SP 9), Fenglong (ST 40), Zusanli (ST 36) and Zhongwan (CV 12) are added; for blood stasis, Geshu (BL 17) and Xuehai (SP 10) are added.

随证配穴：肾虚加肾俞、然谷，若肾阳虚加命门、关元，若肾阴虚加太溪；肝郁加肝俞、太冲、阳陵泉；痰湿加阴陵泉、丰隆、足三里、中脘；血瘀加膈俞、血海。

Performance: Needling is given from the 12th day of the menstrual cycle. For the treatment of kidney asthenia, reinforcing needling technique is used; Mingmen (GV 4) and Guanyuan (CV 4) are needled with warmed needles or applied with moxa-cone or moxa-roll moxibustion. For the treatment of liver depression, mild reinforcing and reducing needling techniques are used; Ganshu (BL 18) is needled with reinforcing technique, Taichong (LR 3) and Yanglingquan (GB 34) are needled with reducing technique. For the treatment of phlegm-dampness syndrome, reducing needling technique is used; Zusanli (ST 36) is needled with reinforcing technique and the rest acupoints are needled with reducing techniques. For the treatment of blood stasis, reducing needling technique is used; Geshu (BL 17) and Xuehai (SP 10) are tapped with cutaneous needles and applied with cupping after needling.

操作：在月经周期第12日开始针刺。肾虚证，针用补法，命门、关元行温针灸或艾条灸或大艾炷灸；肝郁证，针用平补平泻法，肝俞行补法，太冲、阳陵泉行泻法；痰湿证，针用泻法，足三里行补法，余穴用泻法；血瘀证，针用泻法，膈俞、血海用皮肤针叩刺后拔罐。

2. Ear acupuncture

2. 耳针疗法

Prescription: Endocrine (CO_{18}), Internal Genitalia (TF_2), Kidney (CO_{10}), Subcortical (AT_4) and Apex of tragus ($AT_{1,2,4i}$).

处方：内分泌，内生殖器，肾，肝，皮质下，对屏尖。

Performance: Each time 2-3 acupoints are needled with moderate stimulation for 30 minutes. Or Wangbuliuxingzi (Semen Vaccariae) is used for ear acupressure. The two ears are pressed alternatively and the sealed seeds are changed once every 3-4 days. The patient is

操作：每次2～3穴，中等刺激，留针30分钟。或以王不留行籽压耳法，左右交替，嘱病人每日按压3～4次；每3～4日更换1次。

advised to press the acupoints 3 - 4 times a day.

5. 12. 7 Malposition of fetus

[**Introduction**]

Malposition of fetus refers to incorrect position of the fetus 30 weeks after pregnancy. The gravida shows no subjective symptoms and the problem can only be found in the examination. Abnormal fetal position is usually seen in pluripara or gravida with loose abdominal wall. If it is not timely rectified, dystocia will be caused. TCM believes that abnormal fetal position is caused by asthenia of qi and blood, insufficiency of fetal qi or abnormal development of the fetus, weakness of the uterus in contraction or stagnation of qi and blood.

[**Treatment**]

Prescription: Zhiyin (BL 67).

Performance: The clothes are loosened and the gravida sits on a armchair or laying on the bed in a supine position. Zhiyin (BL 67) is moxibusted with moxa-roll for 15 - 20 minutes once or twice a day till the position of the fetus is rectified. The rectification rate is high for those 7 months after pregnancy and low for those 8 months after pregnancy. Sometimes acupuncture or electrical acupuncture is used for rectification of fetal position. But most often moxibustion is used.

七、胎位不正

【**概述**】

胎位不正是指妊娠 30 周后,胎儿在子宫体内的位置不正而言。孕妇本身无自觉症状,经产前检查才能明确诊断,常见于经产妇或腹壁松弛的孕妇,如不及时纠正,分娩时可造成难产。中医称为“胎不正”,由于气血亏虚,胎气不足或胎儿发育异常,子宫收缩无力,或气血阻滞影响胞胎运转而成。

【**治疗**】

处方:至阴。

操作:解松腰带,坐在靠背椅或仰卧床上,以艾条灸两侧至阴穴 15～20 分钟,每日 1～2 次,至胎位转正后为止。以妊娠 7 个月者成功率最高,8 个月以上者次之。也有采用针刺或电针者,但多数用灸法。

5.13 Pediatric diseases

第十三节 儿科疾病

5. 13. 1 Infantile convulsion

[**Introduction**]

Infantile convulsion refers to acute syndrome of the

一、小儿惊厥

【**概述**】

惊厥是小儿时期常见的

central nervous system due to organic or functional abnormal changes. The clinical manifestations are convulsion and coma. This syndrome is divided into acute convulsion and chronic convulsion in TCM. Acute convulsion is marked by sudden onset and high fever accompanied by convulsion and coma due to exogenous seasonal pestilence and sudden fright which lead to internal accumulation of phlegm-heat, consequently resulting in transformation of heat from stagnation of pathogenic factors and production of wind and phlegm from extreme heat. The location of this syndrome is in the heart and liver. Chronic convulsion is marked by slow onset as well as repeated convulsion and coma or paralysis usually seen after severe disease and chronic disease due to prenatal insufficiency or lingering of acute convulsion, asthenia of the spleen and hyperfunction of the liver, or production of wind resulting from asthenia of liver and kidney yin. The location of this syndrome is in the liver, spleen and kidney.

中枢神经系统器质或功能异常的急性病证，以临床出现抽搐、昏迷为主要症状。本病属中医“惊风”范畴，根据其发病情况可分为急惊风和慢惊风。凡来势急骤，以高热伴抽风、昏迷为特征，称为急惊风，因外感时邪、暴受惊恐，内蕴痰热，邪郁化热，热极生风生痰生惊而致，其病位在心肝。凡来势缓慢，以反复抽痉、昏迷或瘫痪为主症者称为慢惊风，多见于大病久病之后，或先天禀赋不足，或急惊风经治不愈等，脾虚肝旺，或肝肾阴虚而生风，病位在肝脾肾。

[Syndrome differentiation]

【辨证】

1. Acute convulsion

The symptoms are coma, upward staring of eyes, lockjaw, stiffness of neck, opisthotonus, convulsion of limbs, or high fever without sweating and dysphoria; or poor appetite, vomiting and sputum rale in the throat; or nervousness, restless sleep and taut and rapid pulse.

1. 急惊风

神志昏迷，两目上视，牙关紧闭，颈项强直，角弓反张，四肢抽搐，或高热无汗，烦躁不安；或纳呆呕吐，喉间痰鸣；或惊恐不安，夜卧不宁，脉弦数。

2. Chronic convulsion

The symptoms are somnolence or coma, occasional convulsion, or tremor of hands and feet, or spasm of limbs, cold limbs, dispiritedness, anorexia, sallow complexion and emaciation, loose stool or stool with indigested food in it, profuse and clear urine as well as deep and weak pulse.

2. 慢惊风

嗜睡或昏迷，时有抽搐，或手足蠕动，或肢体拘挛，四肢厥冷，精神委顿，不思饮食，面黄肌瘦，大便溏薄或完谷不化，小便清长，脉沉弱无力。

[**Treatment**]

1. Body acupuncture

(1) Acute convulsion:

Prescription: Yintang (EX-HN 3), Shuigou (GV 26), Shixuan (EX-UE 11) and Taichong (LR 3).

Modification: For high fever, Dazhui (GV 14) and Quchi (LI 11) are added; for profuse phlegm, Fenglong (ST 40) and Zhongwan (CV 12) are added; for lockjaw, Jiache (ST 6) and Hegu (LI 4) are added.

Performance: The filiform needles and reducing technique are used, moxibustion is not applied. Three-edged needle is used to prick Shixuan (EX-UE 11) and Yintang (EX-HN 3) for bloodletting. Shuigou (GV 26) is needled obliquely upward with rotation in a great range for reducing purpose.

(2) Chronic convulsion:

Prescription: Ganshu (BL 18), Pishu (BL 20), Shenshu (BL 23), Zusanli (ST 36), Qihai (CV 6), Baihui (GV 20) and Yintang (EX-HN 3).

Modification: For loose stool or stool with indigested food in it, Shenque (CV 8) is added for moxibustion; for anorexia, Zhongwan (CV 12) is added.

Performance: Filiform needle and reinforcing technique are used. Baihui (GV 20) and Yintang (EX-HN 3) are needled with mild reducing and reinforcing techniques; the rest acupoints are needled with reinforcing technique or with warmed needle or applied with moxa-roll moxibustion.

2. Ear acupuncture

Prescription: Sympathetic Nerve (AH_{6a}), Ear Shenmen (TF_4), Subcortex (AT_4), Heart (CO_{15}), Liver (CO_{12}), Spleen (CO_{13}) and Kidney (CO_{10}).

Performance: Each time 3 - 4 acupoints are selected according to the pathological conditions. For the treatment

【治疗】

1. 体针疗法

(1) 急惊风:

处方:印堂,水沟,十宣,太冲。

随证配穴:高热加大椎、曲池;痰多加丰隆、中脘;口噤不开加颊车、合谷。

操作:毫针刺用泻法,不灸。印堂、十宣用三棱针点刺出血,水沟向上斜刺行大幅度捻转泻法。

(2) 慢惊风:

处方:肝俞,脾俞,肾俞,足三里,气海,百会,印堂。

随证配穴:大便溏薄或完谷不化加灸神阙;不思饮食加中脘。

操作:毫针刺用补法。百会、印堂施平补平泻法,余穴均用补法,温针灸或艾条灸。

2. 耳针疗法

处方:交感,神门,皮质下,心,肝,脾,肾。

操作:根据病情选用 3～4 穴,急惊风用强刺激,留针

of acute convulsion, strong stimulation is needed and the needle is retained for 60 minutes. For the treatment of chronic convulsion, moderate stimulation is required and the needle is retained for 30 minutes. Or Wangbuliuxingzi (Semen Vaccariae) is used for ear acupressure and press the sealed seeds on the selected ear acupoints 3 - 4 times a day. The sealed seeds are changed once every 3 - 4 days.

60分钟；慢惊风用中等刺激，留针30分钟。或王不留行籽压耳，每日按压3～4次，左右交替；每3～4日更换1次。

5.13.2 Infantile diarrhea

［**Introduction**］

Infantile diarrhea, one of the commonly encountered diseases in pediatrics, is usually due to improper diet, bacterial and viral infection in the intestines. The main clinical manifestations are frequent defecation, abdominal flatulence and borborygmus as well as watery stool. According to TCM this disease is caused by exogenous pathogenic factors, improper diet, hypofunction of the spleen and stomach, dysfunction of the spleen and stomach in transformation and transportation as well as interaction between lucid and turbid materials in the intestines. This disease mainly involves the spleen and stomach. However, prolongation may affect the kidney.

［**Syndrome differentiation**］

1. Diarrhea due to damp-heat

The symptoms are loose stool with yellow color and foul odor, abdominal pain, fever, thirst, burning sensation in the anus, scanty and brownish urine, reddish tongue with yellowish greasy coating as well as slippery and rapid pulse.

2. Diarrhea due to dyspepsia

The symptoms are loose stool with milk clot or food residue and putrid odor like bad egg, crying, anorexia, unpressable abdominal pain, belching or vomiting, light-reddish tongue with thick and greasy or yellowish and

二、婴幼儿腹泻

【概述】

婴幼儿腹泻是儿科常见病之一，多由饮食不当和肠道细菌、病毒感染引起，临床主要表现为大便次数增多，腹胀肠鸣，粪质稀薄如水样。本病属中医"泄泻"范畴，由感受外邪，饮食内伤，脾胃虚弱，脾胃运化失常，清浊相干，并走大肠而成。病变脏腑主要在脾胃，久病可及肾。

【辨证】

1. 湿热泻

泻下稀薄，色黄而秽臭，腹部疼痛，发热口渴，肛门灼热，小便短赤，舌红苔黄腻，脉滑数。

2. 伤食泻

大便稀烂夹有乳片或食物残渣，大便腐臭，状如败卵，吵闹，不思乳食，腹痛拒按，嗳气或呕吐，舌淡红，苔厚腻或

dirty coating.

黄垢。

3. Diarrhea due to yang asthenia

3. 阳虚泻

The symptoms are prolonged diarrhea, loose stool or stool with indigested food in it, or accompanied by prolapse of the anus, cold sensation in the limbs and body, pale complexion, dispiritedness or even cold limbs, light-colored tongue with whitish coating as well as deep and thin pulse.

久泻不愈,大便清稀,或完谷不化,或伴脱肛,形寒肢冷,面色苍白,精神委靡,甚则四肢厥冷,舌淡,苔白,脉沉细。

[**Treatment**]

【**治疗**】

1. Body acupuncture

1. 体针疗法

Prescription: Tianshu (ST 25) and Zusanli (ST 36).

处方:天枢,足三里。

Modification: For damp-heat, Quchi (LI 11) and Neiting (ST 44) are added; for severe fever, Dazhui (GV 14) and Hegu (LI 4) are added; for severe dampness, Yinlingquan (SP 9) is added; for dyspepsia, Zhongwan (CV 12), Neiting (ST 44) and Sifeng (EX-UE 10) are added; for diarrea due to yang asthenia, Pishu (BL 20), Shenshu (BL 23) and Guanyuan (CV 4) are added.

随证配穴:湿热泻加曲池、内庭,热重加大椎、合谷,湿重加阴陵泉;伤食泻加中脘、里内庭、四缝;阳虚泻加脾俞、肾俞、关元。

Performance: Needling without retention of needles is suitable for the treatment of the infants under the age of 4. for the treatment of diarrhea due to damp-heat and dyspepsia, Sifeng (EX-UE 10) is pricked with three-edged needle to let a little yellowish liquid; for the treatment of diarrhea due to yang asthenia, the acupoints are needled with reinforcing needling technique or warmed needle or moxibusted with moxa-roll or Guanyuan (CV 4) is moxibusted with big moxa-cone.

操作:小于4周岁幼儿针刺不留针。湿热、伤食泻针用泻法,四缝用三棱针点刺放出少量黄水;阳虚泻针用补法,温针灸或艾条灸或关元穴大艾炷灸。

2. Moxibustion

2. 艾灸疗法

Prescription: Shenque (CV 8), Guanyuan (CV 4) and Changqiang (GV 1).

处方:神阙,关元,长强。

Performance: Shenque (CV 8) is moxibusted with the cushion of salt; Guanyuan (CV 4) and Changqiang (GV 1) are moxibusted with moxa-roll or moxa-cone once a day. Moxibustion therapy is applicable to the treatment of diarrhea due to yang asthenia.

操作:神阙隔盐灸,关元、长强艾条灸或艾炷灸,每日1次,适用于阳虚泻患者。

5.13.3　Infantile enuresis

［Introduction］

Infantile enuresis refers to involuntary and recurrent urination during sleep among infants over three years old. Enuresis may occur once in several days in mild cases and every night in serious cases, accompanied by lassitude and emaciation. According to TCM, infantile enuresis is caused by insufficiency of kidney qi which fails to consolidate the bladder; or by asthenia of lung and spleen qi that fails to govern the lower energizer; or by stagnation of heat in the liver meridian and disorder of the bladder in transforming qi. This syndrome mainly involves the kidney and bladder.

［Syndrome differentiation］

1. Insufficiency of kidney yang

The symptoms are enuresis during sleep even several times a night, clear and profuse urine, dispiritedness and lassitude, whitish complexion and cold limbs, aching and weakness of the loins and knees, hypomnesis or poor mentality, light-colored tongue and thin pulse.

2. Asthenia of spleen and lung qi

The symptoms are enuresis during sleep, aggravation after fatigue, profuse and frequent urination, frequent spontaneous sweating, poor appetite, shortness of breath and no desire to speak, weakness of limbs, loose stool, light-colored tongue and thin pulse.

［Treatment］

1. Body acupuncture

Prescription: Guanyuan (CV 4), Zhongji (CV 3), Sanyinjiao (SP 6) and Pangguangshu (BL 28).

Modification: For insufficiency of kidney yang, Shenshu (BL 23) and Mingmen (GV 4) are added; for asthenia of spleen and lung qi, Pishu (BL 20), Feishu (BL 13),

三、小儿遗尿

【概述】

遗尿是指3岁以上的小儿睡中小便自遗，醒后方知，并反复出现的一种儿科常见病，轻者数日遗尿1次，重者每夜自遗，伴倦怠，形体消瘦。属于中医“遗溺”范畴，由肾气不足，下元不能固摄；或肺脾气虚，不能约束下焦；或肝经郁热，膀胱气化失常所致，病变脏腑主要为肾与膀胱。

【辨证】

1. 肾阳不足

睡中遗尿，甚者一夜数次，尿清而长，神疲乏力，面白肢冷，腰膝酸软，记忆力减退或智力较差，舌淡，脉细。

2. 脾肺气虚

睡中遗尿，一经劳累，尿床加重，尿频量少，常自汗出，食欲不振，少气懒言，四肢乏力，大便溏薄，舌淡，脉细。

【治疗】

1. 体针疗法

处方：关元，中极，三阴交，膀胱俞。

随证配穴：肾阳不足加肾俞、命门；脾肺气虚加脾俞、肺俞、气海、足三里。

Qihai (CV 6) and Zusanli (ST 36) are added.

Performance: The acupoints are needled with filiform needles and reinforcing technique or warmed needle or moxibustion with moxa-roll. Guanyuan (CV 4) and Zhongji (CV 3) are needled, after urination, obliquely downward with rotation of the needle for reinforcing purpose; Sanyinjiao (SP 6) is needled obliquely upward to direct the needling sensation to transmit upwards.

操作：毫针刺用补法，温针灸或艾条灸。关元、中极穴，于排空小便后向下斜刺，行捻转补法；三阴交向上斜刺使针感上传。

2. Scalp acupuncture

2. 头针疗法

Prescription: Zone of pedal movement and sensation and reproductive zone.

处方：足运感区，生殖区。

Performance: The needles are inserted in the scalp and twirled quickly or attached with electricity. The needles are retained for 30 minutes.

操作：沿皮刺，快速捻转，或用电针，留针 30 分钟。

5.14 Others

第十四节 其 他

5.14.1 High fever

一、高热

[**Introduction**]

Temperature over 39℃ is high fever, usually seen in acute infection, acute infectious disease and heat-stroke, often accompanied by coma and spasm. According to TCM, high fever is caused by exogenous wind-heat that leads to dysfunction of the lung in depuration and pulmonary qi to disperse; or by combat between pathogenic factors and healthy qi due to inner invasion of febrile pathogenic factors unrelieved in the exterior into qi phase, blood phase and the pericardium.

【概述】

一般以体温超过 39℃ 的称为高热，常见于急性感染、急性传染病、中暑等多种疾病中，常伴有昏迷、痉挛等症。本病属中医“壮热”、“实热”范畴，引起高热的原因很多，本节仅介绍外感引起的高热。由外感风热，肺失清肃，卫失宣散；或温邪在表不解，内入气分，内陷营血，内犯心包，邪正相争而成。

[**Syndrome differentiation**]

【辨证】

1. Wind-heat attacking the lung

1. 风热犯肺

The symptoms are cough, slight aversion to wind and

发热咳嗽，微恶风寒，汗

cold, sweating, headache, sore throat, dry mouth and thirst, or vomiting of yellowish sticky fluid, thin tongue fur, floating and rapid pulse.

出头痛，咽喉肿痛，口干而渴，或吐黄色粘液，苔薄，脉浮数。

2. Severe heat in qi phase

The symptoms are high fever, no aversion to cold, aversion to heat, flushed cheeks and red eyes, thirst and desire for cold drinks, cough and chest pain, or constipation, unpressable abdominal flatulence, yellowish dry tongue fur, rapid and full pulse.

2. 气分热甚

高热，不恶寒反恶热，面目红赤，口渴饮冷，咳嗽胸痛，或大便秘结，腹部胀痛拒按，苔黄燥，脉洪数。

3. Invasion of heat into blood phase

The symptoms are high fever worsened in the night, restlessness, even delirium, thirst without desire for drinks, or maculae, or hemorrhage, hematemesis, hematochezia, deep red and dry tongue, thin and rapid pulse.

3. 热入营血

高热夜甚，烦躁不安，甚则神昏谵语，口燥而不渴，或斑疹隐隐，或见衄血、吐血、便血，舌红绛而干，脉细数。

4. Invasion of summer-heat into the heart

The symptoms are high fever, dysphoria, thirst and profuse drinking, dry mouth and lips, burning sensation in the muscles, occasional delirium, even coma and spasm, deep red and dry tongue as well as full and rapid pulse.

4. 暑热蒙心

壮热，心烦不安，口渴引饮，口唇干燥，肌肤灼热，时有谵语，甚则神昏痉厥，舌红绛而干，脉洪数。

[**Treatment**]

Prescription: Dazhui (GV 14) and Quchi (LI 11).

Modification: For invasion of wind-heat into the lung, Chize (LU 5), Yuji (LU 10) and Waiguan (TE 15) are added; for severe heat in qi phase, Hegu (LI 4), Neiting (ST 44) and Guanchong (TE 1) are added; for invasion of heat into blood phase, Quze (PC 3), Laogong (PC 8) and Weizhong (BL 40) are added; for invasion of summer-heat into the heart, twelve Jing-well acupoints are added.

Performance: The acupoints are needled with filiform needles and reducing needling techniques. Moxibustion is not used. Dazhui (GV 14) is needled with the rotation of the needle for reducing purpose; Guanchong (TE 1) and the twelve Jing-well acupoints are pricked by the

【治疗】

处方：大椎，曲池。

随证配穴：风热犯肺加尺泽、鱼际、外关；气分热甚加合谷、内庭、关冲；热入营血加曲泽、劳宫、委中；暑热蒙心加十二井穴。

操作：毫针刺用泻法，不灸。大椎行捻转泻法，关冲、十二井穴用三棱针点刺出血，热甚则于曲泽、委中穴用三棱针点刺放血。

three-edged needle for bloodletting; for severe high fever, Quze (PC 3) and Weizhong (BL 50) are pricked by the three-edged needle for bloodletting.

5. 14. 2 Coma

［**Introduction**］

Coma refers to temporary loss of consciousness for a short period of time due to insufficiency of cerebral blood flow. Usually there is no sequela. However, rehabilitation is difficult to be obtained in some cases and death may be caused eventually. The clinical manifestations are sudden faint, unconsciousness and cold limbs. According to TCM, coma is caused by asthenia of qi and blood or disorder of yin and yang, adverse flow of qi, disconnection between nutrient qi and defensive qi as well as obstruction of the upper orifices due to wind, fire and phlegm.

［**Syndrome differentiation**］

1. Asthenia syndrome

The symptoms are sudden coma, unconsciousness, cold limbs, indistinct respiration, open mouth and spontaneous sweating, pale complexion, deep and thin pulse.

2. Sthenia syndrome

The symptoms are sudden coma, unconsciousness, cold limbs, dyspnea, lockjaw and deep-sthenic pulse.

［**Treatment**］

Prescription: Shuigou (GV 26), twelve Jing-well acupoints and Baihui (GV 20).

Modification: For asthenia syndrome, Neiguan (PC 6), Qihai (CV 6) and Zusanli (ST 36) are added; for sthenia syndrome, Zhongchong (PC 9), Taichong (LR 3), Laogong (PC 8) and Yongquan (KI 1) are added.

二、昏厥

【概述】

昏厥是指一过性脑血流量不足引起突然而短暂的意识丧失,一般昏厥时间较短,醒后无后遗症,但也有一厥不复,而导致死亡者。临床主要表现为突然昏倒,不省人事,四肢厥冷等。相当于中医"厥证"范畴,由气血亏虚或风火痰致阴阳失调,气机逆乱,营卫之气不能顺接,清窍受扰所致。

【辨证】

1. 虚证

突然昏倒,不省人事,四肢厥冷,气息微弱,张口自汗,面色苍白,脉沉细。

2. 实证

突然昏倒,不省人事,四肢厥冷,气壅息粗,四肢僵直,牙关紧闭,脉沉实。

【治疗】

处方:水沟,十二井,百会。

随证配穴:虚证加内关、气海、足三里;实证加中冲、太冲、劳宫、涌泉。

Performance: For the treatment of asthenia syndrome, reinforcing needling technique is used; Shuigou (GV 26), the twelve Jing-well acupoints, Baihui (GV 20) and Neiguan (PC 6) are needled with mild reducing and reinforcing techniques; Qihai (CV 6) and Zusanli (ST 36) are needled with reinforcing technique or with warmed needle or moxibusted with moxa-roll. For the treatment of sthenia syndrome, reducing needling technique is used; the twelve Jing-well acupoints and Zhongchong (PC 9) are pricked with the three-edged needle for bloodletting; Shuigou (GV 26), Laogong (PC 8) and Yongquan (KI 1) are needled with the rotation of the needles for reducing purpose.

操作：虚证针用补法，水沟、十二井、百会、内关针用平补平泻法，气海、足三里针用补法，温针灸或艾条灸；实证针用泻法，十二井、中冲用三棱针点刺出血，水沟、劳宫、涌泉行捻转泻法。

5.14.3 Obstinate hiccup

三、顽固性呃逆

[**Introduction**]

Obstinate hiccup refers to spasm of diaphragm resulting from the stimulation of the diaphragm due to various reasons. The clinical manifestations are constant and involuntary hiccup in the throat affecting talking, chewing, respiration and sleep. According to TCM, hiccup is usually caused by failure of gastric qi to descend, adverse flow of gastric qi over the diaphragm and disorder of qi due to improper diet, or stagnation of liver qi or weakness of spleen yang.

【概述】

顽固性呃逆是多种原因造成膈神经受刺激而引起的膈肌痉挛。临床主要表现为喉间呃呃连声，不能自止，并妨碍谈话、咀嚼、呼吸、睡眠等的一种疾病。中医称“哕”、“呃逆”，俗称“打呃”。多由饮食不节，或肝郁气滞，或脾阳虚弱，等致胃气不降，上逆胸膈，气机逆乱而成。

[**Syndrome differentiation**]

【辨证】

1. Dyspepsia

The symptoms are loud hiccup, distending pain in the chest and abdomen, belching, anorexia, thick and greasy tongue coating, slippery and sthenic pulse.

1. 食积证

呃声洪亮，脘腹胀痛，嗳气厌食，苔厚腻，脉滑实。

2. Qi stagnation syndrome

The symptoms are constant hiccup, distending pain in the chest and hypochondria, dysphoria, thin tongue

2. 气滞证

呃呃连声，胸胁胀满，烦闷不舒，苔薄，脉弦有力。

coating, taut and powerful pulse.

3. Stomach-cold syndrome

The symptoms are slow and strong hiccup, alleviation with warmth, aggravation with cold, discomfort in the epigastrium, normal taste in the mouth, whitish and slippery tongue coating and slow pulse.

[**Treatment**]

1. Body acupuncture

Prescription: Geshu (BL 17), Neiguan (PC 6) and Zhongwan (CV 12).

Modification: For dyspepsia, Neiting (ST 44) and Zusanli (ST 36) are added; for qi stagnation, Danzhong (CV 17) and Taichong (LR 3) are added; for stomach-cold, Weishu (BL 21), Liangmen (ST 21) and Guanyuan (CV 4) are added.

Performance: The acupoints are needled with filiform needles and reducing technique. For the treatment of stomach-cold syndrome, warmed-needle moxibustion or moxibustion with moxa-roll is used.

2. Ear acupuncture

Prescription: Internal Ear (HX_1), Sympathetic Nerve (AH_{6a}), Stomach (CO_4), Liver (CO_{12}) and Spleen (CO_{13}).

Performance: The acuponts are needled with strong stimulation and the needles are retained for 30 minutes. Or embedment of needles is used and the ears are embedded alternatively once 3 - 4 days.

3. 胃寒证

呃声沉缓有力，得热则减，得寒愈甚，胃脘不舒，口中和，苔白润，脉迟缓。

【治疗】

1. 体针疗法

处方：膈俞，内关，中脘。

随证配穴：食积证加里内庭、足三里；气滞证加膻中、太冲；胃寒证加胃俞、梁门、关元。

操作：毫针刺用泻法，胃寒者行温针灸或艾条灸。

2. 耳针疗法

选穴：耳中，交感，胃，肝，脾。

操作：强刺激，留针30分钟；或埋皮内针，左右交替，每3～4日1次。

5.14.4 Stopping smoking

[**Introduction**]

Stopping smoking means to eliminate addiction to tobacco and the abstinence symptoms, such as general weakness and restlessness. According to TCM, smoking affects the functions of the heart, pericardium, lung,

四、戒烟

【概述】

戒烟是指消除吸烟患者对烟叶制品的瘾癖，消除中断吸烟后患者出现的全身软弱无力、烦躁等症状。中医认为

spleen and stomach, especially leading to disorder of pulmonary qi.

吸烟能影响心、心包、肺、脾、胃等脏腑功能，尤其是导致肺气失调。

[**Syndrome differentiation**]

Smoking will make the smokers with addiction feel refreshed and comfortable. Smokers with addiction may smoke several cigarettes a day or several packs of cigarettes a day. Usually smokers with addiction have a history of smoking for half a year or one year, becoming dependent on smoking. Stoppage of smoking may lead to such symptoms as inability to work normally, general weakness, restlessness, discomfort in the throat, constant yawning, blurred vision and bradyesthesia.

【辨证】

吸烟成瘾，吸入后有清醒、欣快感。由每日少则几支多达几包，吸烟量大小不等。一般有半年至1年以上的吸烟史，对烟叶有依赖性，否则难以胜任正常工作，停吸后可出现软弱无力，烦躁不安，咽喉不适，呵欠连作，视觉朦胧，感觉迟钝等一系列临床表现。

[**Treatment**]

1. Body acupuncture

Prescription: Hegu (LI 4), Lieque (LU 7), Zusanli (ST 36) and Kongzui (LU 6).

Modification: For restlessness, Shenmen (HT 7) and Sanyinjiao (SP 6) are added; for discomfort in the throat, Jiache (ST 6) is added; for blurred vision, Jingming (BL 1) and Fengchi (GB 20) are added; for vertigo, Yintang (EX-HN 3) and Baihui (GV 20) are added.

Performance: The acupoints are needled with filiform needles; Hegu (LI 4) and Lieque (LU 7) are needled with the rotation of the needles for reducing purpose; strong stimulation is required when addiction irritates.

【治疗】

1. 体针疗法

处方：合谷，列缺，足三里，孔最。

随证配穴：烦躁不安加神门、三阴交；咽喉不适加颊车；视觉朦胧加睛明、风池；头昏加印堂、百会。

操作：毫针刺用泻法，合谷、列缺行捻转泻法，瘾发时加大刺激量。

2. Ear acupuncture

Prescription: Ear Shenmen (TF_4), Sympathetic Nerve (AH_{6a}), Lung (CO_{14}), Trachea (CO_{16}), Subcortex (AT_4), Liver (CO_{12}) and Stomach (CO_4).

Performance: Each time 2 - 3 acupoints are selected and needled with strong stimulation; or embedment of needles is used or Wangbuliuxingzi (Semen Vaccariae) is

2. 耳针疗法

选穴：神门，交感，肺，气管，皮质下，肝，胃。

操作：每次选2～3穴，中强刺激。埋皮内针或王不留行籽压耳，左右交替，每3～4

used for ear acupressure alternatively on both ears once 3 - 4 days. The patient is advised to press the acupoints 3 - 4times a day to control the irritation of addiction. The sealed seeds are changed once every 3 - 4 days.

日更换1次；嘱病人每日自行按压 3～4 次，以控制烟瘾发作。

Postscript

The Compilation of *A Newly Compiled English-Chinese Library of TCM* was started in 2000 and published in 2002. In order to demonstrate the academic theory and clinical practice of TCM and to meet the requirements of compilation, the compilers and translators have made great efforts to revise and polish the Chinese manuscript and English translation so as to make it systematic, accurate, scientific, standard and easy to understand. Shanghai University of TCM is in charge of the translation. Many scholars and universities have participated in the compilation and translation of the Library, i.e. Professor Shao Xundao from Xi'an Medical University (former Dean of English Department and Training Center of the Health Ministry), Professor Ou Ming from Guangzhou University of TCM (celebrated translator and chief professor), Henan College of TCM, Guangzhou University of TCM, Nanjing University of TCM, Shaanxi College of TCM, Liaoning College of TCM and Shandong University of TCM.

The compilation of this Library is also supported by the State Administrative Bureau and experts from other universities and colleges of TCM. The experts on the Compilation Committee and Approval Committee have directed the compilation and translation. Professor She

后　记

《(英汉对照)新编实用中医文库》(以下简称《文库》)从2000年中文稿的动笔,到2002年全书的付梓,完成了世纪的跨越。为了使本套《文库》尽可能展示传统中医学术理论和临床实践的精华,达到全面、系统、准确、科学、规范、通俗的编写要求,全体编译人员耗费了大量的心血,付出了艰辛的劳动。特别是上海中医药大学承担了英语翻译的主持工作,得到了著名医学英语翻译家、原西安医科大学英语系主任和卫生部外语培训中心主任邵循道教授,著名中医英语翻译家、广州中医药大学欧明首席教授的热心指导,河南中医学院、广州中医药大学、南京中医药大学、陕西中医学院、辽宁中医学院、山东中医药大学等中医院校英语专家的全力参与,确保了本套《文库》具有较高的英译水平。

在《文库》的编撰过程中,我们始终得到国家主管部门领导和各中医院校专家们的关心和帮助。编纂委员会的国内外学者及审定委员会的

Jing, Head of the State Administrative Bureau and Vice Minister of the Health Ministry, has showed much concern for the Library. Professor Zhu Bangxian, head of the Publishing House of Shanghai University of TCM, Zhou Dunhua, former head of the Publishing House of Shanghai University of TCM, and Pan Zhaoxi, former editor-in-chief of the Publishing House of Shanghai University of TCM, have given full support to the compilation and translation of the Library.

专家对编写工作提出了指导性的意见和建议。尤其是卫生部副部长、国家中医药管理局局长佘靖教授对本书的编写给予了极大的关注,多次垂询编撰过程,并及时进行指导。上海中医药大学出版社社长兼总编辑朱邦贤教授,以及原社长周敦华先生、原总编辑潘朝曦先生及全体编辑对本书的编辑出版工作给予了全面的支持,使《文库》得以顺利面世。在此,一并致以诚挚的谢意。

With the coming of the new century, we have presented this Library to the readers all over the world, sincerely hoping to receive suggestions and criticism from the readers so as to make it perfect in the following revision.

在新世纪之初,我们将这套《文库》奉献给国内外中医界及广大中医爱好者,恳切希望有识之士对《文库》存在的不足之处给予批评、指教,以便在修订时更臻完善。

Zuo Yanfu
Pingju Village, Nanjing
Spring 2002

左言富
于金陵萍聚村
2002 年初春

A Newly Compiled Practical English-Chinese Library of Traditional Chinese Medicine

(英汉对照)新编实用中医文库

Basic Theory of Traditional Chinese Medicine	中医基础理论
Diagnostics of Traditional Chinese Medicine	中医诊断学
Science of Chinese Materia Medica	中药学
Science of Prescriptions	方剂学
Internal Medicine of Traditional Chinese Medicine	中医内科学
Surgery of Traditional Chinese Medicine	中医外科学
Gynecology of Traditional Chinese Medicine	中医妇科学
Pediatrics of Traditional Chinese Medicine	中医儿科学
Traumatology and Orthopedics of Traditional Chinese Medicine	中医骨伤科学
Ophthalmology of Traditional Chinese Medicine	中医眼科学
Otorhinolaryngology of Traditional Chinese Medicine	中医耳鼻喉科学
Chinese Acupuncture and Moxibustion	中国针灸
Chinese Tuina (Massage)	中国推拿
Life Cultivation and Rehabilitation of Traditional Chinese Medicine	中医养生康复学